Toxins in Food

Chemical and Functional Properties of Food Components Series

SERIES EDITOR
Zdzisław E. Sikorski

Chemical and Functional Properties of Food Proteins
Edited by Zdzisław E. Sikorski

Chemical and Functional Properties of Food Components, Second Edition
Edited by Zdzisław E. Sikorski

Chemical and Functional Properties of Food Lipids
Edited by Zdzisław E. Sikorski and Anna Kołakowska

Toxins in Food
Edited by Waldemar M. Da̧browski and Zdzisław E. Sikorski

Toxins in Food

EDITED BY

Waldemar M. Dąbrowski Ph.D., D.Sc

Professor
Department of Food Microbiology
Faculty of Food Sciences and Fisheries
Agricultural University of Szczecin, Poland

Zdzisław E. Sikorski Ph.D., D.Sc

Professor
Department of Food Chemistry, Technology and Biotechnology
Faculty of Chemistry
Gdańsk University of Technology, Poland

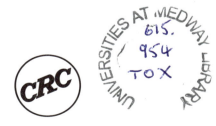

CRC PRESS

Boca Raton London New York Washington, D.C.

Library of Congress Cataloging-in-Publication Data

Toxins in food / edited by Waldemar M. Dąbrowski and Zdzisław E. Sikorski.
    p. cm. – (Chemical and functional properties of food series)
    ISBN 0-8493-1904-8 (alk. paper)
    1. Food–Toxicology. 2. Toxins. I. Dąbrowski, Waldemar M. II. Sikorski,
Zdzisław E. III. Chemical and functional properties of food components series

RA1258.T727 2004
615.9′54–dc22   2004050301

Visit the CRC Press Web site at www.crcpress.com

© 2005 by CRC Press LLC
No claim to original U.S. Government works
International Standard Book Number 0-8493-1904-8
Library of Congress Card Number 2004050301
Printed in the United States of America 1 2 3 4 5 6 7 8 9 0
Printed on acid-free paper

Preface

Globalization, the characteristic trend of the past few decades, affects food through mass production in mega-processing plants and by global distribution of products that once used to be sold locally. The developments in food technology also include very significant improvements in hygiene of food production. Novel systems, such as GMP, HACCP or TFQM, are being introduced to assure a high standard of food quality. However, foodborne poisonings still pose a very serious hazard to consumers' health, both in developed and in developing countries; due in part to a lack of knowledge among some producers and consumers regarding the risks and benefits related to food. Thus, the updating of information on foodborne poisoning agents is an essential element for the improvement of food hygiene.

This book contains a concise, yet well-documented, presentation of the current state of knowledge on the content, chemical properties, modes of action, and biological effects of toxins occurring in food. The first chapter offers a unique introduction, outlining the current toxicological hazards connected with food. Chapters 2, 3, 4, 6, and 7 describe the toxins that occur naturally in raw materials, such as plant and mushroom toxins, biogenic amines, and fish toxins, while chapters 8 to 12 deal with toxic compounds present in foods due to neglect during processing or as a result of environmental or raw-material contamination, such as bacterial toxins, mycotoxins, heavy metals, pesticides, and antibiotics. Toxic substances that may be generated in food during processing, packaging, and storage are presented in chapters 13 and 14. The health aspects of food allergies and the medical impact of toxins in food are discussed in chapters 5 and 15.

In preparing this book, we have been fortunate to work with highly-qualified specialists in the respective areas from the U.S. and Europe, who accepted our invitation and agreed to all reasonable editorial suggestions. The monographic chapters are based on their personal research experience and on critical evaluation of the present knowledge, as presented in the current world literature. We are pleased to acknowledge their collaboration. Thanks to their expertise, this volume may become a valuable source of information not only for food scientists, food technology, biology and biotechnology students, but also for all persons interested in food safety.

We are honored to dedicate this book to Dr. Eleanor Riemer, who heartily promoted the idea of establishing the series *Chemical and Functional Properties of Food Components* and helped the editors to shape the volumes according to the needs of the potential readers. Thank you, Eleanor, for your contribution.

Waldemar Dąbrowski and Zdzisław E. Sikorski

About the Editors

Waldemar Dąbrowski received an M.Sc. degree from the Faculty of Biology and the Earth Sciences at the University of Łódź, Poland, a Ph.D. from the Faculty of Veterinary Medicine at the University of Warmia and Mazury in Olsztyn, Poland, and a D.Sc. from the Medical University of Poznań, Poland. He worked for several years as a lecturer in the Department of Microbiology and Immunology of the Pomeranian Medical University of Szczecin. Later, for almost six years, he was in charge of a microbiological laboratory in Libya. At present, he is a professor in the Faculty of Food Sciences and Fisheries and head of the Department of Food Microbiology at the Agricultural University of Szczecin, Poland. He has published approximately 120 papers, mainly in food microbiology, medical microbiology, and immunology. His research focuses on food microbiology, particularly on the presence and intraspecies diversity of *Listeria monocytogenes* isolates from food and food-processing environments.

Zdzisław E. Sikorski received his Ph.D. and D.Sc. from the Gdańsk University of Technology, and an additional doctorate from the Agricultural University in Szczecin. He gained practical experience in several food industry plants in Poland and Germany, as well as on a fishing trawler. He was organizer and head of the Department of Food Chemistry and Technology. He served for five years as Dean of the Faculty of Chemistry at Gdańsk University of Technology and for seven years as chairman of the Committee of Food Technology and Chemistry of the Polish Academy of Sciences. He worked as researcher/professor in the Department of Agricultural Biochemistry, Ohio State University, Columbus, Ohio; CSIRO in Hobart, Australia; DSIR in Auckland, New Zealand; and National Taiwan Ocean University, Keelung. His research deals mainly with functional properties of food proteins and interactions of food components. He has published approximately 210 journal papers, 14 books (in Polish, English, Russian or Spanish), nine chapters on marine food science and food chemistry in other books, and holds seven patents. In 2003, he was elected a fellow of the International Academy of Food Science and Technology.

List of Contributors

Chapter 1
Waldemar Dąbrowski, Ph.D., D.Sc.
Professor
Department of Food Microbiology,
Faculty of Food Sciences and Fisheries,
Agricultural University of Szczecin, Poland
wm.dabrowski@tz.ar.szczecin.pl

Chapter 2
Kip E. Panter, Ph.D.
Research Animal Scientist
USDA ARS Poisonous Plant Research Laboratory, Logan, UT, USA
kpanter@cc.usu.edu

Chapter 3
Heinz Faulstich, Ph.D.
Professor
Max-Planck-Institut für Zellbiologie, Rosenhof, Germany
hfaulstich@web.de

Chapter 4
Paola Albertazzi, Ph.D.
Senior Lecturer
Centre for Metabolic Bone Disease, Hull, United Kingdom
p.albertazzi@hull.ac.uk

Chapter 5
Elżbieta Kucharska, M.D., Ph.D.
Assistant Professor
Department of Human Nutrition,
Faculty of Food Sciences and Fisheries,
Agricultural University of Szczecin, Poland
kucharska@tz.ar.szczecin.pl

Chapter 6
George J. Flick, Jr. Ph.D.
University Distinguished Professor
Food Science and Technology Department
Virginia Polytechnic Institute
Blacksburg, VA, U.S.A.
flickg@vt.edu
Linda Ankenman Granata, Ph.D.
Food Science and Technology Department
Virginia Polytechnic Institute
Blacksburg, VA, U.S.A.

Chapter 7
Lorraine C. Backer, Ph.D., MPH
National Center for Environmental Health,
Centers for Disease Control and Prevention,
Atlanta, Georgia, U.S.A.
lbacker@cdc.gov
Helen Schurz-Rogers, Ph.D.
National Center for Environmental Health,
Centers for Disease Control and Prevention,
Atlanta, Georgia, U.S.A.
hhs0@cdc.gov
Lora E. Fleming, M.D., Ph.D., MPH
Associate Professor,
NIEHS Marine and Freshwater Biomedical Sciences Center,
Rosenstiel School of Marine and Atmospheric Sciences,
University of Miami, Virginia Key, Florida, U.S.A.
lfleming@med.miami.edu
Barbara Kirkpatrick, Ed.D.
Mote Marine Laboratory, Sarasota, Florida, U.S.A.
bkirkpat@mote.org
Janet Benson, Ph.D., DABT,
Lovelace Respiratory Research Institute, Albuquerque, New Mexico, U.S.A.
jbenson@irri.org

Chapter 8
Waldemar Dąbrowski, Ph.D., D.Sc.
Professor
Department of Food Microbiology,
Faculty of Food Sciences and Fisheries,
Agricultural University of Szczecin, Poland
wm.dabrowski@tz.ar.szczecin.pl
Dagmara Mędrala, Ph.D.
Department of Food Microbiology,
Faculty of Food Sciences and Fisheries,
Agricultural University of Szczecin, Poland
duska@tz.ar.szczecin.pl

Chapter 9
Ana M. Calvo, Ph.D.
Assistant Professor
Department of Biological Science,
Northern Illinois University
DeKalb, Illinois, U.S.A.
amcalvo@niu.edu

Chapter 10
Mikołaj Protasowicki, Ph.D., D.Sc.
Professor
Department of Toxicology,
Faculty of Food Sciences and Fisheries,
Agricultural University of Szczecin, Poland
promik@tz.ar.szczecin.pl

Chapter 11
Carl K. Winter, Ph.D.
Director, Food Safe Program and
Extension Food Toxicologist
Department of Food Science and Technology
University of California
Davis, California, U.S.A.
ckwinter@ucdavis.edu

Chapter 12
Stanley K. Katz, Ph.D.
Department of Biochemistry and Microbiology,
New Brunswick, New Jersey, U.S.A.
sekatz@aesop.rutgers.edu
Paula-Marie L. Ward, Ph.D.
Department of Biochemistry and Microbiology,
New Brunswick, New Jersey, U.S.A.
plward@aesop.rutgers.edu.

Chapter 13
Zdzisław E. Sikorski, Ph.D., D.Sc.
Professor
Department of Food Chemistry, Technology and Biotechnology,
Gdańsk University of Technology, Poland
sikorski@chem.pg.gda.pl

Chapter 14
Barbara Piotrowska, Ph.D.
Department of Food Chemistry, Technology and Biotechnology,
Gdańsk University of Technology, Poland
karolina@chem.pg.gda.pl

Chapter 15
Elżbieta Kucharska, M.D., Ph.D.
Assistant Professor
Department of Human Nutrition,
Faculty of Food Sciences and Fisheries,
Agricultural University of Szczecin, Poland
kucharska@tz.ar.szczecin.pl

Table of Contents

1

Introduction

Waldemar Dąbrowski

CONTENTS

1.1 TOXINS IN FOOD – THE PAST AND THE PRESENT

Air, water, soil, and food are all unavoidable components of the human environment. Each of those elements influences the quality of human life, and each of them may be contaminated. Food is not only the elementary source of nutrients, but may also contain natural chemical substances with toxic properties, e.g., cyanogenic glycosides (many plants), solanine (green parts of potatoes, sprouted potatoes, and potatoes stored in light), industrial pollutants (heavy metals), biogenic amines (fish), or mycotoxins (moldy foodstuffs).

Poisons have been used since the dawn of civilization, especially at royal courts, to eliminate opponents and to put condemned prisoners to death. They also have been used for hunting (e.g., curare) or for ritual ceremonies in primitive tribes. Hemlock (*Conium maculatum* L.) is one of the oldest poisons known. In 399 B.C. Socrates was condemned to death by the Athenian court and forced to drink hemlock. Both Caligula and Cleopatra were known to have eliminated their victims by using poisoned food or giving poisoned flower garlands to guests. In the Middle Ages poisoning was the most popular form of convincing a political antagonist of one's rights. The Renaissance Italian family of Borgia was suspected of the most sophisticated murders, committed with arsenic added to foods, candle wicks, or book paper, although this is not confirmed by historians. Historical sources say that the fear of poisoning caused Henry IV of France to eat only eggs that he had cooked himself and to drink only water that he had drawn himself from the Seine river.

A significant historical discovery was that an antidote to arsenic poisoning is the ingestion of gradually increasing doses of the poison: rather than accumulating in the human body, the higher doses of arsenic are excreted in the stool. Similarly, a habit of taking arsenic with foodstuffs developed about 200 years ago among the uplanders in northern Syria and in the Austrian Tyrol. This did not lead to fatal poisonings, but caused an illusive feeling of energy boost that could be used to overcome exhaustion. In the same way, since the 16th century, old horses were fed with small amounts of arsenic to temporarily improve their vitality and energy in order to deceive buyers at horse markets.

These anecdotes show the truth in the statement by Paracelsus, that "*All things are poison and nothing is without poison. Dosage alone determines poisoning.*" This phenomenon is fundamental for homeopathy, a branch of alternative medicine, which suggests treating particular syndromes by using minimal doses of medicines that in higher amounts would trigger the same disease symptoms among healthy individuals ('*similia similibus curantur*').

In the 21st century the term 'food terrorism' was coined, which highlights the possibility of deliberate use of food as a vector for orally-ingested toxins in terrorist attacks.

As well as being used for intentional poisonings, toxic substances present in plants or spoiled foods have been the causes of accidental poisonings, frequently epidemic and leading to death. Medieval examples include ergot poisonings, known as *ignis sacer* (holy fire) or *ignis Sancti Antonii* (St. Anthony's fire) (a French outbreak in 994 A.D. led to over 40 000 deaths), while contemporary poisonings may be caused by, for example, preserves containing *Clostridium botulinum* spores, poisonous mushrooms being mistaken for edible *Agaricus campestris*, or fish contaminated with mercury compounds (the Minamata disease outbreak in Japan in 1958).

1.2 FOOD CONTAMINATION

Food may be contaminated directly or indirectly. Direct contamination occurs when a toxic substance is present in raw food materials, whereas indirect contaminants get into food during processing, storage, handling, or preparation. Indirect contaminants also include substances that become toxic and harmful to people due to food processing practices. Indirect contamination is most frequently the result of ignorance, lack of education of food handlers, inadequate space, poor facility design, or improper handling practices.

Contrary to popular belief, application of chemical substances, such as pesticides or fertilizers, in food production is not as harmful as rumors and urban myths would seem to indicate. Pesticides eliminate pests that would otherwise be a frequent cause of poisoning of grains, vegetables, and fruit due to the toxic products of their metabolisms. Chemically synthesized fertilizers are more easily detectable in food than their natural substitutes, which facilitates their adoption for use on food products (Moghissi 1998).

1.3 THE EFFECTS OF FOOD COMPONENTS ON HUMANS

Pathogenic actions of food components on the human body may manifest as intoxication, allergy or intolerance. In developed countries, between 300 and 1000 kg of food annually passes through the intestinal tract of an adult person. If toxic compounds are present, even in low concentrations, they may result in a cumulative effect that leads to disease symptoms.

Results and symptoms of foodborne poisonings may have acute, subacute, or mild courses. Patients with mild and subacute symptoms of poisonings usually do not seek or do not need medical treatment, therefore such cases are not registered by health services and so statistics often do not show actual rates of occurrence.

Symptoms of poisoning may affect all or only few individuals in a particular population. Symptoms may be divided into early, late, and delayed; early symptoms occur a few hours after toxin ingestion, late symptoms up to several days after, and delayed symptoms affect patients after some weeks, or even months. The most dangerous situation involves delayed, subacute symptoms that do not affect all individuals in an analyzed population. In such a cases, a relationship between consumed food and disease symptoms is practically impossible to confirm and may lead to a misdiagnosis.

The control of dangerous reactions to components in foods is not as widely conducted as is the monitoring of side effects caused by pharmaceuticals. This problem results mainly from the complexity of food matrices, and from the limited possibilities for attributing specific effects to particular food components.

1.4 WHAT AFFECTS FOOD SAFETY ISSUES TODAY?

Modern food toxicology is defined by changes within the population and changes in food production. Consumer requirements transform the food market and lead indirectly to progress in the food-processing industry. However, an increasing gap is observed in Europe between innovations in food technology and consumers' competence in handling food, which may lead to the development of a food-illiterate population that neglects food-hygiene risks and does not understand food-related health problems (Oltersdorf, 2003).

1.4.1 POPULATION CHANGES

Changes currently affecting populations include changes to demographic structure and to health conditions. In developed countries, an increase in the number of elderly, immunocompromized (including AIDS affected patients), allergic, and diabetic people, as well as patients receiving prolonged treatment with corticosteroids or cytotoxic medicines, has become a new trend for populations. Elderly and sick people require specific diets, which impact on patterns of food consumption. There is clear evidence that the impacts of medical progress and improved environmental conditions lead to better health in human populations in developed countries.

In developing countries, however, where the low quality of life, poor sanitary conditions, poor standards of food processing, storage and handling, and poor-quality drinking water obtained from contaminated sources, increase morbidity in diseases acquired via the gastrointestinal tracts.

Food poisonings also occur endemically, and concern food that is produced and consumed locally, e.g., Japanese fish *fugu*, or particular mushroom species.

Lifestyle changes caused by urbanization in industrial countries also lead to changes in food processing methods. People eat more frequently in restaurants, cafeterias, canteens, or fast-food chains, where food is processed in large quantities, even before it is needed, and a decline in the number of home-prepared meals is also observed. These factors do not seem to increase the actual number of foodborne disease outbreaks, but rather make the consequences of each outbreak more severe – mass production of food means that an outbreak may affect many more people than would an outbreak caused by food served at a home dinner table.

Changes in populations' lifestyles make new demands on food producers. Producers now have to try to meet requirements for food products for diabetics or people with allergies (so called 'functional foods,' including foods for special dietary use, medical foods, and dietary supplements), as well as having to expand their offering of food products for people who prefer heat-and-serve food or so-called 'organic' (practically non-processed) food. New classes of food products are being developed constantly to fulfil specific demands of particular segments of the consumer market. These developments can, however, have an impact on food safety. In the example of meeting consumers' demands for refrigerated ready-to-eat products, one result has been an increase in intoxication caused by enterotoxins of opportunistic pathogens, such as *Clostridium perfringens*, the spores which may survive such drastic conditions as cooking at 100°C for one hour (Novak and Juneja, 2002).

Additionally, 'population heterogeneity' causes some subpopulations to be more susceptible 'target groups' than others, and, more significantly, to some of the most natural and basic components of foods. Nuts are an example of a food that was consumed without any health risk for years, but which now triggers an increasing number of acute anaphylactic reactions among consumers. Another example was the ingestion of the aminoacid tryptophan in the 1980s, which was used as an antidepressant and by bodybuilders but led to muscle degradation or acute eosinophilic-myalgia syndrome (EMS), resulting in 37 deaths and 1500 permanent injuries. The problems were due to presence of PAA (3-phenylaminoalanin) and EBT (1.1′-ethylidenebistryptophan) in the preparations that were sold. The outbreak did not affect all people taking tryptophan to the same degree, which led to a hypothesis that the disease developed within a subpopulation characterized by a particular metabolic pathway (Lazarus, 1996; Simat et al., 1996).

1.4.2 Trends in Food Production

Novel foods, which include artificially-synthesized or genetically-modified foods, create a challenge for food safety monitoring. Even if novel foods pass standard safety assessments, they may generate delayed risks that result in problems which appear suddenly in a susceptible subpopulation. To take population heterogeneity into account, it is possible that in the future the safety of novel foods will be tested by human trials, as is standard practice in pharmacological research on new medicines (Lazarus, 1996).

Novel foods are the extreme example of changes in food production. Other innovations include extending the shelf life of products by using novel packaging materials or through use of new food additives.

Product packaging is not only attractive to consumers, but also enables the extension of shelf life for its content by protecting against microbiological, biological, and chemical alterations. Presently, over 30 different plastics are being used as packaging materials to meet the requirements of producers and consumers. In addition, different types of additives – such as antioxidants, stabilizers, lubricants, and anti-static and anti-blocking agents – have been developed to improve performance, either during the processing and production of the foods, or during application of the polymeric packaging materials. There is clear evidence that the packaging and storage of food can lead to product contamination; components of the packaging materials can migrate into the food (Lau and Wong, 2000). The toxicological aspects of packaging materials are exhaustively described in Chapter 13 of this volume.

Toxicological studies on direct food additives have revealed toxic and harmful actions. Food dyes and preservatives have been used since ancient Roman times to improve the color of wine or to disinfect wine containers. The development of chemistry led to many unwise experiments, such as the dying of food with copper, chrome, lead, mercury, arsenic, and cadmium salts. In the U.S. in 1906, over 300 food dyes were officially tested, of which only seven passed and were allowed to be used in food. Only two of them – erythrosine and idigotine – are permitted now. The lists of preservatives are also constantly modified in different countries. Quite recently, formic acid, which is used to preserve semi-products, was banned in Poland due to its deleterious effects.

Deleterious effects can also be exerted by components which have pharmacotherapeutic properties but which are perceived not to be harmful, e.g., niacin. In 1983, 14 people suffered from acute onset of rash, pruritis, and sensation of warmth after consumption of pumpernickel bagels. Studies revealed that the pumpernickel flour was enriched with large amounts of niacin, containing 60 times the normal level. Each bagel contained approximately 190 mg of niacin, whereas the recommended daily intake is about 13 mg per day for the average adult (Sevchick et al., 1983). Patterson et al. (1983) highlighted the fact that chronic use of excessive doses of niacin by persons taking large amounts of vitamins may lead to hepatitis.

Indirect food additives, which are the most frequent sources of poisoning-like diseases, are not natural food components. They enter food as contaminants from the environment during processing, packaging, and storage. Antibiotics given to farm animals, pesticide residues, or chemicals that migrate from food packaging are examples of such indirect additives. An example of an illegal indirect additive is the deliberate application of nitrofuran drugs (synthetic antibiotics banned in the 1990s due to their mutagenic, tumorigenic, and cytotoxic properties) in pig, poultry, and fish production. This use was revealed by new analytical methods, and abuse of these drugs has been shown to be a global problem that affects countries ranging from Thailand, via China, to Romania (Draisci et al., 1997; MacCracken and Kennedy, 1997; MacCracken et al., 2000; Kennedy, 2003). It would be difficult not to agree with those who say that "animal feed must not serve as the dustbin for waste producers," especially after Europe's latest food contamination incident – synthetic progesterone was found in products ranging from animal feed to soft drinks (Rogers, 2003).

It also appears that traditional forms of food processing may not be as safe as expected. The example of the formation of acrylamide in different heat-processed foods may be cited (see Chapter 13 of this volume). However, there are no incontrovertible answers to the questions: is acrylamide in food harmful for consumers?, and what is the average intake? The American Council on Science and Health states that there is "no credible evidence that acrylamide in foods poses human cancer risk." New Zealand food safety experts, using a 'no observable adverse effect level' for acrylamide of 0.1 mg per kg bodyweight, also estimate that people eating fried potatos and crisps (products suspected to contain the largest amounts of acrylamide) are a very low risk of cancer from this source. European Union experts decided that the risk of exposure to polyacrylamide in food remains undetermined (Sharp, 2003).

The possibility of aluminum migration and its perniciousness were noticed at the beginning of 1980s. Aluminum is widely distributed in foodstuffs, at concentrations higher in plant than in animal food. Orally-consumed aluminum is increasingly considered to be a contaminant of the food chain, playing a role in the etiology of neurodegenerative diseases such as Morbus Alzheimer and amyotrophic lateral sclerosis. In the past, aluminum has been always considered as harmless, even if it was present in the environment. The main sources of orally-consumed aluminum are food materials, food additives, containers, kitchen utensils, packaging containing aluminum, and drinking water (Müller et al., 1998). A very high level of aluminum was also detected in chewing gum (from 3.5 to 4.5 mg per 5 g stick) (Kupchella and Syty, 1980; Varo et al., 1980). However, it turned out that during chewing, only from 0.01 to 0.046 mg of aluminum per stick is released (Lione and Smith, 1982). Even though high doses of aluminum are present in foods consumed only rarely and in small quantities (e.g., cocoa, cocoa products, spices, black tea leaves), the population that is susceptible to aluminum (e.g., patients with chronic renal failure who cannot excrete aluminum via the renal pathway and so accumulate it at toxic levels) cannot be ignored as such a syndrome affects 5% of the population. Because the role of aluminum in etiology of neurodegenerative diseases is unknown, its presence in food cannot be neglected.

1.5 FOOD ALLERGY OR FOOD INTOLERANCE?

Between 12 and 20% of Americans, British and Dutch people complain about food allergies. In fact, problems are more likely to be due to food intolerance rather than actual allergy. This has been confirmed by skin-prick tests, analysis of immunoglobulin E level in serum, and enzyme-linked immunosorbent assay (ELISA) tests which found food intolerance in 2 to 5% of adults and 6 to 13% of children (age 1 to 6) in Europe. Challenge-proved adverse reaction to food is one tenth of that perceived and allergic reactions to chemicals and additives in food are even more rare. A similar ratio occurs in Asia. The dietary habits in different countries determine the observed rates of food sensitivities. Sensitivity to fish occurs frequently in Scandinavia, to rice in Japan, to peanuts in the U.S. and the U.K., and to seafood and milk in Italy. It also means that communities not exposed to particular allergens are not affected as frequently by various forms of sensitivities, e.g., allergy to peanuts is rare in Scandinavia where peanuts are not a popular snack, and allergy to seafood is uncommon in populations separated from bodies of water (Samartin et al., 2001). Artificial additives, industrial pollutants, and other chemicals present in contemporary food are often blamed for the increasing rates of food allergies (Halstensen et al., 1997). In the draft proposal for European Council and Parliament Directive III/5909/97 (16 January, 1998), a so-called 'hit list' of major serious allergens (MSAs), which contains ten food ingredients or substances that have to be indicated as allergenic or incompatibility inducing, was presented. Foods and ingredients that are recognized as being responsible for increased allergenic sensitivity, and which have to be declared on lists of ingredients, include:

- cereals containing gluten and their products
- crustaceans and their products
- eggs and their products
- fish and fish products
- peanuts and peanut products
- soybeans and their products
- milk and milk products (including lactose)
- tree nuts and nut products
- sesame seed
- sulfite at concentration of 10 mg per kg or more

Because such components may be inactivated during food processing and lose their potential allergenic properties, e.g., refined peanut oil, problems for both legislation (to label such food or not?) and analysis (how to detect antigens in processed food?) will most certainly occur soon. A precise threshold value for each allergenic food product or substance (the level at which adverse effects are produced) will inevitably be needed to replace the use of the 5% maximum level for allergic components in foods (suggested by Codex Alimentarius). Unfortunately, this will require novel analytical tools and equipment and will definitely lead to an increase in the prices of 'allergen-free' products.

1.6 LINKS BETWEEN FOOD AND HEALTH – TRACING A HUMAN GENOME

A new perspective on the practical approach to food toxicology will soon be given by the ability to determine exact relationships between the occurrence of particular diseases, diet, and major histocompatibility complexes (MHCs). Uncovering the secrets of the human genome will support the determination of such links. Although it sounds like an idea from fiction, it is possible that in the future each consumer will be provided with advice such as 'avoid this and that product or you will get sick', based on knowledge of his own specific genotype and prepared at, or even before, birth.

The link between diet and occurrence of insulin-dependent diabetes mellitus (IDDM) has already been confirmed. There is also a connection of a poligenic character between MHC II genes and IDDM. The MHC encoded on a short arm of chromosome 6 is a main marker, but the syndrome also depends on the insulin gene located on chromosome 11. It has been confirmed that about 90% of patients suffering from IDDM have human leukocyte antigen (HLA) DR4 or DR3 pattern, or both. It is probable that despite genetically-encoded predisposition to IDDM, viral infections and food factors (e.g., cow milk, nitroso compounds, nitrates, and nitrites) also have an impact. A nitrosamine-rich diet in pregnant women and during bottle-feeding of children is blamed for the occurrence of IDDM among children (Akerblom et al., 1997). Conversely, elimination of selected components from diet caused an improvement among 30 to 40% of patients suffering from rheumatoid arthritis (RA). In some cases the improvement was so significant that it led to discontinuation of prescribed medicines. RA may be triggered by sporadically consumed food, most frequently milk, cheeses, shrimp, or maize (Gamlin and Brostoff, 1997).

Studies revealed that homozygotic individuals with a particular genetic variation in the *PRNP* gene (encoding the normal form of the prion protein), which causes the presence of methionine at position 129, are particularly prone to variant Creutzfeldt-Jakob disease (vCJD), a human form of transmissible spongiform encephalophaty. Heterozygosity at this position appears protective. Suppositions are made that also show that HLA pattern may be a marker of vCJD morbidity (Partanen, 2003). If the assumptions are confirmed, it would be logical to warn consumers with such a genetic make-up against eating beef.

Scientists recently announced that a sialic acid Neu5Gc (*N*-glycolyneuraminic acid), normally present in red meat but not in humans, may be incorporated into the tissues of meat consumers and accumulate there, leading the consumers' bodies to produce antibodies directed against it and which destroy a body's own tissues. As the occurrence of Neu5Gc was also detected in the courses of cancers, there is now a discussion on whether it may contribute to development of cancer diseases as well as cardiovascular disease and diabetes. The possible connections have not been proven so far (Tangvoranuntakul et al., 2003), yet it may turn out that diet style, i.e., excessive consumption of red meat, is responsible for more severe diseases than we could expect. This reinforces the observation that food does not have to contain substances commonly regarded as toxic to exert a negative effect on human health.

1.7 CONCLUSIONS

Everything changes. Changes affect the environment, society, and food – its processing and its packaging. Changes cause foods and processes that used to be safe, healthy, and validated by years of tradition to be safe no longer. The free-market economy, aimed at immediate profits boosted by competition and multinational corporations, exposes producers to the temptations of illegal practices, with consequent impacts of food quality and consumer safety. Grob et al. (1999) concludes quite pessimistically that *"Everybody emphasizes quality, but behind the high quality design of the packing there is often a product which is just shaped by the need to reduce costs."*

Nowadays, food has become more of an economic and political issue than ever before, and inevitably it is no longer the concern only of food technologists and food producers. A strong consumer lobby also now impacts on the food industry. Rational opinion and expectations of consumers should not be ignored, however public perceptions are unfortunately not always in agreement with the results of scientific analyses. For example, although there is no clear evidence that genetically-modified (GM) food is dangerous for humans, public objections may result in the prohibition of further studies and GM farm production, just by making it economically unprofitable. The definite bias against GM food that is expressed by society is explained by previous failure by politics to communicate risk and uncertainty, which led to distrust of scientists and government organizations (Berry, 2003).

If the causes of current problems affecting food quality are understood, we will be able to foresee and predict future problems. If food quality is not controlled by the actions and compromises forced by the free-market economy, or included as part of political 'game', everybody will benefit.

1.8 REFERENCES

Akerblom, H.K., Knip, M., Hyöty, H., Rejijonen, H., Virtanen, S., Savilahti, E. and Ilonen, J. (1997). Interaction of genetic and environmental factors in the pathogenesis of insulin-dependent diabetes mellitus, *Clinica Chimica Acta*, 257, 143–156.

Berner, L.A. and O'Donell, J.A. (1998). Functional foods and health claims legislations: applications to dairy foods, *Int. Dairy J.*, 8, 355–362.

Berry, S. (2003). Food safety: communicating the risks, *BioMedNet, News and Features Magazine*, 27 October.

Draisci, R., Giannetti, L., Lucentini, L., Palleschi, L., Brambilla, G., Serpe, L. and Gallo P. (1997). Determination of nitrofuran residues in avian eggs by liquid chromatography – UV photodiode array detection and confirmation by liquid chromatography – ionspray mass spectrometry. *J. Chromatogr., A*, 777, 201–211.

Gamlin, L. and Brostoff, J. (1997). Food sensitivity and rheumatoid arthritis, *Environ. Toxicolo. Pharmacol.*, 4, 43–49.

Grob, K., Spinner C.H., Brunner, M. and Etter R. (1999). The migration from the internal coatings of food cans; summary of the findings and call for more effective regulation of polymers in contact with foods: a review. *Food Add. Cont.*, 16, 579–590.

Halstensen, T.S., Løvik, M., Alexander, J. and Smith, E. (1997). Environmental chemicals and food allergy/intolerance, a synopsis, *Environ. Toxicol. Pharmacol.*, 4, 179–185.

Hey, G.H. and Luedemann, G.B. (2001). Food legislation and the protection of allergic and hypersensitive persons: an overview, *J. Chromatogr. B*, 756, 337–342.

Kennedy, G. (2003). *FoodBRAND and global nitrofuran abuse*. PolFood Workshop, Poznań, Poland, 1–2 December.

Lau, O.W. and Wong, S.K. (2000). Contamination in food from packaging material. *J. Chromatogr. A*, 882, 255–270.

Lazarus, N.R. (1996). Population heterogeneity and its impact on the risk management of food safety. *Environ. Toxicol. Pharmacol.*, 2, 89–91.

MacCracken, R.J. and Kennedy, D.G. (1997). Determination of the furazolidone metabolite, 3-amino-2-oxazolidinone, in porcine tissues using liquid chromatography-thermospray mass spectrometry and the occurrence of residues in pigs produced in Northern Ireland, *J. Chromatogr. B*, 691, 87–94.

MacCracken, R.J., MacCoy, M.A. and Kennedy, D.G. (2000). Furazolidone residues in pigs: criteria to distinguish between treatment and contamination, *Food Additives Contaminants*, 17, 75–82.

Moghissi, A.A. (1998). Food safety and diet, *Environ. Int.*, 24, 821–822.

Müller, M., Anke, M. and Illing-Günther, H. (1998). Aluminium in foodstuffs, *Food Chem.*, 61, 419–428.

Novak, J.S. and Juneja, V.K. (2002). *Clostridium perfringens*: hazards in new generation foods, *Innovative Food Sci. Emerging Technol.*, 3, 127–132.

Oltersdorf, U., Developments in food processing and increasing gaps in consumers competence of food handling – the challenge for nutrition policy in Europe, *J. Food Eng.*, 56, 163–169.

Partanen, J. (2003). Genetic susceptibility to variant Creutzfeldt-Jakob disease, *Lancet*, 361, 447.

Patterson, D.J., Dew, E.W., Gyorkey, F. and Graham, D.Y. (1983). Niacin hepatitis, *South Med. J.*, 76, 239–242.

Rogers, A. (2003). EU promises reforms after another food scandal, *Lancet*, 360, 857.

Samartin, S., Marcos, A. and Chandra, R.K. (2001). Food hypersensitivity, *Nutr. Res.*, 21, 473–497.

Sevchick, J., Guerrette, M., George, E., Campana, J., Redmond, S., Nitzkin, J.L., Reiffler, C., Martin, K., Eiseman, D., Guzewich, J. and Rothenberg, R. (1983). Niacin intoxication from pumpernickel bagels – New York, *MMWR*, 32, 305.

Sharp, D. (2003). Acrylamide in food, *Lancet*, 361, 361.

Simat, T. et al. (1996). Unerwünschte Nebenprodukte in biotechnologisch hergestelltem L-Tryptophan. *GIT Fachzeitschrift für das Laboratorium*, 339–344.

Tangvoranuntakul, P., Gagneu, P., Diaz, S., Bardor, M., Varki, N., Varki, A. and Muchmore, E. (2003). Human uptake and incorporation of an immunogenic nonhuman dietary sialic acid. *Proc. Nat. Acad. Sci. U.S.A.*, 100, 12045–12050.

2

Natural Toxins of Plant Origin

K.E. Panter

CONTENTS

2.1 INTRODUCTION

Poisonous plants and the natural toxins therefrom cause significant economic losses to livestock industries throughout the world. Using 1989 figures, it was estimated that poisonous plants cause losses of over $340 million annually to the livestock industry in the seventeen western states of the U.S. (Nielsen and James, 1992; Frandsen and Boe, 1991). Applying a 3% annual inflation rate, this figure would have exceeded $500 million in 2003. This estimate only includes losses caused by the deaths of cattle and sheep and does not include increased management costs, lost forage and grazing opportunities, additional health care, etc. Other livestock species and wildlife are also affected by poisonous plants, further increasing losses. As a recent illustration, in the spring of 1997 over 4000 calves either died or were destroyed because of lupine-induced 'crooked calf syndrome' in a single county of eastern Washington state (Panter et al., 1999). The direct losses to ranchers in this area exceeded $1.7 million (calf losses only). This figure did not take into account losses due to cow deaths, extensive culling of cows without calves, heifer replacement costs, increased cost of veterinary care, increased management, etc. Furthermore, this dollar amount does not take into account the economic impact on other businesses in the area supported by the cattle industry. The overall cost of poisonous plants to rural communities, and especially the livestock industry, is enormous.

While poisonous plants on grazing lands have a significant impact on livestock production throughout the world, the natural toxins (secondary metabolites) in the plant may have multiple and diverse functions, not only for the plant world but also for the benefit of mankind. Many current pharmaceuticals have been chemically optimized from natural toxins of plant origin. New plant compounds and familiar compounds with renewed interest, e.g., nutraceuticals, herbal preparations, nutritional supplements, etc, are increasingly finding their value in human nutrition and health.

Given the significance of plant compounds to people and animals, the primary function of secondary metabolites in plants remains a topic of extensive discussion and research. It has been argued for decades that many of these compounds serve as a defense mechanism to protect plants against herbivory, predation or disease (reviewed in Wink, 1999). Secondary compounds can protect a plant in various ways: by imparting bitterness or causing discomfort or some other negative cue to inhibit herbivory, or they may be overtly toxic thus killing or debilitating the predator or causing an inherent aversion to the plant.

Secondary compounds produced by plants may have other significant survival roles, such as signals to attract insects, birds, or other animals to enhance pollination or seed dispersal. In addition to any potential functions, secondary compounds may concomitantly serve a physiologic function, such as protection against ultraviolet (UV) light or frost, or provide a function in nitrogen transport and storage. In several instances, compounds can serve multiple functions in the same plant. Anthocyanins or monoterpenes can be insect attractants in flowers, but are insecticidal and antimicrobial at the same time in leaves (Wink, 1999). Similarly, insects and other organisms have evolved alongside plants thereby utilizing the plant's protective mechanism.

The relationship between milkweeds and the monarch butterfly demonstrates a synergistic relationship between a plant and an insect (Harborne, 1993). The larvae of the monarch butterfly feed on milkweeds and accumulate cardenolides. Birds feeding on the caterpillars, pupae, or adults, will vomit and subsequently become averted and thus avoid the monarch butterflies. Interestingly, other butterflies, such as viceroy, which do not feed on milkweed, have evolved with nearly identical color pattern (mimicry), so birds avoid these nontoxic insects as well.

There are numerous other examples of plants, insects, large herbivores, and other organisms playing synergistic roles in nature's balance. Multiple functions are typical of plant compounds and do not contradict in any way their main role as chemical-defense and signal-induction compounds. A trait that serves multiple functions in a given plant or animal is more likely to survive the rigors of natural selection.

In general, plant organs that are important for survival and reproduction, such as flowers and seeds, will concentrate defense compounds. Consequently, compounds may be more rapidly synthesized or stored at certain stages of critical growth, i.e., in buds, young tissue or seedlings. While most wild plant species contain secondary compounds, many plants have evolved additional protection, such as thorns, spikes, glandular organs, stinging hairs, or an impenetrable bark (as do many trees). Many of these species rely on secondary compounds during early growth phase or seed phase, but during vegetative and mature stages are protected by mechanical or morphological adaptations. Although plants have a limited capacity to replace or regenerate parts that are eaten, diseased, or damaged, secondary compounds are of major importance for promoting survival. The capacity for open growth and regeneration, which is prominent in perennials, allows for a margin of tolerance towards herbivores and microbes. While the role of secondary compounds in plant evolution is significant for survival, their impacts on the health and well-being of people and animals may be beneficial or deleterious.

Over 100,000 secondary compounds have been identified, and categorized into one of two major classes:

1. Nitrogen-containing compounds, that include alkaloids, glycosides, proteins, polypeptides, amines and non-protein amino acids.
2. Nitrogen-free compounds, that include some organic acids, alcohols, polyacetylenes, resinous toxins and mineral toxins.

For thousands of years, people have used some of these compounds as flavors, dyes, fragrances, insecticides, hallucinogens, nutritional supplements, animal or human poisons, and therapeutic or pharmaceutical agents. While secondary compounds are an evolutionary adaptation in plants, they serve multiple functions for mankind.

Many volumes have been written on the natural toxins of plants. While the negative effects of plant toxins on people and the impact of plant toxins on livestock producers have been the most publicized, the diversity of these toxins and their potential as new pharmaceutical agents for the treatment of diseases in people and animals has received widespread interest in modern society. Scientists are actively screening plants from all regions of the world for bioactivity and potential pharmaceuticals for the treatment or prevention of many diseases.

This chapter will focus on plants and their toxins that have been researched at the USDA-Agricultural Research Service's Poisonous Plant Research Laboratory, in Logan, Utah, but will also mention other relevant toxins affecting animals and people.

2.2 NITROGEN-CONTAINING PLANT TOXINS

2.2.1 ALKALOIDS

An alkaloid is a basic, nitrogen-containing compound generally found in higher plants. Pelletier (1983) suggested that "an alkaloid is a cyclic compound containing nitrogen in a negative oxidation state which is of limited distribution in living organisms". Pelletier's definition includes alkaloids with nitrogen as part of a heterocyclic system and extracyclic bound nitrogen. A basic characteristic is no longer a prerequisite for the definition of an alkaloid.

Several thousand alkaloids have been identified and characterized in plants. Over 20% of higher-plant families contain alkaloids, thus alkaloids are the most ubiquitous and significant class of plant toxins (Blackwell, 1990). Although it has been suggested that alkaloids are waste by-products of plant metabolism, they may play a role in binding ionic nitrogen needed by seedlings. Alkaloids were initially associated with the plant kingdom, but more and more alkaloid compounds are being discovered in microorganisms, fungi, marine invertebrates, insects, and higher animals (Roberts and Wink, 1998). Many of these alkaloids have led to the discovery of new pharmaceuticals and new treatments for diseases in humans and animals.

Quinine, strychnine and brucine are extremely bitter alkaloids. Bitter alkaloids may have evolved a universal role in plant chemical defense, as a feeding deterrent. However, there are little data on animal/plant relationships that show bitterness is the only controlling factor in preventing herbivore ingestion of poisonous plants. There are many examples of animals eating plants that, in human terms, are "bitter as gall". Wink et al. (1993) partially disproved the bitterness theory in a feeding trial with geese in which the birds avoided essential oils but tolerated bitter alkaloids. In a recent study, cattle grazed bitter lupines, but only late in the season when more palatable grasses had become senescent and dry and the lupines remained green (Ralphs, 2003).

Bitterness remains a major issue for study. In particular, what drives livestock's consumption of poisonous plants? The cause of willful consumption of poisonous plants, albeit bitter tasting, by livestock has been debated for decades and is a significant focus of research at the Poisonous Plant Research Laboratory. Roitman and Panter (1995) recently published a review of plant alkaloids that cause livestock poisoning.

2.2.1.1 Piperidine Alkaloids

Piperidine alkaloids are widely distributed in nature, mostly in plants, but also in lower animals. Of the hundreds of piperidine alkaloids known, most are derived by one of three biosynthetic pathways in the plant, using the building blocks of lysine, acetate, or mevalonate as precursors (reviewed in Panter and Keeler, 1989). The common nucleus of all piperidine alkaloids is the piperidine ring (Figure 2.1). Some of the simple-structure piperidines follow the lysine and acetate pathways, while the more complex ones use mevalonate. Acetate-derived piperidine alkaloids are common in nature in plants and lower animals. For example, the simple piperidines in poison-hemlock – γ-coniceine and coniine – are acetate pathway derived. Likewise, anabaseine, also acetate pathway derived and a known tobacco alkaloid, has been identified as a poison gland product of *Aphaenogaster* ants and various 2,6-disubstituted piperidine alkaloids have been isolated from the fire ant (*Solenopsis saevissima*) in which these alkaloids function as attractants (Roberts and Wink, 1998). More than 100 different alkaloids (many of them piperidine) have been isolated from neotropical frogs of the Dendrobatidae family and others have been identified in numerous microorganisms.

The piperidine alkaloids are historically significant because of the ancient Greek practice of executing criminals with tea made from poison-hemlock (*Conium maculatum* L.). Early literature refers to human poisoning more frequently than animal poisoning. One of the most famous historical accounts of poison-hemlock is the execution of the philosopher Socrates, who was sentenced to death by drinking hemlock tea after he was convicted of introducing new divinities into the philosophy of the day. A recent historical account of Socrates' death was published by Daugherty in 1995.

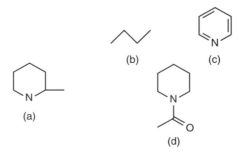

FIGURE 2.1 Piperidine ring (a) and three functionalities of three carbons or larger that impart teratogenic activity; (b) coniine, (c) anabasine, and (d) ammodendrine.

Even today, accidental human poisonings occasionally occur; however most current reports involve ingestion by livestock species. An incident of human poisoning was reported by Frank et al. (1995) in which a six-year-old boy and his father were successfully treated for accidental poison-hemlock poisoning. After ingesting young poison-hemlock leaves, the boy became unresponsive and was then hospitalized. After identification of the plant and appropriate hospital treatment, the boy recovered completely.

In ancient times, poison-hemlock seed was collected green, dried and stored to be used medicinally as a sedative. The dried leaf and juice of *Conium maculatum* L. (Hemlock) were listed in pharmacopoeias of London and Edinburgh from 1864 to 1898, and the last official record appeared in Great Britain in the British Pharmaceutical Codex of 1934. Interest in the medicinal value of poison-hemlock has declined because of the unpredictability of its effects. The unpredictability is now understood, the toxin profile and concentration in the plant and green seed can vary dramatically because of environmental factors or, even, diurnally.

Poison-hemlock also has historical significance to researchers because coniine was the first alkaloid discovered, in 1827, and was first synthesized in 1886 (Landenburg, 1886, reviewed in Panter and Keeler, 1989).

Poison-hemlock contains three major and five minor alkaloids. The toxicity and teratogenic effects of the three major alkaloids have been compared (Figure 2.2). γ-Coniceine usually predominates in early vegetative stages of plant growth and coniine and *N*-methyl coniine usually predominate in seed and mature plant. γ-Coniceine is the precursor to all the other poison-hemlock alkaloids. γ-coniceine is seven to eight times more toxic in a mammalian bioassay compared with coniine, which is one and a half to two times more toxic than *N*-methyl coniine (Figure 2.2). The pharmacological activity is similar among these alkaloids but varies in potency because of structural differences. Pharmacological studies with conium alkaloids have demonstrated that they act as neuromuscular blocking agents. Peripheral actions on smooth muscle are initiated by ganglionic stimulation and subsequent blockade, which explains some of the early clinical signs of stimulation to the gastrointestinal (GI) tract and urinary system. Spinal reflexes are later blocked, which has been attributed to the increased membrane permeability to potassium ions.

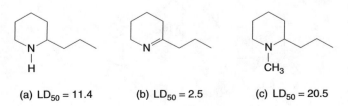

(a) $LD_{50} = 11.4$ (b) $LD_{50} = 2.5$ (c) $LD_{50} = 20.5$

FIGURE 2.2 Three piperidine alkaloid teratogens from *Conium maculatum* (poison-hemlock); (a) coniine, (b) γ-coniceine, and (c) *N*-methyl coniine, with accompanying LD_{50} as determined in a mouse bioassay.

Pharmacologically, the properties of all three alkaloids are very similar, except γ-coniceine is more stimulatory to autonomic ganglia and *N*-methyl coniine has a greater blocking effect (Fodor and Colasanti, 1985).

The teratogenic effects of poison-hemlock are well known and have been described in cattle, sheep, goats, and pigs (Figure 2.3; Panter et al., 1999). Numerous field cases of poisoning and subsequent malformations have been reported. The birth defects, susceptible stages of pregnancy and description of toxicoses have been evaluated in laboratory studies, thus implicating the individual alkaloids responsible. Skeletal system contractures generally manifest in the limbs, neck, and lower spinal column, e.g., arthrogryposis, scoliosis, torticollis, etc. Additionally, cleft palate has been shown to occur in a relatively high percentage of cases. The mechanism of action, susceptible stages of pregnancy, and detailed descriptions of the teratogenic effects have been reviewed by Panter et al. (1999).

Nicotiana species and certain lupine species also contain potent toxic and teratogenic piperidine alkaloids (Figure 2.4). All teratogenic piperidine alkaloids have specific structural characteristics that are responsible for induction of birth defects. Their molecular structures include a piperidine ring, with a side chain of at least three carbons or larger attached adjacent to

(a)   (b)

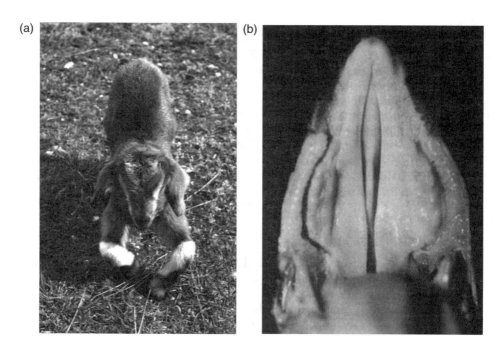

FIGURE 2.3 (a) Skeletal defects and (b) cleft palate induced in a newborn goat by maternal ingestion of coniine (*Conium maculatum*), anabasine (*Nicotiana glauca*) or ammodendrine (*Lupinus formosus*).

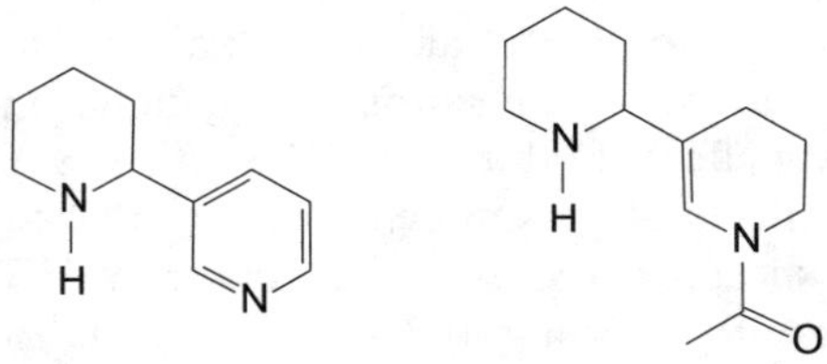

(a) $LD_{50} = 1.6$ (b) $LD_{50} = 134.4$

FIGURE 2.4 Piperidine teratogens; (a) anabasine from *Nicotiana glauca*, and (b) ammodendrine from *Lupinus formosus*.

the nitrogen atom (Figure 2.1). The structural characteristics were first proposed by Keeler and Balls in 1978 and all experiments since that time have supported this theory. Teratogenicity is thought to occur because the structure of these alkaloids means they compete with acetylcholine at the binding sites of the neuromuscular junction. Fetal clinical effects include a significant reduction in fetal movement during critical stages of gestation. Just as fetal movement helps to prevent skeletal contracture malformations, fetal movement is critical in the prevention of cleft palate. The stage of gestation when the fetus is exposed to alkaloids is related to the type of malformation manifested. For example, in goats (the animal model selected for mechanism research) the susceptible stage of pregnancy for cleft palate induction is 35 to 41 days of gestation, and when this period is extended to day 60 skeletal malformations also occur. Malformations and mechanisms of action are the same for all piperidine alkaloids possessing the structural characteristics discussed above.

In addition to lupines, poison-hemlock and Nicotiana spp., other plant species of the genera Genista, Prosopis, Lobelia, Cytisus, Sophora, Pinus, Punica, Duboisia, Sedum, Withania, Carica, Hydrangea, Dichroa, Cassia, Ammondendron, Liparia, and Colidium contain potentially toxic and teratogenic piperidine alkaloids. Many plant species or varieties from these genera may be included in animal and human diets (Keeler and Crowe, 1984).

2.2.1.2 Quinolizidine Alkaloids

Quinolizidine alkaloids are mainly found in genera of the Fabaceae (legume) family. This family is very large and commercially important, and contains hundreds of quinolizidine alkaloids. More than 150 quinolizidine alkaloids have been structurally identified and characterized in lupines alone (Kinghorn and Balandrin, 1984). Significant genera containing quinolizidine alkaloids include *Lupinus, Laburnum, Cytisus, Thermopsis* and *Sophora*. Most of these contain the teratogen anagyrine (Figure 2.5).

The common structural feature of quinolizidine alkaloids is a decalin ring system with a nitrogen at one vertex. Often a second or third nitrogen atom is

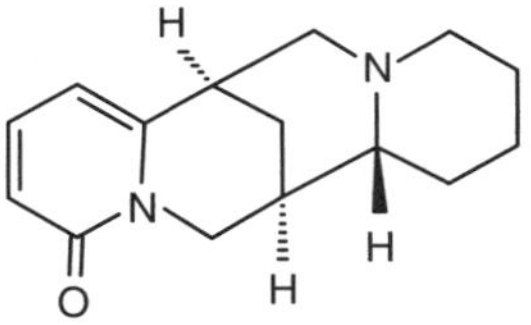

Figure 2.5 Anagyrine, teratogenic quinolizidine alkaloid from *Lupinus* spp.

incorporated into additional six-membered rings. Bicyclic, tricyclic, tetracyclic and even more complex alkaloids with five to ten rings have been characterized (Keeler, 1989). Interestingly, anagyrine appears to be the only quinolizidine alkaloid known at this time with teratogenic activity in cattle.

2.2.1.2.1 Lupinus *Spp.*

Lupinus spp. (lupines) contain both quinolizidine and piperidine alkaloids that are toxic and teratogenic. Lupines have caused large losses to the sheep and cattle industries in the past, and they continue to cause significant losses to the cattle industry in the western U.S. Recent calf losses due to congenital birth defects ('crooked calf syndrome', Figure 2.6) have been reported in Oregon, Idaho, Utah, California, Nevada, Montana, Washington and western Canada from 1992 to 2003 (personal communications, 1992–2003). Eighteen lupine species from the western U.S. have been reported to contain the teratogen anagyrine (Figure 2.5) with 14 of these containing teratogenic levels (Davis and Stout, 1986). Two species, *L. formosus* and *L. arbustus*, contain teratogenic levels of the piperidine alkaloid ammodendrine (Figure 2.4; Panter et al., 1998a). Lupine alkaloids are produced by leaf chloroplasts and are translocated via the phloem and stored in epidermal cells and in seeds (Wink et al., 1995).

Quinolizidine alkaloid content and profile varies between lupine species and also varies between individual plants depending on environmental conditions, season and stage of plant growth (Wink and Carey, 1994). Alkaloid content may be highest during early growth stages, decreasing through the bud stage, and concentrating in the flowers and maturing seeds. Seed pods grazed by sheep were responsible for catastrophic losses in the early 1900s. Seed pods contain high protein levels and high concentrations of alkaloids. Unfortunately, seed pods occur at a time when grasses and other desirable forbs senesce and lupine preference increases (Ralphs, 2003). Toxic and teratogenic effects depend on the amount of plant ingested, the concentration of toxic alkaloids in the plant, and how rapidly alkaloids are absorbed.

The effects of site and elevation on alkaloid content have been described by Carey and Wink (1994). Total alkaloid content decreases as elevation increases, and was shown to be six times higher in plants at 2700 m versus plants collected at 3500 m. This phenomenon persisted even when seedlings from the highest and lowest elevations were grown under identical greenhouse conditions, thus

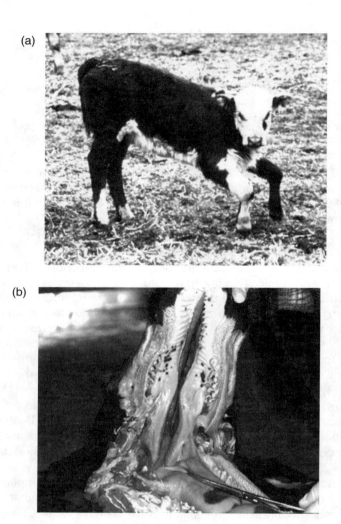

FIGURE 2.6 'Crooked calf syndrome' with (a) arthrogryposis, and (b) cleft palate. Other skeletal malformations not shown here include scoliosis, torticollis, lordosis and kyphosis.

suggesting evolutionary genetic differences. For many lupines, the time and degree of seeding varies from year to year. Many lupines possess high nutrient qualities and would be considered good range forage if the toxic/teratogenic alkaloids were not present. In some circumstances, lupine may be grazed relatively safely.

Livestock deaths have generally occurred under conditions in which animals consume large amounts of pods or toxic plants in a brief period of time. Most losses happen when hungry livestock are driven through an area of heavy lupine growth, or are trailed through an area where the grass is covered by snow but the taller lupines are exposed. Poisoning has occurred when animals are unloaded into an area of lupine infestation after having been transported long distances. Frequently, animals are forced to graze lupines because of overgrazing and lack of other forage. A naive or unaware management decision can result in large, sometimes catastrophic, losses.

Teratogenicity
Lupine species containing the teratogenic alkaloid anagyrine present significant risks to cattle producers when pregnant cows are allowed to graze on infested pastures during susceptible stages of gestation. The defects are characterized as one or more of the following: arthrogryposis (contracture and malalignment defects of the limbs), scoliosis (spinal column twisting), torticollis (deformed neck), kyphosis (spinal depression) and cleft palate (Figure 2.6). While bone and joint development appears to be normal, defects are believed to be contracture-type defects resulting from abnormal tendon, muscle and ligament tension induced by a lack of fetal movement during susceptible periods of gestation.

The susceptible periods of gestation have been defined in cattle. The severity and type of malformations also depend on the alkaloid dosage ingested, the stage of pregnancy when the plants are eaten, and the length of time ingestion takes place. The most critical gestational period for exposure in cattle is 40 to 70 days, with susceptible periods extending to 100 days. The cleft palate induction period in cattle was narrowly defined to within gestation days 40 to 50 (Panter et al., 1998a).

Livestock Species Differences
The syndrome 'crooked calf disease', associated with lupine ingestion, was first reported in the late 1950s. It includes various skeletal contracture-type birth defects and occasional cleft palate (Figure 2.6). Epidemiologic evidence and chemical comparison of teratogenic and non-teratogenic lupines has determined that the quinolizidine alkaloid anagyrine (Figure 2.5) is the teratogen (reviewed in Panter et al., 1999). A second teratogen, ammodendrine, was found in *Lupinus formosus*, *L. arbustus* and other species and induced similar types of skeletal birth defects (Keeler and Panter, 1989). Further research determined that the anagyrine-containing lupines only caused birth defects in cattle and were not teratogenic in sheep or goats (Panter et al., 1999). However, no breed predilection or genetic susceptibility to the lupine-induced condition has been determined in cattle. The piperidine-containing lupines caused birth defects in experimentally treated cattle and goats (Keeler and Panter, 1989; Panter et al., 1994). Other piperidine alkaloids and piperidine-containing plants also cause contracture-type birth defects and cleft palate in cattle, sheep, pigs, and goats (Panter et al., 1998b, 2000). These studies led to the hypothesis that possible metabolism or absorption differences occur between cattle, small ruminants and non-ruminants. It was originally hypothesized that cattle might metabolize the quinolizidine alkaloid anagyrine to a complex piperidine, meeting the structural characteristics determined for the simple teratogenic piperidine alkaloids in poison-hemlock (Keeler and Panter, 1989; Figures 2.1,

2.2, 2.4, and 2.5). There are multiple ways that the ring structure of anagyrine can be opened, thus meeting the criteria for teratogenicity proposed by Keeler and Panter (1989). The change in ring structure hypothesis was supported by feeding trials with other piperidine alkaloid-containing plants, extracts, and pure compounds. Even though comparative studies supported the hypothesis that cows may convert the quinolizidine alkaloid anagyrine to a complex piperidine by ruminal metabolism, more recent evidence reporting the absorption and elimination patterns of many of the quinolizidine alkaloids, including anagyrine, in cattle, sheep, and goats did not support this theory (Gardner and Panter, 1993).

Mechanism of Action
The proposed mechanism of action for lupine-induced malformations and cleft palate in cattle has been elucidated using a goat model. Panter et al. (1990) hypothesized that the mechanism for induced contracture defects and cleft palate involves a chemically-induced reduction in fetal movement such as one would expect with a sedative, neuromuscular blocking agent, or anesthetic. The proposed mechanism of action was supported by experiments using radio ultrasound imaging. A direct relationship was recorded between reduced fetal activity and severity of contracture-type skeletal defects and cleft palate in sheep and goats. Further research suggests that this inhibition of fetal movement must be over a protracted period of time during specific stages of gestation.

Ultrasonographic studies (Panter et al., 1990) demonstrated that strong fetal movement occurs in the untreated goat beginning at about day 35 of gestation, with extension-type movements of the fetal head and neck. Under the influence of certain teratogenic alkaloids through days 35 to 41 of gestation, fetuses remained tightly flexed with their chin on the sternum and there were no extension-type movements. Subsequently, the newborn goats from affected does had cleft palates but no other birth defects. Panter and Keeler (1992) suggested that these cleft palates were caused by an alkaloid-induced mechanical interference by the tongue between the palate shelves during programmed palate closure times (day 38 in goats; between days 40 and 50 in cows).

Biomedical Application
The establishment of appropriate animal models for biomedical application is essential if new techniques and procedures are to be applied to human conditions. Briefly, the syndrome of plant-induced cleft palate and contracture skeletal malformations in livestock ('crooked calf syndrome'), as described above, is the same whether it is induced by *Lupinus*, *Conium* or *Nicotiana* spp. Likewise, the malformations are described as the same in cattle, sheep, goats, and pigs. While the development of a small ruminant model (goat) was primarily to study the mechanism of action of 'crooked calf syndrome' in cattle, interest in the induced congenital cleft palate and the goat model led to biomedical applications (Panter et al., 2000a).

Cleft palates induced by toxic plants in the goat model closely mimic the human cleft condition (Weinzweig et al., 1999a, b). This model is also useful for histological comparison of the prenatal and postnatal repaired cleft palate and comparison of craniofacial growth and development. Therefore, the goat model provides an ideal congenital model for studying the etiology of cleft palate in humans, for development of fetal surgical techniques *in utero*, and for comparing palate histology after prenatal or postnatal repair. The biomedical application of these plants and the specific animal model selected has evolved over time and occurred because of the discovery of specific biological effects in the goat and their relationship with similar conditions in humans (Panter and Keeler, 1992; Weinzweig et al., 1999a, b; Panter et al., 2000b).

As research in craniofacial abnormalities evolved, two key factors surfaced in the study of the mechanism of action and advancement of the biomedical research on the human cleft palate condition:

1. the goat as a preferred animal model
2. *Nicotiana glauca* and anabasine as a preferred test plant/alkaloid

With availability of these two factors, the advancements in studying the human cleft palate condition are rapidly progressing (Weinzweig et al., 1999a, b, 2002).

Recent research has focused on the privileged period of fetal scarless healing and development of *in utero* surgical procedures to repair human cleft palates early in gestation. To emphasize the significance of this research, Dr. Jeff Weinzweig, M.D. (plastic surgeon, Brown University, Providence, RI) stated:

> Children born with cleft palate often undergo a series of operations to correct the ensuing deformities, only the first of which is the actual palate repair at the age of six to twelve months. For many children, speech remains a major problem as well as craniofacial development. Our goal, of course, is to eliminate the need for any of these reconstructive procedures by performing the cleft palate repair *in utero*. Never, more than now, in the age of fetal surgery has this been a real possibility. Despite this, what is truly exciting is that we now have a congenital goat model of cleft palate as well as the model of *in utero* cleft repair.

Therefore, the biomedical value of the goat model using *N. glauca* plant or anabasine-rich extracts to induce cleft palates has been applied to human medicine (Weinzweig et al., 1999a, b, 2002).

While the benetifs of fetal surgical intervention in life-threatening circumstances have been demonstrated, the role of fetal intervention (surgery) in the treatment of non-life-threatening congenital anomalies remains a source of much debate. Recently, Weinzweig et al. (2002) described and characterized a congenital model for cleft palate in the goat, presented the methodology and techniques used to successfully repair congenital cleft plates *in utero*, and demonstrated successful scarless palatal healing and development after repair.

This model closely simulates the etiopathogenesis of the human anomaly. Thus, *in utero* cleft palate repair early in gestation (on or before day 85 in the goat) is feasible and results in scarless healing of the soft and hard palates. Furthermore, this congenital cleft palate goat model is highly reproducible with little variation, representing an ideal animal model.

In summary, this research has significant implications in the management of fetal cleft palates in humans and application in the study of the etiology and treatment for agricultural research. Understanding the periods of fetal susceptibility, elucidating teratogenic plants and toxins therefrom, and understanding mechanisms of action will provide information for livestock managers whereby losses might be reduced.

2.2.1.3 Steroidal Alkaloids and Steroidal Glycoalkaloids

Steroidal alkaloids and steroidal glycoalkaloids are common toxins found in the Liliaceae and Solanaceae families respectively. *Veratrum* spp. (false hellebore) and *Zygadenus* spp. (death camas) from the lily family, and *Solanum* spp. (nightshades, potato, eggplant, and Jerusalem cherry) and *Lycopersicon* (tomato) from the Solanaceae family, are reported to be toxic, and some are teratogenic (Gaffield and Keeler, 1994). Over 1100 steroidal alkaloids have been characterized and toxicity information is known for many of these. These alkaloids are generally divided into solanum and veratrum or jerveratrum classes, based on structural features and biological activity. Table 2.1 illustrates the relative potency of 13 of these alkaloids in a hamster bioassay (Gaffield and Keeler, 1994).

2.2.1.3.1 Solanum Glycoalkaloids

Solanum spp. are distributed worldwide and have been responsible for numerous livestock and human cases of poisoning. Because of their importance as food plants, particularly the potato, there have been numerous studies to assess the distribution and concentration of glycoalkaloids in different plant parts. The chemistry of the potato, including tubers, vines, and sprouts, has been reported by Sharma and Salunkhe (1989). For example, the flesh of the tuber is the lowest at 12 to 50 ppm, followed by the skins at 300 to 600 ppm, the leaves at 400 to 1000 ppm and sprouts and flowers at 2000 to 5000 ppm (values represented as total glycoalkaloid). As would be expected, the photosynthesizing parts contain the highest concentration of the glycoalkaloids and for this reason vines and green and sprouted potatoes are usually removed from human food supply. However, these green culled potatoes, and occasionally the vines, are fed to livestock, especially when regional feed sources have become scarce. This practice has caused severe poisoning and death.

The structural features of the solanum alkaloids are based on two primary skeletal configurations: solanidane, with or without glycoside functionalities, as featured by the toxic and teratogenic steroidal alkaloids α-chaconine and α-solanine with the indolizidine type E–F ring (Figure 2.7a); and the spirosolane

Table 2.1
Steroidal alkaloids found in *Veratrum* spp. and *Solanum* spp. with their relative teratogenic potency, as determined in a hamster bioassay.

Alkaloid	Teratogenicity
Tomatidine	0
Tomatine	1
5α,6-Dihydrosolasodine	4
Solasodine	6
5α,6-Dihydrosolasodine	10
Solanidine	35
α-Solanine	35
Cyclopamine	35
5α,6,12β,13α-Tetrahydrojervine	40
α-Chaconine	50
12β,13α-Dihydrojervine	60
Jervine	100

Source: Adapted from Gaffield, W. and Keeler, R.F. (1994), *Pure and Appl. Chem.* **66**, 2407–2410.

configuration, represented by the non-teratogenic alkaloids tomatine or tomatidine with spirofused E and F rings (Gaffield and Keeler, 1994; Figure 2.7b). Both classes are represented by alkaloids with or without glycoside functionality. A number of *Solanum* spp. has caused poisoning in livestock. *Solanum fastigiatum*, *S. kwebense*, and *S. dimidiatum* have induced cerebellar degeneration in cattle, including progressive degeneration and vacuolation of Purkinje cells (Cheeke, 1998). The lesions appear as a lysosomal storage disease

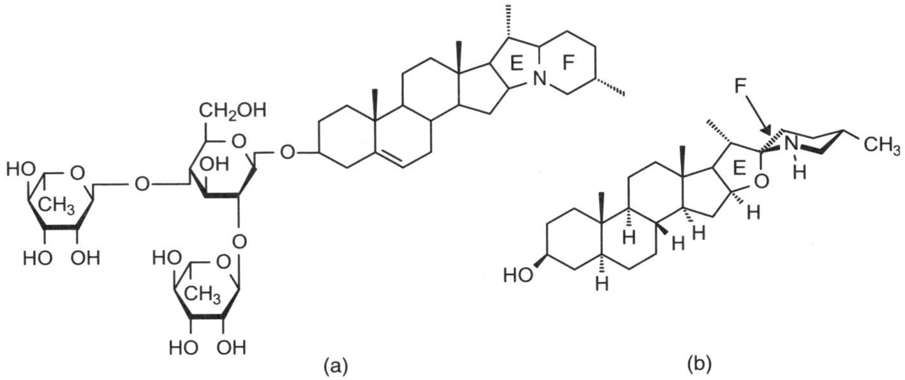

FIGURE 2.7 Two steroidal alkaloids from *Solanum* spp.; (a) α-chaconine, with teratogenic activity, and (b) tomatidine, non-teratogenic alkaloid.

similar to that caused by locoweeds. These plants contain the solanidane-type alkaloids with the indolizidine configuration of the E–F rings, similar to that found in locoweeds (Figure 2.7b; see Section 2.2.6).

Few data have been reported on the alkaloid profiles or concentrations of the wild *Solanum* spp. (nightshades). Livestock poisoning has been reported from black nightshade (*S. nigrum*), climbing nightshade (*S. dulcamara*), and silverleaf nightshade (*S. eleagnifolium*). Clinical effects from ingestion of these species include gastrointestinal upset and associated problems, such as diarrhea and reduced feed intake. A neurological effect from the inhibition of acetylcholinesterase has also been reported (reviewed in Beasley, 1997).

Other plants of the nightshade family, including *Atropa belladonna* (deadly nightshade), *Hyoscyamus niger* (black henbane), and *Datura stramonium* (Jimson weed), contain atropine-like toxins that are anticholinergic, blocking the muscarinic receptors. An incidence in southern Utah of cattle poisoned on black henbane, with many death losses, was recently reported (Pfister, 2003). Atropine and atropine-like alkaloids are discussed Section 2.2.1.7.

2.2.1.3.2 *Veratrum and Zygadenus Alkaloids*

Steroidal alkaloids found in the Liliaceae family, primarily *Veratrum* and *Zygadenus*, have been responsible for large losses in livestock. Human and livestock deaths have occurred from accidental ingestion of death camas (Panter et al., 1987). Thousands of lambs have died or been destroyed because of *Veratrum*-induced malformations, most notably a craniofacial defect called cyclopia (Binns et al., 1965; James, 1999; Figure 2.8). Tracheal stenosis, skeletal malformations and early embryonic death are also common (Keeler and

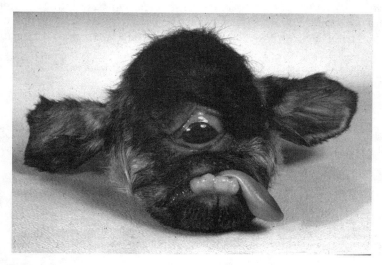

FIGURE 2.8 Congenital cyclopia induced by maternal ingestion of *Veratrum californicum* (or the steroidal alkaloid cyclopamine) on day 14 of gestation.

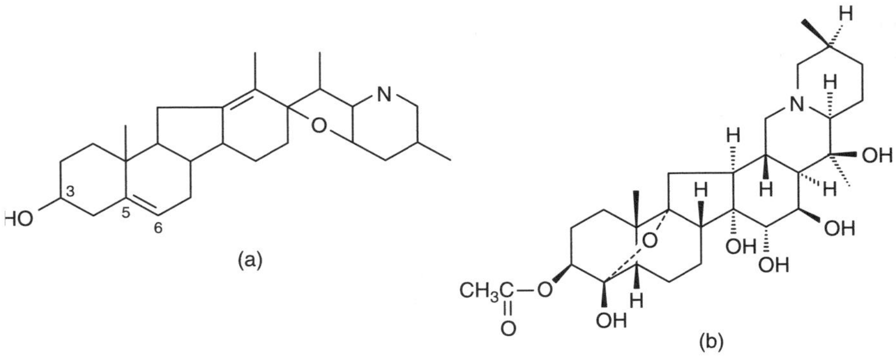

FIGURE 2.9 (a) Cyclopamine, steroidal alkaloid teratogen from *Veratrum* spp., and (b) zygacine, non-teratogenic alkaloid from *Zygadenus* spp.

Young, 1986). *Zygadenus* has caused overt poisoning in sheep and cattle, however no teratogenic effects have been reported.

The steroidal alkaloids in *Veratrum* and *Zygadenus* are divided into two classes; the jerveratrum and ceveratrum types (Figure 2.9). These alkaloids have a modified cyclopentanoperhydrophenanthrene ring structure (steroid skeleton) with C-nor-D-homo with a contracted C-ring and an expanded D-ring (Gaffield, 2000). Jerveratrum alkaloids have alkamines with one, two or three oxygen atoms, and occur as such or as monoglycosides. Ceveratrum alkaloids have seven, eight or nine oxygens and occur as free alkamines or esters of simple aliphatic or aromatic acids. They do not occur as glycosides. Several structural variations around the nitrogen portion of the veratrum alkaloids are found in the plant including the highly bioactive teratogens jervine, cyclopamine and the glucose glycoside cycloposine.

Veratrum Alkaloids
Jerveratrum alkaloids were responsible for multiple congenital defects (Figure 2.8) in sheep when pregnant ewes grazed *Veratrum* plants during specific stages of gestation (Keeler, 1986). Because of the *Veratrum*-induced anomalies and their relationship to human conditions, the steroidal alkaloids have become important tools or probes for studying developmental processes involving craniofacial, limb, and foregut morphogenesis. During gastrulation, the embryo undergoes several morphogenetic events that lead to differentiation of the three primary germ layers: the gut (endoderm); the muscles, bones and connective tissue (mesoderm); and the skin and nervous tissue (ectoderm; reviewed by Gaffield, 2000).

The Sonic hedgehog gene and the Hedgehog (Hh) family of secreted proteins play key roles in developmental processes, ranging from bone morphogenesis to neurological differentiation (reviewed in Gaffield, 2000). Sonic hedgehog directs the intercellular signals between germ layers at the time of differentiation and has been shown to be responsible for the induction of the grotesque cyclopic malformation in sheep. The link between *Veratrum*-induced cyclopia in sheep and the inhibition of the Sonic hedgehog gene pathway resulted from research on mouse embryos that lacked functional copies of Sonic hedgehog, resulting in several forms of holoprosencephaly. Subsequently, cyclopamine and jervine were shown to inhibit specifically the Sonic hedgehog gene pathway, causing the various forms of holoprosencephaly.

Two research groups have concluded that the jerveratrum alkaloids induce their primary teratogenic effect on developing embryos by selectively blocking Sonic hedgehog signal transduction. Sonic hedgehog also regulates other processes controlled by genes downstream and is intimately involved in the development of limbs, skin, eye, lung, teeth, nervous system, and differentiation of sperm and cartilage (Hammerschmidt et al., 1997).

Zygadenus Alkaloids
Zygadenus spp. (death camas) contain several steroidal alkaloids of the ceveratrum type (with seven, eight or nine oxygens and the nitrogen incorporated into a quinolizidine ring; Figure 2.9b). The most known alkaloids are zygacine and zygadenine. While the alkaloids are similar in structure to *Veratrum* alkaloids, they are not thought to be teratogenic and they impart a different clinical toxicosis. All parts of the plant are toxic, especially the bulb. The alkaloids decrease blood pressure, slow heart rate, and may cause pulmonary congestion before death. Poisoning generally occurs in sheep but cattle, horses, pigs, and humans have all been poisoned (Panter et al., 1987).

Potential Biomedical Applications of Cyclopamine
A variety of diseases and clinical disorders result from mutations in the human Sonic hedgehog gene and associated pathways. Hedgehog is known to regulate downstream genes called Patched, Smoothened or Gli (Hammerschmidt et al., 1997). Since cyclopamine selectively inhibits the hedgehog pathway, it makes perfect sense that *Veratrum* alkaloids (cyclopamine) could provide tools or probes for investigating hedgehog-associated diseases in humans. Among the associated diseases are not only holoprosencephaly and various tumors, but also several forms of polydactyly derived from genetic defects in hedgehog network genes. Holoprosencephaly syndrome in humans is relatively common in early embryogenesis, occurring in 1 of 250 spontaneous abortions and 1 in 16,000 live births (Matsunaga and Shiota, 1977). Cyclopamine's ability, both to induce holoprosencephaly in experimental animals and to strongly inhibit Sonic hedgehog signal transduction, offers the potential to enhance understanding of human brain and spinal cord development at the cellular and molecular levels (Gaffield, 1996).

Other genetic disorders have been associated with the hedgehog gene and the downstream genes (Patched, Smoothened or Gli) that are positively or negatively regulated by the hedgehog proteins (reviewed in Gaffield et al., 2000). For example, Patched, Smoothened and Gli have been implicated in basal cell nevous syndrome, rhabdomyosarcoma, medulloblastomas, and primitive neuroectodermal tumors. These genes are regulated downstream from Sonic hedgehog. In addition, Patched mutations have been identified in breast carcinoma, a meningioma, esophageal squamous carcinoma, and trichoepithelioma. Activating mutations in Smoothened are often found in sporadic basal cell carcinomas and primitive neuroectodermal tumors. Cyclopamine and its derivatives, because of their ability to regulate hedgehog genes, have been proposed as 'potential mechanism-based' therapeutic agents for the treatment of tumors arising from disruption of components of the Hedgehog pathway. Hedgehog inhibitors, such as cyclopamine, might be effective in controlling the onset or progression of certain lesions or disease states in non-pregnant adults because of the low toxicity of drug levels that are effective in blocking Sonic hedgehog (Taipale et al., 2000).

Cyclopamine also interferes with cholesterol metabolism that results in decreased cholesterol synthesis and the accumulation of late biosynthetic intermediates. Cyclopamine was evaluated as an inhibitor of multi-drug resistance in tumor cells. Intrinsic or acquired resistance of tumor cells to cytotoxic drugs is a major cause of failure of chemotherapy. Both cyclopamine and the spirosolane alkaloid tomatidine from tomatoes act as potent and effective chemosensitizers in multidrug-resistant cells (Lavie et al., 2001). Therefore, plant steroidal alkaloids, such as cyclopamine and tomatidine, or their analogs, may serve as chemosensitizers in combination with chemotherapy and conventional cytotoxic drugs for treating multidrug-resistant cancers.

Pancreatic development in the embryo was enhanced upon exposure to cyclopamine. Cyclopamine inhibition of Sonic hedgehog signaling apparently permits expansion of portions of the endodermal region of the foregut where Sonic hedgehog signaling does not occur, resulting in pancreatic differentiation in a larger area of the foregut endoderm (Kim and Melton, 1998), thus providing a tool in the treatment of pancreatic diseases and development of cell-replacement therapies or an artificial pancreas.

Future Research
Research models using cyclopamine as a probe or tool could provide insight into understanding the etiologic role of environmental agents in various human birth defects. Clarification of the Sonic hedgehog network might further reveal how this network interacts with other signal transduction pathways. Cyclopamine and other steroidal alkaloids will be used to further define human anomalies, and will be particularly useful in treatment of certain human diseases, including some cancers.

2.2.1.4 Norditerpenoid Alkaloids

Over 40 norditerpenoid alkaloids have been reported in species of larkspurs. Data on toxicity in a mammalian system have been reported for 25 of these by the Poisonous Plant Research Laboratory (reviewed in Panter et al., 2002). The commonality among all the wild larkspur species is the presence of norditerpenoid alkaloids, which are responsible for poisoning livestock, particularly cattle. These alkaloid toxins are of three general classes, based on chemical structural features (Figure 2.10a–c):

1. lycoctonine type
2. 7,8-methylene-dioxylycoctonine (MDL) types (e.g. deltaline)
3. N-(methylsuccinimido)-anthranoyllycoctonine (MSAL) types (e.g. MLA)

These distinct structural features have been correlated to their toxic activity. The MSAL-type alkaloids (Figure 2.10c), in particular methyllycaconitine (MLA), nudicauline (NUD) and 14-deacetylnudicauline (14-DAN), are the toxic alkaloids responsible for the majority of poisonings by larkspurs. Deltaline (Figure 2.10b) of the MDL type, though much less toxic, is prevalent in most larkspur populations, and if present in high enough concentrations will exacerbate the toxic effects of the MSAL-type alkaloids. Deltaline by itself would not be a significant threat to livestock unless toxic levels of the MSAL-type alkaloids are present. The lycoctonine type alkaloids (Figure 2.10a) are the least toxic and are found in variable concentrations in larkspurs.

The MSAL-type alkaloids are potent neuromuscular poisons in mammals, acting at the post-synaptic neuromuscular junction. Variations in structural features of each norditerpenoid alkaloid can exacerbate or reduce toxicity. While the mechanism of action of the norditerpenoid alkaloids involves blocking of neuromuscular transmission at the $\alpha 1$ nicotinic acetylcholine receptors, relative toxicity of individual alkaloids is observed to change with variations in the structural characteristics of the alkaloids (Dobelis et al., 1999). In comparison with the lycoctonine and MDL-type alkaloids, the high toxicity

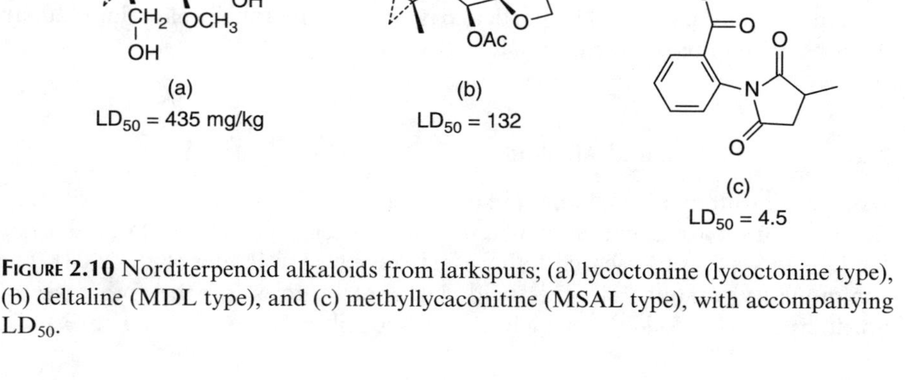

FIGURE 2.10 Norditerpenoid alkaloids from larkspurs; (a) lycoctonine (lycoctonine type), (b) deltaline (MDL type), and (c) methyllycaconitine (MSAL type), with accompanying LD_{50}.

of the three MSAL-type alkaloids (NUD, 14-DAN, MLA) can be associated with the presence of a methylsuccinylanthranoyl ester at C18 (Figure 2.10c). Removal of the ester functionality from MLA, thereby forming lycoctonine (Figure 2.10a), eliminates the neuromuscular activity.

The active core of the norditerpenoid alkaloids is the lycoctonine skeleton, and the quaternary amine element of all the diterpene alkaloids is an important component of the neuromuscular blocking effects. The methylsuccinylanthranoyl ester functionality at C18 imparts potency to the alkaloids via orientation and/or binding affinity to the nicotinic receptors. The C14 functionalities and the pattern of oxygenation and the electronic nature of the oxygen bearing functionalities enhance the physiological manifestations and potency of toxicity. The structural features of the norditerpenoid alkaloids, mainly NUD, MLA, and 14-DAN, are potent competitive antagonists of acetylcholine at the skeletal neuromuscular junction. Recent comparisons of binding affinities of MSAL and MDL alkaloids using lizard muscle nAChR showed distinct differences (Dobelis et al., 1999). Differences in binding affinity and toxicity among MSAL norditerpenoid alkaloids and between MSAL and MDL alkaloids are related to the structural characteristics of the alkaloids, i.e., nudicauline > 14-deacetylnudicauline > MLA > > barbinine > > > > deltaline. In mice and rats, high doses of MLA elicit central nervous system (CNS) effects (Stegelmeier et al. 1998).

The larkspur (*Delphinium*) species are generally divided into three categories (Nielsen and Ralphs, 1987; Majak et al., 2000):

1. Tall larkspurs (*D. barbeyi, D. occidentale, D. glaucescens, D. brownii,* and *D. glaucum*), 1 to 2 m in height, generally growing in moist, high mountain habitats above 2400 m.
2. Intermediate larkspurs (*D. geyeri*; plains larkspur), 0.6 to 1 m tall and present on the short grass prairies of Wyoming, Colorado and Nebraska.
3. Low larkspurs (*D. andersonii* and *D. nuttallianum*) which generally grow on the desert/semi-desert, foothill or low mountain ranges and are less than 0.6 m tall.

Larkspur poisoning has been a major cause of cattle losses on western rangelands for many years (Cronin and Nielsen, 1979) and continues to be the most serious poisonous plant problem on western U.S. high mountain rangelands (Ralphs et al., 1997). Some of the first range improvements on Forest Service allotments were 'poison fences' to keep cattle away from larkspur. Even today, the presence of tall larkspur dictates when and how some of these ranges are utilized. Larkspur populations should be tested during the flowering and pod stages of growth for MSAL-type alkaloid concentration. Whenever the concentrations exceed 3 mg/g during the flowering stage, when cattle often initiate consumption, the cattle should be removed and not returned until pods shatter later in the season (Pfister et al., 2002). If the concentration of the MSAL-type alkaloids exceeds 3 mg/g in the pods, risk will be moderate to high if cattle are eating the pods. Larkspurs containing lower concentration of the MSAL-type alkaloids (< 3 mg/g) in the leaves, flowers, or pods are usually safe for grazing throughout the grazing season because cattle would need to ingest very large quantities for fatalities to occur.

2.2.1.5 Pyrrolizidine Alkaloids

Pyrrolizidine alkaloids (PAs) are common in three plant families, Fabaceae (*Crotalaria* spp.), Asteraceae (*Senecio* spp.), and Boraginaceae (*Amsinckia, Borago, Cynoglossum, Echium, Heliotropium,* and *Symphytum*). There are over 1200 *Senecio* spp. throughout the world, with many containing toxic PAs (Cheeke, 1998). Over 250 species of *Senecio* are endemic to South Africa (Kellerman et al., 1988), 128 to Brazil (Habermehl et al. 1988), and over 200 to Chile (Smith and Culvenor, 1981). Pyrrolizidine alkaloid poisoning in animals and humans is a worldwide problem. It is a significant impediment to international trade because of contaminated or potentially contaminated animal feeds and human foods (Huxtable and Cooper, 2000; Edgar and Smith, 2000). Pyrrolizidine alkaloids can enter the human food chain via contaminated grains, milk, honey, eggs, and other foods or herbal products. In 1992, the German Federal Health Bureau established intake limits for PAs. Regulations specified 0.1 μg as the maximum daily intake limits for hepatotoxic pyrrolizidine alkaloids and their *N*-oxides from herbal plants or plant extracts. Prescribing herbal products containing PAs to pregnant or lactating women is strictly prohibited. Intake limitations and restrictions of use have created trade restrictions with various countries.

Human poisonings have been common throughout the world and numerous cases have been reported (Huxtable and Cooper, 2000). These cases are generally veno-occlusive disease, manifest as abdominal distention due to ascitic fluid. Pulmonary disease, vertigo, and vomiting have also been reported. Human cases of one or two, or up to 50 or 60, individuals are common, but larger death losses have been reported. Such cases include over 3900 deaths in Tadjikistan in 1993 and 7200 in Afghanistan in 1976 from *Heliotropium*, several hundred in the West Indies from *Crotalaria* and *Senecio* in 1954, and over 200 in Uzbekistan in 1950 from *Trichodesma* are reported. Some PAs and the pyrroles are carcinogenic.

PAs contain two fused five-member rings with a nitrogen at one of the vertices (necine base; Figure 2.11a) and one or more branched carboxylic acids attached as esters to one or two of the necine hydroxyl groups (Figure 2.11b, c). The PAs in toxic plants are of three general classes; monoesters, noncyclic diesters, and cyclic diesters. Most hepatotoxic PAs are esters of the base retronecine or heliotridine, and diastereomers of each other with opposing configuration at the C7 position of the pyrrolizidine nucleus (Figure 2.11b). Cyclic diesters (Figure 2.11c) are the most toxic, noncyclic diesters are of intermediate toxicity, and monoesters the least toxic (Cheeke, 1998). The heliotridine esters are more reactive than the retronecine esters.

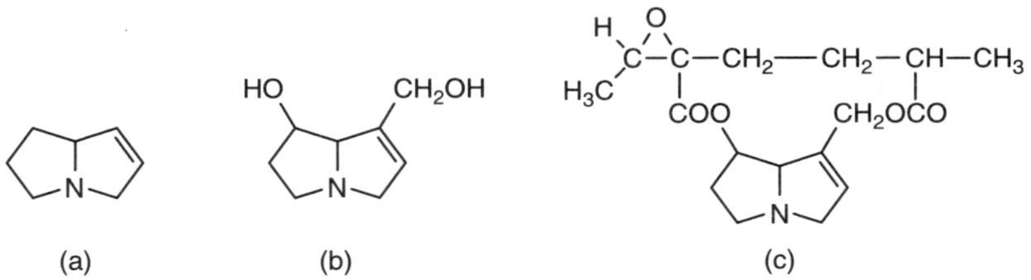

FIGURE 2.11 Pyrrolizidine alkaloid toxins including; (a) the pyrrolizidine nucleus, (b) retronecine, a less toxic monoester, and (c) jacobine, a highly toxic cyclic diester.

For PAs to be toxic, certain key structural features must be present; a double bond in the 1,2 position of the PA nucleus, and branching in the ester group. The PAs that are more easily hydrolyzed by esterases produce fewer toxic pyrroles upon liver activation. However, PAs with more branching in the side chains produce more toxic pyrroles because hydrolysis is hindered, allowing the PA to get to the liver where toxic activation occurs. These toxic pyrroles are powerful alkylating agents and will react with many tissues. Small amounts of pyrroles may escape hepatic circulation and can cause lesions in the lungs, heart, kidneys, GI tract, or brain. Minimal toxic activation of some PAs may occur in these tissues, although the level of microsomal enzyme activity in these tissues is not fully understood. Damage from PAs found in *Senecio*, *Heliotropium*, and *Echium* is generally confined to the liver, while *Crotalaria* intoxication induces significant pulmonary lesions.

There are significant differences in toxicity of PAs in different animal species. Cattle and horses are considered among the most sensitive, with cattle nearly twice as sensitive. Relative sensitivity to pyrrolizidine alkaloid toxicity was reported by Cheeke (1998) as: cattle > horse > rat > chicken > rabbit > guinea pig > goat > sheep > hamster > Japanese quail > gerbil. To put this relationship in perspective, the lethal dose of PA as a percent of body weight is 3.6% for cattle versus 3640% for gerbils. Resistance or sensitivity to pyrrole activation in the liver is largely a reflection of the microsomal enzyme activity in the liver, rather than the gut microbes, although gut metabolism can not be ignored (Cheeke, 1998).

The hepatotoxic element of pyrrolizidine alkaloid toxicosis in cattle often has a latent period between ingestion and manifestation of the disease. The PA found in the plant is generally not toxic, but requires metabolic activation in the liver by microsomal enzymes to the reactive pyrrole or pyrrolic dehydroalkaloids (DHAs; Figure 2.12). Once the toxic pyrrole is formed it binds to DNA (crosslinks) and is believed to remain in the liver or hepatic circulation, further exacerbating liver disease. Metabolism and toxicity of pyrrolizidine alkaloids were reviewed by Huxtable and Cooper (2000). Often, this chronic poisoning was recognized in cattle in the northwest when cattle would graze tansy ragwort (*Senecio jacobea*; Molyneux et al., 1991a). Cattle would show some early signs of poisoning, such as depression and lethargy, and if blood samples were drawn, liver enzyme levels would be seen to be

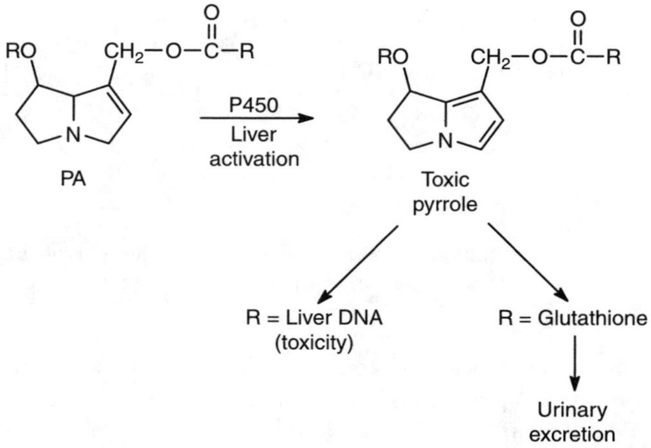

FIGURE 2.12 Metabolic activation by the liver of pyrrolizidine alkaloid to the toxic pyrrole (liver bound and highly toxic) and the glutathione conjugate (excretion metabolite).

elevated. Animals would recover, appearing relatively normal for a period of time, until some stress-related incident, such as cold weather, pregnancy, onset of lactation, shipping, or other disease condition, would trigger a 'hepatic crisis'. It is believed that this 'crisis' results in further liver damage, the animal becomes sick and often dies from liver failure. Hepatic crisis is known to occur months or even years after exposure to PA-containing plants. While PAs are primarily liver toxins, there are PAs that are extrahepatic in their pathology. Pulmonary, neurological, and other organ damage have been reported, but it is not clear whether it results from toxic metabolism in those tissues or from circulating toxic pyrroles that have escaped the hepatic circulation after activation. Peracute and acute poisoning have been reported in experimental settings where relatively high single doses have been administered. Peracute and acute poisoning are not of the hepatic type, but rather involve pulmonary function and neurological function which are seldom observed in the field or with chronic poisoning. Occasionally, peracute poisoning has been diagnosed in humans eating highly-contaminated foods or when pregnant women drink comfrey tea containing high levels of PAs.

Daily ingestion of relatively low amounts of PAs over weeks or months will often not result in any outward clinical signs of poisoning. However, pathologically, the hepatocytes will gradually enlarge, bile ducts proliferate, and lobular atrophy will occur. Central and sublobular veins are often occluded by fibrous tissue. The large hepatocytes (megalocytosis) are generally pathogneumonic for PA poisoning. Hepatocyte enlargement is generally accompanied by an absence of cell division (antimitotic activity).

Pyrrolizidine alkaloid poisoning continues to be a significant problem in the U.S. and throughout the world, and is a focus of research at the USDA Poisonous Plant Research Laboratory.

2.2.1.6 Indolizidine and Polyhydroxy Alkaloids

Indolizidine alkaloids are defined by an indane ring system with nitrogen at one vertex, as represented by the locoweed toxin swainsonine (Figure 2.13). Since swainsonine's discovery in the late 1970s and early 1980s, first by Dorling et al. (1978) from the Darling pea (*Swainsona*) in Australia and then by Molyneux and James (1982) in the *Astragalus* and *Oxytropis* locoweeds, many other glycosidase-inhibitory alkaloids have been discovered (Molyneux et al., 2002). In Australia, Darling pea poisoning was called 'peastruck', and in the U.S. a similar disease called 'locoism' has been induced by ingestion of *Astragalus* spp. and *Oxytropis* spp. Initially only represented by swainsonine, the broader class of compounds called 'polyhydroxy alkaloids' now includes indolizidine, pyrrolizidine, and tropane alkaloids and some of the pyrrolidine and piperidine analogs. Because of similar biological activity and chemical features (all contain multiple hydroxyl groups), these alkaloids are often discussed together as polyhydroxy alkaloids.

Interest in swainsonine was high from the outset as its potent and specific inhibition of α-mannosidase was key in explaining the mechanism of action of certain genetic disorders and the plant-induced locoism in livestock. Since swainsonine's discovery it has been used as a biochemical tool for studying numerous biochemical processes in the cell, such as glycoprotein processing and synthesis, glycoprotein modification and storage, specific glycoprotein disorders, T-lymphocyte function, and cancer metastasis (reviewed in James et al., 2004).

Similarly, discovery of other polyhydroxylated indolizidine alkaloids that possess glycosidase inhibitory properties, such as castanospermine, lentiginosine, and their derivatives, have been reported (Molyneux et al., 1991b). Castanospermine, the major alkaloid in Moreton Bay chestnut (*Castanospermum australe*), has also been associated with livestock poisoning. Castanospermine is a potent competitive inhibitor of β-glucocerebrosidase and lysosomal α-glucosidase and, like swainsonine, interferes with glycoprotein processing, although in a slightly different way. Interest in castanospermine was stimulated when it was discovered to inhibit tumor growth, viral replication and HIV syncytium formation (reviewed by Roitman and Panter, 1995). An epimer of castanospermine, 6-epicastanospermine, is a potent inhibitor of amyloglucosidase but does not inhibit β-glucosidase or α- or β-mannosidase. These alkaloids have a high degree of specificity for individual enzymes, yet they only differ slightly in chemical structure.

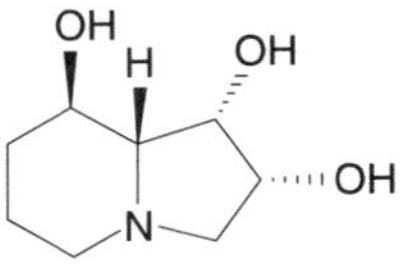

FIGURE 2.13 The indolizidine alkaloid toxin swainsonine (a potent inhibitor of α-mannosidase), responsible for locoweed toxicosis.

A second pair of dehydroxyindolizidine alkaloids (also epimers of each other) was isolated from locoweeds. Lentiginosine is a potent inhibitor of amyloglucosidase, but the 2-epilentiginosine epimer is not, thus demonstrating again the unique specificity of these compounds to inhibit only specific enzymes. Lentiginosine and its epimer are present in some locoweeds as minor components, however they are potent inhibitors of cellular enzyme function and most likely contribute to the emaciated condition of animals severely poisoned on locoweed.

Locoweed poisoning has been a major focus of research at the USDA Poisonous Plant Research Laboratory since the very early 1900s (James et al., 1981). In 1909, C.D. Marsh published a bulletin describing locoweed poisoning of the western plains. Only species of *Astragalus* and *Oxytropis* that contain swainsonine are true locoweeds (Marsh, 1909). Since discovering swainsonine as the toxin in locoweeds in 1982, many species of *Astragalus* and *Oxytropis* in the U.S., South America, and China have been confirmed as locoweeds (Molyneux et al., 1994). Recently, swainsonine was isolated from *Ipomoea carnea*, a member of the morning glory family, which has been responsible for a locoweed-like syndrome in sheep and goats in Australia and South Africa. In addition to swainsonine, *A. lentiginosus* contains minor amounts of N-oxide derivative and lentiginosine and 2-epilentiginosine, two structurally related dihydroxy alkaloids that undoubtedly contribute to the reported toxicoses.

Although the toxin content of locoweeds is generally low (0.2% of dry weight), it is found in all above-ground parts of the plant, but is more concentrated in the flowers and seeds. Because of its exceptional potency, it has been calculated that levels greater than 0.001% can cause poisoning if the plant is consumed over a sufficient period of time. The alkaloid appears to be remarkably stable, even dead plants as much as two years old retain enough of the toxin to cause locoism. The potential hazard of any particular plant species to livestock can be assessed by analysis of a representative plant sample for the presence of swainsonine.

The isolation of swainsonine from *Swainsona* species resulted from the observation that the poisoning induced in livestock by these plants was biochemically, morphologically, and clinically similar to the genetic disease 'mannosidosis', which, like locoism, results from an insufficiency of the enzyme α-mannosidase. It was therefore hypothesized that the toxin was an inhibitor of α-mannosidase. This enzyme was used as a probe for bioactivity and ultimately for the separation and purification of the active compound (Dorling et al., 1978; Colegate et al., 1979). The chemical structure of swainsonine is not complex and has many similarities to the simple sugar mannose (which it mimics). It suppresses the action of the enzyme α-mannosidase, which is essential for proper functioning of all animal cells. The enzyme trims sugar molecules from complex, but abnormal, molecules known as glycoproteins within the cell. Once the correct number of sugars have been trimmed, the smaller molecules can be targeted for other functions. Failure of the trimming process results in an accumulation of complex molecules within the cell, resulting in vacuolation. After a sufficient number of cells have been damaged from over accumulation of these compounds, signs of poisoning appear. Since all cells depend on proper functioning of α-mannosidase, many different organs can be damaged, including the brain, heart, liver, pancreas, thyroid, reproductive system, etc. (Stegelmeier et al., 1999).

Like simple sugars, swainsonine is water-soluble and therefore distributed to many parts of the body. It is rapidly excreted, primarily in the urine, but in lactating animals a portion of it is transferred to the milk (James and Hartley, 1977). This fast excretion rate suggests that occasional consumption of locoweeds for short periods is unlikely to have serious effects, but continuous consumption, even at low levels, results in poisoning. Short intensive grazing episodes have been used as a management tool for grazing pastures heavily infested with locoweed (Ralphs et al., 1984).

By recognizing swainsonine as an inhibitor of α-mannosidase, and its ability to interact with receptor sites for mannose substrates on the enzyme, other structurally similar alkaloids were proposed to have similar properties. One such alkaloid, castanospermine, was isolated from seeds of the Moreton Bay chestnut (*Castanospermum australe*), an Australian rainforest tree. The leguminous seeds, which litter the ground beneath the trees, are toxic to livestock. When tested, castanospermine was found to be a potent inhibitor of α- and β-glucosidase, enzymes that are essential for glycoprotein processing (especially in digestion). The discovery of the biochemical activity of this alkaloid suggested a close analogy to locoweed poisoning, although the signs of poisoning are different with pronounced gastrointestinal disturbances and no discernable neurological damage.

A chemical analysis of *C. australe* seeds resulted in the identification of several structurally-related indolizidine alkaloids, differing from castanospermine only in the orientation of specific hydroxyl groups around the ring system. These include some pyrrolizidine alkaloids, which were named australines. These alkaloids inhibited α- and β-glucosidases to a greater or lesser extent, but were present at significantly lower levels than castanospermine. The identification of swainsonine, castanospermine, and australine, together with isomers differing in their stereochemistry, suggests that other similar compounds capable of mimicking sugars might exist in nature as glycosidase inhibitors (Molyneux et al., 1994)

This reasoning has led to the identification of several hydroxylated alkaloids belonging to the tropane class, known as calystegines, which inhibit α- and β-galactosidase and β-glucosidase. At present, this group consists of 14 alkaloids differing by the number, disposition, and stereochemistry of the hydroxyl groups, with calystegines B2 and C1 being the most commonly found. Various combinations of these alkaloids have been discovered in several plant families, including Convolvulaceae, Solanaceae, and Moraceae (Molyneux et al., 1993).

A syndrome in livestock occurs with respect to *Ipomoea* species, which have been found to poison sheep in Australia and goats in Africa (Molyneux et al., 1995). The analysis of *I. calobra* and *I. polpha* from Queensland showed that these plants contain not only calystegines B2 and C1, but also swainsonine. An analogous pattern of alkaloids was detected in *I. carnea* from Mozambique (de Balogh et al., 1999). The toxicity of these plants results from the effect of the toxins on at least three different enzymes and many of the symptoms (neurological) have been correlated with locoism induced by α-mannosidase inhibition, and GI dysfunction exacerbated by inhibition of α-galactosidase and β-glucosidase.

The fundamental cellular function of glycoprotein processing is that it affects glycoproteins that are involved in numerous essential physiological functions, especially cell–cell recognition reactions critical to pathogenesis, inflammation, parasitism, development, cell adhesion, and symbiosis. The polyhydroxy alkaloids exhibit a diversity of biological effects, including insecticidal, herbicidal, antimicrobial, and therapeutic activity. The discovery and isolation of many of the alkaloids have been a result of observations of the ultimate clinical effects that result from the consumption by animals of plants containing these bioactive compounds.

Biomedical Applications
Humans and animals are affected by genetic diseases that occur as a result of inhibition of glycoprotein-processing enzymes (reviewed by James et al., 2004). These diseases are collectively known as lysosomal storage diseases. The animal diseases, genetic or induced, have counterparts in humans. For example:

1. Pompe's disease
2. Gaucher's disease
3. Fabry's disease
4. genetic mannosidosis

Pompe's disease is a generalized glycogenosis caused by a deficiency of the lysosomal enzyme α-1,4-glycosidase, resulting in abnormal storage of glycogen in skeletal muscles, heart, liver, and other organs. Gaucher's disease is a chronic familial deficiency of a glucocerebroside-cleaning enzyme, resulting in abnormal storage of cerebrosides in reticuloendothelial cells and characterized by spenomegaly, hepatomegaly, skin pigmentation, pinqueculae of the scleras, and bone lesions. Fabry's disease (*angiokeratoma corporis diffusum universale*) is an inherited disorder of glycolipid metabolism due to a deficiency of a ceramide trihexosidase-cleaving enzyme.

Genetic mannosidosis has been described in man, Angus cattle and Murray Gray cattle, and is characterized by a deficiency of α-mannosidase leading to storage of excess mannose-rich oligosaccharides in lysosomes. Pathologically, there is vacuolation of reticuloendothelial cells in the liver and lymph nodes, pancreatic exocrine cells, and neurons. Affected cattle are ataxic, uncoordinated, fail to thrive, and die in the first year of life.

Locoweed poisoning mimics exactly the genetic mannosidosis. Thus, the availability of specific inhibitors (plant toxins) of these enzymes provides a mechanism for induction of phenocopies of these genetic diseases in animal models. As an example, feeding experiments with castanospermine in rats resulted in vacuolation of hepatocytes and skeletal myocytes, and glycogen accumulation, consistent with Pompe's disease. Young rats treated with swainsonine developed axonal dystrophy in the CNS as a consequence of lysosomal storage of incompletely processed mannosides, which has a parallel in genetic mannosidosis and locoweed poisoning. Experiments using the indolizidine alkaloids described and other alkaloids have the potential to provide useful information for early diagnosis and possible methods of intervention to interrupt the progression of such diseases.

Although mammalian toxicity of the polyhydroxy alkaloids is an obvious medicinal concern, the capability to disrupt the general cellular function of glycoprotein processing leads to the expectation that these compounds should have therapeutic potential for the treatment of various disease states. Although many drug candidates have significant toxicity, it is well recognized that an appropriate dose–response relationship that minimizes harmful side-effects can often be achieved. Moreover, adverse effects, such as the neurological damage caused by swainsonine, often develop quite slowly and appear to be reversible if ingestion of the alkaloid is terminated, as would be the situation with most drug regimens. Investigation of these alkaloids for therapeutic potential has so far concentrated on four major disease states, namely the treatment of cancer, inhibition of metastasis, anti-viral treatments, and anti-parasitic therapy. Structurally related compounds have also been investigated as anti-diabetes drugs.

Swainsonine has received particular attention as an anti-metastatic agent, and this effect has been shown to be due to enhancement of natural killer T-cells to cancerous cells. *In vivo* experiments with mice have shown that animals provided with drinking water containing 3 µg/ml swainsonine for 24 hours prior to injection with B16-F10 murine melanoma cells had an 80% reduction in pulmonary colonization. Pharmacokinetic studies indicate that the levels of alkaloid and period of administration would be insufficient to produce neurological damage. It has been suggested that post-operative metastasis of tumor cells in humans could be suppressed by intravenous administration of the alkaloid prior to and following surgery. Administration of swainsonine in clinical trials in humans with advanced malignancies showed that lysosomal α-mannosidases and Golgi mannosidase II were inhibited, and improvement in clinical status occurred.

Castanospermine suppresses the infectivity of a number of retro viruses, including the human immunodeficiency virus (HIV), responsible for AIDS. This effect is a direct consequence of glycoprotein processing inhibition, resulting in changes in the structure of the glycoprotein coat of the virus. Cellular recognition of the host is prevented and syncytium formation is suppressed. In spite of this effect, the alkaloid suffers from the disadvantage that it is highly water-soluble and therefore rapidly excreted. This limitation has been partially dealt with by optimization, to give a lipophilic derivative. This has undergone clinical trials against AIDS in humans, either alone or in combination with AZT, with the only significant side-effect being gastro-intestinal disturbances, as might be predicted (Dennis et al., 1993).

The ability of polyhydroxy alkaloid glycosidase inhibitors to prevent cellular recognition has resulted in their use in studies of clinical situations where suppression of an immune response would be desirable, or for use against parasitic diseases. *In vivo* experiments have shown that castanosper-mine can be used as an immuno-suppressive drug, promoting heart and renal allograft survival in rats. Parasitic diseases may also be controlled by altering cellular recognition processes. Swainsonine has been demonstrated to inhibit the association of *Trypanosoma cruzi* (the cause of Chagas' disease) with the host cell by formation of defective mannose-rich oligosaccharides on the cell surface. Castanospermine provides protection against cerebral malaria by preventing adhesion of *Plasmodium falciparum* to infected erythrocytes.

Polyhydroxy alkaloids have considerable potential for treatment of a variety of disease states in humans and animals. The challenge to using them as commercial drugs is to minimize their toxicity and enhance the specificity of their beneficial effects.

2.2.1.7 Tropane Alkaloids

Tropane alkaloids are primarily found in the Solanaceae family and include Jimson weed (*Datura stramonum*), henbane, (*Hyoscyamus niger*), mandrake (*Mandragora*), *Atropa belladonna* (deadly nightshade), *Brugmansia* spp., and *Solandra* spp. They also appear in other plant families, including Convolvulaceae, Brassicaceae, Protaceae, Euphorbiaceae, Moraceae, Oleaceae, Rhizophoraceae, and Erythroxylaceae. *Brugmansia* is native to the Andes Mountains and is very similar to *Datura* spp. (at one time both were included in *Datura* and both have the given name 'angel's trumpet' because of their large, pendulous, trumpet-like, five-toothed flowers). Jimson weed is unpalatable to animals, as are most plants containing the tropane alkaloids, although poisoning of most classes of livestock and humans have been reported in the literature (Kingsbury, 1964; Burrows and Tyrl, 2001). Ingestion of fresh plant material, contaminated hay or silage, and seeds have produced toxicoses. Clinical signs in animals and humans include intense thirst, restlessness, pupillary dilation, increased heart rate, dyspnea, dry mucous membranes, aberrant behavior, and death. In cattle, bloat may occur, and in horses, colic.

Species of *Datura*, *Hyoscyamus* and other tropane-containing genera are of more risk to humans than animals. These plants and their seeds have been used for religious or social functions with ritualistic emphasis. Numerous cases of bizarre and often aggressive behavior have been reported in people using seeds or teas from these plants (Burrows and Tyrl, 2002). As recently as October of 2003, a report appeared at *CNN.com* of four teenagers who ate Jimson weed seeds. All hallucinated and had to be hospitalized. Two were sedated and placed on life-support to prevent danger to themselves and others. The same press release reported that Centers for Disease Control and Prevention recorded 1072 poisonings, including one death, in 2002 from Jimson weed and similar plants.

The tropane alkaloids are divided into two main groups; the Solanaceous tropane alkaloids, including atropine, scopolamine, hyoscyamine, norhyoscyamine, etc. (Figure 2.14a); and the coca tropane alkaloids, including cocaine (Figure 2.14b), cinnamoylcocaine, ecgonine, and other coca derivatives (Harborne and Baxter, 1996). Calystegins are a class of tropane alkaloids that have received recent interest because of their potent enzyme inhibition, as discussed in Section 2.2.1.6.

Calystegin B2 was first isolated from *Calystegia sepium*, and given the name calystegin. It has also been isolated from field bindweed (*Convolvulus arvensis*). Calystegins resemble the indolizidine alkaloids, swainsonine and castanospermine, and are potent inhibitors of glycoprotein enzymes (Molyneux et al., 1993). Calystegin C1 is a potent and specific inhibitor of β-glucosidase; calystegin B1 and B2 inhibit α-galactosidase and β-glucosidase. Whether calystegins are important toxins to humans and animals is yet to be fully determined, but a condition in horses characterized by colic, weight loss, intestinal thickening and fibrosis, and vascular sclerosis has been linked to tropane alkaloids in field bindweed (*C. arvensis*)(Knight and Walter, 2001).

2.2.2 GLYCOSIDES

Glycosides are the second most ubiquitous and important group of plant toxins, after alkaloids (see reviews by Cheeke, 1998; Burrows and Tyrl, 2001; Knight and Walter, 2001). Glycosides are defined as: two-part molecules containing a non-carbohydrate moiety (aglycone) joined by an ether bond to a carbohydrate functionality (such as D-glucose). The non-sugar portion of the glycoside (aglycone) is often the active portion, which imparts toxicity and is released through enzymatic action when the plant tissue is damaged. Glycosides are relatively non-toxic when the two parts of the molecule are

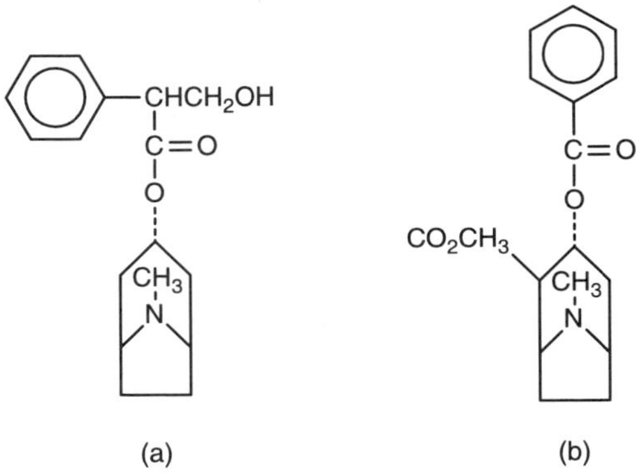

(a)   (b)

FIGURE 2.14 Two common tropane alkaloids in *Solanum* spp.; (a) atropine (*Datura*), and (b) cocaine (*Erythroxylon coca*).

connected; however, hydrolysis in the GI tract of animals, especially ruminants, liberates the aglycone, resulting in toxicity. There are many different classes of glycosides, including cyanogenic, steroidal, nitropropanol, calcinogenic, estrogenic, coumarin, goitrogenic, and others. Vicine from fava beans, carboxyatractyloside from cocklebur and anthraquinones in senna and *Aloe* spp. are also glycosides.

2.2.2.1 Cyanogenic Glycosides

The cyanogenic glycosides occur in many plant genera and species, including *Prunus* (wild cherry), *Hydrangea*, *Sambucus* (elderberry), *Linum* (flax), *Sorghum* (sorghum, sudangrass, johnsongrass), *Manihot* (cassava), and *Bambusa* (bamboo). The aglycone is cyanide or hydrogen cyanide (HCN), referred to as prussic acid. Cyanide is cytotoxic, blocking activity of specific enzymes (cytochrome oxidase) at the terminal stage of the cellular respiratory pathway (Cheeke, 1998; Knight and Walter, 2001). When cytochrome oxidase is blocked, ATP production stops and the cellular organelles in tissue cease to function. Death is rapid. Labored breathing (dyspnea), excitement, gasping, staggering, convulsions, and coma are clinical effects. The mucous membranes and blood are bright cherry red as oxygen is supplied to the tissues but cannot be utilized. Cherry-red blood is diagnostic for cyanide poisoning.

Cyanide is readily hydrolyzed from the sugar in ruminants, or in plants that have been damaged through wilting, frost, trampling, bruising, drought, or chewing. Cellular damage in the plant brings the non-toxic glycoside into contact with the cytosolic enzymes (glucosidases and lyases) that are responsible for the rapid release of free HCN. Ruminant microorganisms also contain these enzymes, and the reaction is optimum at neutral pH. Therefore ruminants are more susceptible than non-ruminants to cyanogenic glycoside poisoning because of rapid liberation of free cyanide. This potent cellular toxin acts very quickly and if high enough doses are ingested, death quickly occurs from cyanosis and asphyxia.

A chronic form of cyanide poisoning is manifest in humans as a neurological disease called tropical ataxic neuropathy. This has been reported in the tropics of west Africa, where cassava is a dietary staple. Clinical effects are the result of demyelinization of the optic, auditory, and peripheral nerve tracts. Goiter is also frequently reported, and results from interference of iodine transport by thiocyanate formation as a detoxification product. In animals, chronic cyanide ingestion also causes degeneration of the nerve tracts, resulting in posterior ataxia, urinary incontinence and cystitis, and can cause birth defects (arthrogryposis) in the fetus. Urinary incontinence and cystitis (equine sorghum cystitis–ataxia syndrome) is common in horses fed sudan grass hay or sorghum fodder for long periods. The cystitis–ataxia syndrome results from demyelinization of the peripheral nerves caused by the lathyrogen T-glutamyl β-cyanoalanine, a metabolite of cyanide glycoside conversion. The lathyrogen interferes with neurotransmitter activity in peripheral nerves and the CNS. Animals may slowly recover if the source of the toxic aminonitrile is removed before nerve damage becomes too severe (Knight and Walter, 2001).

Cyanide is readily detoxified in animals as all animal tissues contain the thiosulfate sulfurtransferase enzyme rhodanese. Rhodanese readily converts cyanide to the thiocyanate which is excreted in the urine.

$$\underset{\text{Thiosulfate}}{S_2O_3^{2-}} + CN^- \omega \xrightarrow{\text{rhodanese}} \omega \ SO_3^{2-} + \underset{\text{Thiocyanate}}{SCN^-}$$

Acute poisoning only occurs when the detoxification mechanism is overwhelmed. This reaction is enhanced by giving sodium thiosulfate and sodium nitrate intravenously as 20% solutions in a 3:1 ratio, which is a recommended antidote for acute cyanide poisoning. It is the thiocyanate metabolite that causes chronic disease when cyanide forage is ingested over an extended period.

2.2.2.2 Steroidal and Triterpenoid Glycosides

In steroidal glycosides, the sugar moiety is joined to the cyclopentanoperhy-drophenanthrene (steroid) nucleus. Steroidal glycosides include the cardenolides (cardiac glycosides) and saponins (sapogenic glycosides).

2.2.2.2.1 Cardiac Glycosides
Toxic cardiac glycosides are found in 11 plant families and more than 34 genera (Knight and Walter, 2001). There are two groups of glycosides in plants, cardenolides and bufadienolides, both of which affect cardiac function. The cardenolides are the best understood, and comprise toxins containing the parent glycosides of digitalis (such as digoxin and digitoxin). Bufadienolides are similar to the cardenolides, but differ in the functionality at C-17 on the D ring. Bufadienolides are prevalent in South African plant species, and are more important in plant poisoning of livestock than the cardenolides (Botha et al., 1998). They are found in three genera of Crassulaceae (*Cotyledon*, *Tylecodon* and *Kalanchoe*). *Kalanchoe* spp. are popular garden- and house-plant varieties and so can be a significant threat to children and pets.

The dogbane family (Apocynaceae) comprises 180 to 200 genera, including *Apocynum*, *Strophanthus*, *Nerium*, *Pentalinon* and others, of which there are over 1500 species that contain cardiac glycosides. There are three general types of intoxications caused by members of the Apocynaceae family: GI irritation, neurotoxicity and cardiotoxicoses. The most toxic species are those that produce the cardenolides. These glycosides, like glycosides in general, are composed of an aglycone (the cardiotoxic portion) and one or more sugars. While the sugars do not cause toxicity, they can alter potency by enhancing absorption and metabolism, depending on which sugar is present.

Some of the most well-known cardenolides include digitoxin from *Digitalis purpurea* (foxglove), convallarin from *Convallaria* (lily-of-the-valley), ouabain from *Strophanthus* and *Acocanthera*, many digitoxin-like cardenolides from

Asclepias (milkweeds), and cardiotoxic genins from *Nerium* (oleander)(Knight and Walter, 2001).

The cardiotoxic activity of glycosides is due to inhibition of ATPase transport and to the increase of myocardial contractility in the same manner as the digitalis pharmaceuticals. Cardiac glycosides given in therapeutic doses can increase the contractility of the heart muscle and slow the heart rate, thereby regulating cardiac output in patients suffering from acute or congestive heart failure. Toxic doses (often only slightly higher than therapeutic) may cause depression, excess salivation, vomiting, diarrhea, weakness, bradycardia, cardiac arrhythmia, and cardiac arrest and death.

2.2.2.2.2 Saponin Glycosides

Plants of the Liliacea family are common sources of steroidal saponins or sapogenins. Sapogenic glycosides are not as toxic as the cardenolides. Saponins contain a polycyclic aglycone (steroid or triterpenoid), and a side chain of sugars attached by an ether bond. Ingestion of saponins often results in gastric irritation and GI upset. Saponins are soap-like substances that cause profuse foaming, producing a distinctive honey-combed, stable foam when shaken in an aqueous solution. This same action will cause bloat in ruminants. Sapogenins are widely distributed in plants, and especially prevalent in forage legumes, making them particularly important in animal nutrition. They are bitter compounds and may decrease palatability and therefore feed intake, and may, for example, exhibit growth-depressing properties in poultry and swine. Saponins are not readily absorbed into the bloodstream, but once the aglycone is absorbed hemolysis may occur. Some saponins, such as those in *Yucca schidigera*, have beneficial effects in animals and are used as food additives (Cheeke, 1998).

2.2.2.3 Nitropropanol Glycosides

Many *Astragalus* species, such as timber milk vetch (*Astragalus miser*, thus the name miserotoxin), Emory milk vetch (*A. emoryanus*) and crown vetch (*Coronilla* spp.) are toxic because of the nitropropanol glycosides of 3-nitro-1-propanol (3-NPOH) and 3-nitropropionic acid (3-NPA)(Majak and Pass, 1989). These compounds, especially 3-NPOH, are acutely toxic, producing methemoglobinemia. The glycosides of 3-NPOH are of greater toxicologic importance in livestock than those of 3-NPA. *Astragalus canadensis* and *A. falcatus* are known to contain high levels of 3-NPA and are very toxic. Cattle are more susceptible to *Astragalus* nitro poisoning than sheep. Miserotoxin, which is the β-D-glucoside of 3-nitro-1-propanol, is the most important 3-NPOH type. Other 3-NPA derivatives include cibarian, corollin, coronarian, coronillin, and karakin. These parent compounds are hydrolyzed to the free aglycones 3-NPA and 3-NPOH by esterases and β-glucosidases in the rumen or gut of herbivores. They are both readily absorbed; 3-NPOH more rapidly than 3-NPA, and also more toxic. 3-NPA is of lesser toxicologic importance because it is more readily degraded in the digestive tract before absorption.

2.2.2.4 Calcinogenic Glycosides

Plants that contain calcinogenic glycoside include *Cestrum diurnum*, *Solanum malacoxylon*, and *Trisetum flavescens* (Knight and Walter, 2001). The toxin is a glycoside of 1,25-dihyroxycholecalciferol which is hydrolyzed to the active vitamin D$_3$. The consumption of these plants by cattle and horses results in excessive calcium absorption and the calcification of soft tissues, such as tendons, arteries, and kidneys. There is approximately 30,000 IU equivalent of Vitamin D$_3$ per kg of plant material, resulting in increased calcium absorption and increased calcium-binding protein. The glycoside in *C. diurnum* is less water-soluble than the glycoside in *Solanum malacoxylon*, and therefore causes less extensive calcification of soft tissues. The resulting dystrophic calcification is especially noticeable in the horse, as manifested by bony prominences on the legs, face, etc., tense abdominal muscles, stiffness with a noticeable short choppy gait, reluctance to move, and eventual recumbency and death. There may be pain upon palpation of tendons and ligaments. *Cestrum* spp. and *S. malacoxylon* also contain cardenolides that may induce similar cardiotoxicity as ouabain. There are other glycosides in some of these species, including carboxyparquin and parquin, which are responsible for hepatic necrosis. These are closely related to the carboxyatractylosides found in cocklebur seedlings.

2.2.2.5 Estrogenic Glycosides (Isoflavones, Coumestans)

Estrogenic glycosides include isoflavones and coumestans in plants that exhibit estrogenic activity. Many of these phytoestrogens are also phenolics. These phytoestrogens induce reproductive dysfunction in animals that graze them for long periods of time. Phytoestrogens are particularly important in subterranean clover (*Trifolium subterran*) and red clover (*T. pratense*), with a history of causing infertility in sheep (clover disease)(Cheeke, 1998). Sheep that graze subterranian clover pastures do not exhibit normal seasonal breeding cycles or estrus cycles and develop cystic ovaries. Wethers exhibit teat enlargement when chronically exposed to phytoestrogens. Fertility returns once ewes are removed from clover pastures, although long-term reduction in fertility has been reported in flocks that are repeatedly affected.

The phytoestrogens (isoflavones) contain a flavone nucleus. Examples of isoflavones are genistein, formononetin and coumestrol, all with potent estrogenic activity. Soybean isoflavones are a concern in human nutrition because of their estrogenic benefits.

2.2.2.6 Coumarin Glycosides

Coumarin glycosides are found throughout the plant kingdom (Burrows and Tyrl, 2001). Seeds of *Aesculus glabra* (Ohio buckeye) contain the coumarin esculin, which is a mild neurotoxin. Sweet clovers (*Melilotus* spp.) contain coumarins that are considered harmless unless moldy conditions exist, in which fungal activity produces the double coumarin dicoumarol. Dicoumarol is a powerful anticoagulant that causes internal hemorrhage and was responsible for extensive losses of cattle in the 1920s in the midwest and Canada. Of benefit to human medicine are the dicoumarol medications (Coumadin7; Warfarin Sodium, etc.) used to thin blood and control clotting in patients with cardiovascular disease. A Warfarin (dicoumarol) derivative is the main ingredient in some rodenticides used as rat and mouse poisons (DeconJ).

Other coumarin-related compounds include furans, found in moldy sweet potatoes, and the furan coumarin complexes (furanocoumarins) found in parsnip leaves (psoralens). They are photoreactive compounds (primary photosensitizers) that exacerbate sunburn to psoralen exposed skin.

2.2.2.7 Goitrogenic Glycosides

Goitrogens decrease production of thyroid hormones by inhibiting their synthesis by the thyroid gland. Consequently, the thyroid enlarges to compensate for reduced thyroxin output, producing a goiter. These compounds are collectively called glucosinolates and are commonly found in *Brassica* spp., such as broccoli, kale, cabbage, cauliflower, rape, etc. (Cheeke, 1998). The glucosinolates are hydrolyzed by glucosinolases to β-D-glucose and derivatives of the aglycone, including isothiocyanates, nitriles, and thiocyanates. The glucosinolate enzymes are released from plant tissues by chewing and by rumen microflora activity. Glucosinolates (mustard oil glycosides) are common in the *Brassica* family and are mild GI irritants if ingested in excess. The thiocyanates and isothiocyanates may interfere with iodine metabolism and contribute to thyroid gland enlargement (goiters). Recent research has shown that glucosinolates found in cruciferous vegetables are degraded into isothiocyanates with strong inhibitory properties for phase I enzymes, and inducers of phase II enzymes with strong potential as cancer chemopreventors (Zhang and Talalay, 1998).

2.2.2.8 Other Glycosides

Anthraquinone glycosides found in senna (*Cassia fistulosa*) and *Aloe* spp. have been included in some commercial cathartics. Vicine is a glycoside in fava beans (*Vicia faba*), and causes hemolytic anemia in people who have a genetic deficiency of glucose-6-phosphate dehydrogenase activity in their red blood cells. Fava beans are grown as a protein supplement for livestock.

A glycoside called carboxyatractyloside has been identified as the toxin in cocklebur (*Xanthium strumarium*). The toxin is in high concentration in seeds and cotyledons, but rapidly diminishes as true leaves develop. Carboxyatractyloside produces hepatic lesions, convulsions and severe hypoglycemia, which is thought to be the result of uncoupling of oxidative phosphorylation. In the U.S., pigs seem to be the livestock most frequently poisoned. Signs of toxicity include depression, reluctance to move, nausea, vomiting, weakness and prostration, dyspnea, paddling, convulsions, coma, and death. Severe hypoglycemia occurs when normal blood glucose levels drop tenfold, thus causing sudden death (Cheeke, 1998).

2.2.3 Proteinaceous Compounds, Polypeptides and Amines

2.2.3.1 Proteinaceous Compounds

Proteins are generally not thought of as overtly toxic, but instead considered to be a group of beneficial compounds that are essential building blocks of cells and cellular function in plants and animals. However, there are numerous examples of harmful proteins found in nature, e.g., bacterial toxins, insect and snake venoms, and toad and fish toxins. The number of harmful or toxic proteinaceous substances occurring naturally in plants is relatively small, especially when compared with alkaloidal or glycoside groups. However, there are proteinaceous plant toxins of significance because of their potent cellular toxicity and for their research potential in molecular neurosurgery.

Toxic lectins include ricin from *Ricinus communis* (castor bean), abrin from *Abrus precatorius* (rosary pea or precatory bean), modeccin from *Adenia digitata*, volkensin from *Adenia volkensii*, and saporin from *Saponaria officinalis*. These lectins are potent cytotoxins that act as proteolytic enzymes, thus preventing protein synthesis at the cellular level (ribosomes)(Wiley, 2000). Ricin and abrin are extremely toxic if ingested and a few seeds chewed up and ingested can be fatal. Both toxins are more toxic when injected. The minimum lethal dose of ricin is 0.00000001% of body weight. These plant toxins have been used to make highly-selective neural lesions for animal models for studying neurodegenerative diseases, such as Alzheimer's and Parkinson's disease (Wiley, 2000).

2.2.3.2 Polypeptides

Toxic polypeptides are found in several species of fungi belonging to the *Amanita* genera (Powell, 1990). *Amanita phalloides* (death cap) and its close relatives contain the cyclopeptides amatoxin, phallotoxin, and phalloidin. These toxins interfere with RNA-polymerase, thereby inhibiting protein synthesis. Cellular degeneration occurs in the intestines, liver, kidney, and heart. *Amanita* is the genus of mushroom most often involved in fatal mushroom poisoning in humans. Blue-green algae (cyanobacter) also contains cyclopeptides that cause GI tract upset and liver damage in cattle. This is a common problem in livestock in late summer or early fall after significant algal bloom (Beasley, 1997).

2.2.3.3 Amines

Toxic amines are common in the *Lathyrus* genera (vetches and sweet peas), mistletoe berries (*Phorandendron* spp.), and *Leucaena* spp. The toxic amines in *Lathyrus* cause degeneration of motor tracts of the spinal cord, resulting in paralysis, and even death. The condition called lathyrism was common in certain human populations before the discovery of the cause and identification of the toxins. The toxins are derivatives of aminopropionitrile. In mistletoe the toxins are phenylethylamine and tyramine. Clinical signs of poisoning include acute GI tract inflammation, decreased blood pressure and cardiovascular collapse.

Leucaena spp. contain mimosine, which is degraded to 3-hydroxy-4(1*H*)-pyridone (3,4-DHP; see Section 2.2.4 for more detail). *Leucaena*, while toxic to unadapted ruminants, is a good source of protein and minerals for many livestock species in some countries. However, if *Leucaena* is ingested as 50% or more of the diet it will depress growth, cause hair loss, and reduce reproductive performance. Mimosine is a toxin that animals may become adapted to. Ruminal adaptation can be transferred from animal to animal, suggesting a specific set of rumen organisms are capable of detoxifying this amine.

2.2.4 NON-PROTEIN AMINO ACIDS

Almost 300 non-protein amino acids have been isolated from or identified in plants. Of these about 20 have been implicated in toxicoses in humans and animals (Hegarty, 1978; Cheeke, 1998).

Hypoglycin A from the fruit of *Blighia sapida*, a tree that grows in Jamaica and Africa, causes hypoglycemia and vomiting in animals and humans. Fatalities, which have occurred, were attributed to a sudden drop in blood sugar.

The lathyrogenic amino acids include β-*N*-(γ-L-Glutamyl) aminopropioni-trile from the sweet pea (*Lathyrus odoratus*) and α-Amino-β-oxalylamino-propionic acid, diaminobutyric acid and oxalyl diaminopropionic acid from the flat pea (*Lathyrus sylvestris*). The lathyrogenic amino acids are responsible for a disease complex called lathyrism. The complex has been divided into two diseases with differing etiology: osteolathyrism, characterized by skeletal abnormalities, and neurolathyrism, characterized as a neurological disease affecting humans, horses, and cattle.

Mimosine is a toxic amino acid, structurally similar to tyrosine, in *Mimosa pudica* and *Leucaena leucocophala*, both legumes. *Leucaena* is a shrub legume which is an important pasture plant in the tropics and subtropics. In St. Croix, U.S. Virgin Islands, *Leucaena* is a significant grazing plant for sheep and cattle in the region (personal communication, 2001). It is vigorous, rapidly growing, drought tolerant, palatable, and high yielding, and its leaves contain from 25 to 35% crude protein. Little or no toxicoses are reported in ruminants that have become adapted to the plant. This adaptation is from ruminal organisms that can degrade the mimosine and mimosine-metabolites 3,4-DHP (3-hydroxy-4(1*H*)-pyridone) and 2,3-DHP (2,3-dihydroxy pyridine) to non-toxic products. The mimosine degrading microflora have been artificially transferred from resistant goats to susceptible cattle, thus imparting the ability to degrade mimosine to the cattle. Nonruminants are more sensitive to mimosine, apparently because of the lack of degrading microflora (Cheeke, 1998).

Mimosine toxicoses include hair loss in horses, cattle, and laboratory animals and fleece loss in sheep. Cataracts and reproductive problems have also been reported in rodent models. Prolonged ingestion of *Leucaena* by cattle in northern Australia resulted in low weight gains, hair loss and goiter.

The effects of leucaena and mimosine on nonruminants can be reduced to some extent by diet supplementation with ferrous sulfates. Mimosine forms a complex with iron, which is excreted in the feces. Zinc supplementation has reduced the toxicity in cattle and it is believed that copper and zinc ions bind more strongly to mimosine than most other amino acids.

2.3 NITROGEN-FREE PLANT TOXINS

Numerous nitrogen-free toxins occur in plants. As discussed in the introduction to this Chapter, many of these compounds are believed to be for the protection of the plant from herbivory. However, because there is such a diversity in plant compounds, there are other functions they serve, e.g., insect attractants for pollination, and protection against environmental factors, such as UV light, low or high temperatures, drought, etc.

2.3.1 ORGANIC ACID TOXINS

This class of compounds is relatively rare in plants, but is significant when livestock poisoning is considered. The most common example is oxalic acid and its soluble salts, sodium oxalate and potassium acid oxalate. Plants known to contain toxic levels of oxalate include *Halogeton glomeratus*, a range plant introduced into Nevada, Idaho and Utah, which was responsible for extensive losses in sheep in the desert areas of those states in the mid 1900s (James, 1978; Young et al., 1999). Other plants of the *Atriplex*, *Bassia*, *Chenopodium*, *Salsola*, *Rumex*, *Oxalis*, and *Spinacia* genera also contain soluble oxalates, although generally not in concentrations considered to be toxic.

The clinical signs of poisoning are associated with hypocalcemia as the oxalate generally binds blood calcium. This may result in the presence of calcium oxalate crystals in the walls of the gut, blood vessels, and certain organs, such as the kidneys. Other plants, including jack-in-the-pulpit, dumbcane, caladium, etc., contain oxalate crystals as the solid form in plant tissues. These household plants can, if eaten, cause tissue damage and inflammation to the mouth, tongue, and lips, and are considered dangerous for children and pets (Beasley, 1997).

2.3.2 ALCOHOLS AND POLYACETYLENES

Although few alcohol-based toxins are naturally occurring in plants, there are two groups of significance to man and animals. The first is the cicutoxin-like compounds (long-chain diols) found in water hemlock (*Cicuta* spp.; cicutoxin) of North America and *Oenanthe* spp. (oenanthotoxin) of Europe (King et al., 1985). The second is the tremetone class of toxins, found in white snakeroot

(*Eupatorium rugosum*) of the midwest and rayless goldenrod (*Haplopappus heterophyllus*) of the southwest (Cheeke, 1998). Both are highly toxic to humans and animals and numerous poisonings have occurred.

The cicutoxin-like compounds are known for their extreme and violent toxicity. There are other plant species that contain these polyacetylene type compounds, however none are as toxic as cicutoxin and oenanthotoxin. These species all come from the Umbelliferae family and include *Falcaria vulgaris*, *Sium sisarum*, *Carum carvi*, *Aegopodium podagraria* and *Daucus carota*. *Daucus carota* is the common carrot and it contains a similar cicutoxin-like compound, caratotoxin, but is less toxic ($LD_{50} = 100$ mg/kg i.v. in mice) than cicutoxin. Caratotoxin is found in minute amounts in carrots and is not considered a health concern for humans (Crosby and Aharonson, 1967).

The diols (cicutoxin and oenanthotoxin, $C_{17}H_{22}O_2$) are C-17 complex linear structures, containing two trienes and three dienes in differing order, and are the most toxic, whereas the alcohol derivatives ($C_{17}H_{22}O$) are relatively non-toxic (Figure 2.15). Eleven similar polyacetylene compounds have been described in *Cicuta virosa* in Europe. While toxicity has not been determined for each of these compounds, the diols are believed to be the most dangerous. The toxic diols are unstable when exposed to air, thus making detection in tissue samples for diagnostic purposes difficult.

Cicutoxin causes grand mal seizures and death in its victims. The mechanism of action is at the CNS level, causing seizures resembling those induced by picrotoxin from the East Indies shrub *Anamirta coculus*. The pharmacologic action of picrotoxin is known to act at the cerebrospinal axis of the brain stem, with most prominent effects on the mid brain and medulla. No appreciable effect is seen until the dose is high enough to induce seizures (narrow threshold). The signs of poisoning for cicutoxin are similar. As with picrotoxin, barbiturate therapy will prevent seizures and death if administered in a timely manner (Panter et al., 1996).

Pathologic lesions are skeletal- and heart-muscle damage, with accompanying elevation in serum enzymes. Lesions result from strong muscular contractions during repeated seizure activity. Administration of pentobarbital therapy before, or at the beginning of, seizures will prevent grand mal seizures, pathological changes, and death. The powerful and rapid action of cicutoxin

$$\overset{}{HO}-CH_2CH_2CH_2C\equiv C-C\equiv C-CH=CH-CH=CH-CH=CH\overset{\overset{\displaystyle OH}{|}}{C}HCHC_3H_7$$

(a)

$$HO-CH_2CH_2CH_2C\equiv C-C\equiv C-CH=CH-CH=CH-CH=CHCHC_3H_8$$

(b)

FIGURE 2.15 Nitrogen-free toxins from *Cicuta* spp.; (a) the highly toxic cicutoxin, and (b) the less toxic cicutol.

requires quick action to prevent death. Even at lethal doses, treatment can be very successful with anticonvulsants, especially barbiturates. Treatment is required within minutes of poisoning to avoid death.

The second alcohol toxin of significance is tremetol, the toxin found in white snakeroot in the midwest and rayless goldenrod in the southwest. Tremetol is an oily extract of the plant and was first associated with the toxic effects, and named appropriately by Couch in 1927. Tremetol is a mixture of methyl ketone benzofuran derivatives, including tremetone, dehydrotremetone, and hydroxytremetone (Beier and Norman, 1990).

Diseases referred to as 'trembles' in cattle and 'milk sickness' in humans have significant historical interest because of large losses to cattle and humans as the settlers moved into the midwest during the 19th Century (reviewed in Burrows and Tyrl, 2001). The disease was especially severe in the Mississippi and Ohio River valleys, Indiana, Illinois, Kentucky, North Carolina, Ohio, and Tennessee. In areas of Indiana and Ohio, one-fourth to one-half of all the deaths in the early 1800s were attributed to milk sickness. Abraham Lincoln's mother (Nancy Hanks Lincoln), and many of her relatives and neighbors and their animals, died during an epidemic of milk sickness in 1818 in Pigeon Creek, Indiana. Hindustan Falls, a thriving settlement on the White River of southern Indiana, fell victim to what was referred to at the time as a mysterious malady. Much of the livestock and a substantial portion of the human population died of what is now known to be white snakeroot poisoning. The settlement was abandoned, although the cause at the time was unknown. While it was not confirmed that white snakeroot (*Eupatorium rugosum*) was the cause until 1910, it was suggested in the 1830s by Anna Pierce and John Rowe, but ignored.

The effects of white snakeroot are cumulative and small amounts ingested for several weeks may be as toxic as large amounts eaten over several days. All livestock species are susceptible, although there are species differences in the manifestation of the disease. This species difference may be due to metabolic differences (activation by microsomal enzymes). The toxin, originally identified as a ketone called tremetone, is not the toxic agent, but must be activated by cytochrome P_{450} for toxicity to occur (Beier and Norman, 1990). In horses there are significant heart lesions, in addition to the muscle pathology found in all species. In goats, severe, acute hepatic necrosis accompanied by photo-sensitization occurs. Experimentally, a single dose of 5 mg/kg b.w. in Angora and Spanish goats caused severe centrilobular hepatic necrosis, with head pressing, paddling seizures, depression, anorexia, and photosensitization (Reagor, unpublished data). Muscle tremors, which are common in other animals and people, were not observed in goats. Dairy cattle are especially vulnerable when grazed in wooded areas of the Midwest, and because the toxin is transferred through the milk, humans and pets became equally susceptible. Lactating animals are often affected less than non-lactating animals, thus making the young nursing animals, pets, and humans especially vulnerable.

Pathologically, lesions are most distinct in the horse, with pale areas of grayish myocardial streaks with ventricular dilation (Smetzer et al., 1983). In other species, the gross and microscopic lesions are nonspecific with passive congestion of the brain, liver, and kidney, with some degree of fatty liver and subepicardial hemorrhages.

2.3.3 RESINOUS AND PHENOLIC COMPOUNDS

The catch-all classification for other toxins falls in this group. Generally, these compounds are diverse and often chemically unrelated. As diverse as their chemical natures are, so are the diversity of their effects in mammals when ingested or when physical contact is made. Phenolics are one major component of this group, and are themselves very diverse. The definition of a phenolic is an alcohol or hydroxy group coupled to an aromatic ring.

The most familiar phenolic compound is tetrahydrocannabinol (THC), the narcotic drug found in marijuana (*Cannabis sativa*). Over 60 cannabinoids have been isolated from *C. sativa* (Knight and Walter, 2001). Although initially introduced into the U.S. as a fiber-producing plant for rope making, the practice ended in the 1950s. Because of the euphoric effect this plant has when the leaves are smoked and its street value, determined by the illicit drug market, more potent biotypes of *Cannabis* have been selected in tropical countries for importation into the U.S. Grades of marijuana cultivated in other parts of the world have high potency and the female parts from the flowers of Arabian cannabis are known specifically as hashish. While legalization of marijuana in the U.S. is still being debated, the medicinal uses for treating various diseases, such as glaucoma, chemotherapeutic-induced nausea during cancer treatment, and antibacterial effects, are well-documented (Physicians Desk Reference, *PDR for Herbal Medicines*, 2000).

Tannins are polyhydroxyphenolic toxins found in the oak (*Quercus*) family (Cheeke, 1998; Knight and Walter, 2001). Approximately 60 oak species grow in North America, in a wide range of habitats. Two common species in western U.S. that are associated with livestock poisoning are scrub oak (*Quercus gambelii*) and shinnery oak (*Q. havardii*). These species contain gallotannins, which are hydrolyzed in the rumen of cattle to smaller active compounds, including gallic acid, pyrogallol, and resorcinol. Most severe lesions occur in the kidneys, liver, and GI tract. In small quantities, rumen microflora can detoxify tannins and it is when this detox mechanism is overwhelmed that poisoning occurs. Goats and wild ruminants are able to detoxify tannic acid because they have a tannin-binding protein in their saliva which prevents toxicosis. Goats have been used effectively for brush control, to slow the spread of oak. Oak is poisonous at all stages of growth, but buds, new growth, and green acorns are especially toxic. Cattle, sheep, pigs, and horses are susceptible to oak poisoning. Clinical signs of poisoning will vary depending on the amount eaten. Signs begin with depression, feed refusal, and intestinal stasis, progressing to abdominal pain, dehydration, diarrhea, or constipation, and death 5 to 7 days later. Pathologically, liver necrosis, kidney necrosis, hemorrhagic gastroenteritis, and marked elevation in serum liver enzymes occur.

Other significant phenolic resin compounds include the mixture of urushiol variants, immunogenic compounds causing severe dermatitis from the *Rhus* spp. (poison ivy, poison oak and poison sumac).

Hypericin from St. John's wort is another phenolic compound with multiple rings and multiple double bonds. This compound readily absorbs UV light and is a primary photosensitizing agent that will result in severe sunburn in species that either ingest the plant or come in contact with plant dust or leaf extracts.

Gossypol is a phenolic compound found in the pigment glands of cottonseed (*Gossypium* spp.)(Yu et al., 1993). In addition to gossypol, there are 15 other phenolic compounds in cotton seed. Cotton seed is used for oil production and meal for livestock feed. During the oil-extraction process, processors leave most of the gossypol in the meal by heat treating, which causes gossypol to bind to the meal. The main concern for animal feed is free gossypol, as the bound compound is physiologically inactive.

Research studies concluded that diets containing 200 ppm or less of free gossypol as cotton-seed meal was safe for Holstein calves. At 400 ppm, there was an increase in cardiovascular and lung lesions, leading to increased calf losses. Mature beef cows can be safely fed cotton-seed meal as their entire protein supplement as this is generally kept relatively low, whereas dairy cows should not receive more than 3.6 kg/head/day (reviewed by Cheeke, 1998).

Ruminants are more tolerant to gossypol than nonruminants because of further protein binding in the rumen. The biological effects of gossypol are cumulative, with toxicosis being manifested abruptly after prolonged feeding of cottonseed meal to nonruminants, especially pigs. Gossypol reacts with minerals and especially iron. If fed to laying hens, egg yolks turn green because of the gossypol/iron complex that transfers to the egg protein. Anemia is one of the clinical signs of poisoning because of iron deficiency due to the complexing of iron with gossypol. Gossypol-induced lesions include edema, liver damage, ascites, cardiovascular lesions, and kidney damage.

Gossypol has gained interest in society as a male contraceptive because of its infertility properties, yet does not reduce libido. Sperm counts are depressed and spermatozoa are immotile. Extensive damage has been shown to occur to the germinal epithelium in bulls and rams, thus cotton-seed meal should only be fed at low levels or not at all during the breeding season. Testosterone levels in growing bulls are not affected by gossypol, but testicular morphology changes occurred.

Other phenolic compounds of commercial importance include the terpenoids, including mono, di, tri, and sesquiterpenes. While most of these are used as essential oils, fragrances, and flavors in various products, they are toxins in certain species. For example the sesquiterpene lactones of the *Centaurea* species cause an irreversible Parkinson's-like condition in horses called nigro-pallidal encephalomalacia. This is a lethal condition and the prognosis for recovery is grave; in most cases, affected horses should be euthanized before reaching the terminal stages.

2.3.3.1 Pine Needle Abortion

A significant group of resin compounds (labdane resin acids) with biological activity in cattle have been identified in pine, juniper, and other related species. Cattle grazing ponderosa pine needles, lodgepole pine needles, Monterey cypress, and juniper species are known to abort their calves, especially when grazed in the last trimester of pregnancy (James et al., 1989; Gardner and James, 1999). The labdane resin acid, isocupressic acid (ICA), was isolated from ponderosa pine needles and determined to be the putative abortifacient in cattle (Figure 2.16a). Pine needle abortion is a major area of research at the Poisonous Plant Research Laboratory and one of considerable interest to the livestock community in many parts of the world. Other derivatives and metabolites have now been identified with known abortifacient activity (Figure 2.16b, c).

Cattle readily graze ponderosa pine needles, especially during the winter months in the western U.S. Pine needle consumption increases during cold weather, with increased snow depth, and when other forage is reduced or unavailable (Pfister and Adams, 1993). Twenty-three other tree and shrub species found throughout the western and southern U.S. were analyzed for ICA (Gardner and James, 1999). Significant levels (> 0.5% dry weight of the needles) were detected in *Pinus jefferyi* (Jeffrey pine), *P. contorta* (lodgepole pine), *Juniperus scopulorum* (Rocky Mountain juniper), and *J. communis* (common juniper), and from *Cupressus macrocarpa* (Monterey cypress) from New Zealand and Australia. Abortions were induced when lodgepole pine and common juniper containing 0.7% and 2.5% ICA, respectively, were experi-

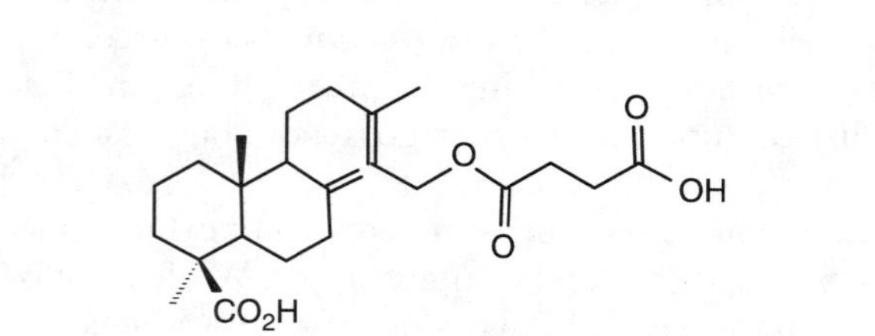

FIGURE 2.16 Three labdane resin acid compounds; (a) isocupressic acid, (b) the acetyl derivative acetlisocupressic, and (c) the succinyl derivative succinylisocupressic, found in certain pine, juniper and cypress trees and which are abortifacient in late-term pregnant cattle.

mentally fed to pregnant cows, inducing abortions in 9 and 3.5 days, respectively (Gardner et al., 1998). This research confirmed field reports of lodgepole pine needle abortion in British Columbia, Canada (France, 1997). Monterey cypress is known to cause abortions in cattle in New Zealand and Southern Australia and contained ICA levels of 0.89% to 1.24%. Korean pine (*Pinus koraiensis*) caused abortion in native Korean cattle, but ICA levels were not reported (Kim et al., 2003). The level of ICA in ponderosa pine needles is generally in the range of 0.5% to 1.7% (Gardner et al., 1994).

Toxicoses from pine needles have been reported in field cases, but are rare and have only occurred in pregnant cattle. No toxicity other than abortion in cattle has been demonstrated from ICA or ICA derivatives. However, the abietane-type resin acids in ponderosa pine needles (concentrated in new growth pine tips) have been shown to be toxic, but not abortifacient at high doses, when administered orally to cattle, goats, and hamsters. Pathological evaluations of intoxicated animals includes nephrosis, edema of the CNS, myonecrosis, and gastroenteritis (Stegelmeier et al., 1996). While abietane-type resin acids may contribute to the occasional toxicoses reported in the field, they do not contribute to the abortions. Most cow losses in the field are associated with difficult parturition or post abortion toxemia due to retained fetal membranes.

2.3.4 MINERAL TOXINS

Mineral toxins are rather unique and probably unrelated to the plant protection theories reviewed in the introduction. These are minerals or metals that the plant usually takes up because of soil conditions, the mineral being in high concentration in the root zones of plants. Occasionally, plants can take up lethal quantities of mineral toxins, such as selenium. While selenium is an essential micronutrient, in excess it is toxic and causes a host of chronic and acute disease conditions. Chronic poisoning can result when livestock ingest plants containing a few ppm of selenium over a long period of time. Clinical effects include hair, tail and mane losses, hoof growth abnormalities, and reproductive problems in some species. While acute selenium poisoning from plants is rare, it can occur and was recently the cause of large losses of sheep on mining reclamation sites (personal communications, 2003). While most acute selenium poisoning has been attributed to indicator plants, such as *Astragalus* and some asters, etc., there are a number of species that are known to take up selenium in toxic levels when selenium is available in the soil. Species of the Brassica family, aster family, and legume family are known to accumulate large levels of selenium. These species also act as selenium pumps, drawing selenium from lower soil horizons to the surface where grasses and other shallow rooted forbs can take up selenium and accumulate toxic levels. Plant species that take up large quantities of selenium include *Medicago* (alfalfa; 1100 ppm), *Grindelia nana* (gum weed; > 6000 ppm), *Aster eatonii* (aster; > 4000 ppm) and *Symphyotrichum* spp. (> 6500 ppm)(Hall, 2003). It was determined that as little as 30 to 60 g of fresh plant was enough to be lethal to sheep grazing in this area. It was also observed that the sheep preferred the gum weed before the alfalfa.

Other striking examples of plants that take up minerals or heavy metals can be found in plants growing on similar mine tailing sites. For example, sheep fescue (*Festuca ovina*) and fine bent (*Agrostis tenuis*) rapidly colonized tailings of heavy-metal mining (Harborne, 1988). *Agrostis* spp. can successfully grow on soils containing as much as 1% lead.

Plants have the ability to rapidly adapt to different soil conditions, however the mechanism for adaptation is not fully understood. Phytochelatins (metal-binding peptides produced in plants) were discovered in the 1980s. While the exact role of these phytochelatins in heavy-metal detoxification in plants is not fully understood, the fact remains that these chelatins provide a plant mechanism whereby metals enter the root system and are transported to the vegetative portions of the plant. *Deschampsia caespitosa* accumulates zinc; *Hybanthus floribundus* accumulates nickel and is an indicator plant for soil nickel and can accumulate up to 22% of its ash as nickel. *Eriogonum ovalifolium* is an indicator of silver deposits in Montana, and certain *Astragalus* species are indicators of selenium and uranium in western states. *Phacelia sericea* will accumulate gold as the cyanide derivative, up to 21 ppb gold in leaves. *Leptospermum scoparium* is a chromium accumulator and *Anthoxanthum odoratum* will accumulate lead. While frequent cases of selenium poisoning from plant uptake from the soil have been reported, no documented cases of poisoning from silver, lead, gold, chromium, etc., have been reported (Harborne, 1988).

Molybdenum concentration can be unusually high in forages growing on soils where there is a naturally high content in the soils. Molybdenum:copper ratios (1:2) are important in animal health, especially in sheep. Molybdenum toxicoses in cattle from plant ingestion has been reported to cause depigmentation of the hair, anemia, depressed growth, and bone disorders.

Nitrate-nitrite toxicity occurs when plants or water (or both) containing high levels of nitrates are consumed. Many crop plants, pasture grasses and weeds may contain high levels of nitrate during certain times of the year. Environmental conditions may also play a role in nitrate accumulation in plants and subsequent toxicoses. Primarily a problem in cattle, nitrate is reduced in the rumen to nitrite which is readily absorbed causing toxicosis (Cheeke, 1998). Plants, hay (dry weight), or water containing 1% or more nitrate (10,000 ppm) are toxic and should be diluted with non-nitrate-containing feed or water. Turnips, oats, kale, sugar beet tops, silage, rye grass, white clover, red root pigweed, variegated thistle, and others have all been implicated in nitrate poisoning (Knight and Walter, 2001). Nitrate levels in plants may vary considerably depending on the plant species, soil nutrient levels (nitrogen, phosphorus, sulfur, and molybdenum), weather, stage of plant growth, etc. Cool, cloudy weather will enhance nitrate accumulation in plants. Nitrate levels are highest at night and early in the morning because the nitrate reducing enzymes are most active during photosynthesis. Stalks are generally higher in nitrate than leaves; nitrates do not accumulate in flowers or fruits.

The nitrite ion readily oxidizes the ferrous ion in hemoglobin to produce methemoglobin. Methemoglobin cannot bind oxygen, thus the animal becomes hypoxic. Clinical signs of poisoning may occur when methemoglobin levels reach 30 to 40%, and death occurs at levels of 80 to 90%.

Abortion in pregnant cattle is frequently reported but exact amounts and mechanism of action is not fully understood. The fetus is particularly susceptible to hypoxia induced by the methemoglobinemia. Fetal death and abortion may occur at any stage of pregnancy because of the decreased fetal oxygen and the limited ability of the fetus to metabolize nitrate (Knight and Walter, 2001).

2.4 CONCLUSION

The poisonous plants and the toxins therefrom discussed in this chapter are only a few of what are to be found in nature and have been reported in the literature. Entire volumes have been dedicated to individual classes of compounds (e.g., Kingsbury, 1964; Cheeke, 1989; Burrows and Tyrl, 2001; Knight and Walter, 2001). Research into poisonous plant is ongoing in many university and government laboratories throughout the world, research which provides new information and tools to better manage livestock grazing systems, thus reducing losses and enhancing the quality of animal products.

Additional spin-off benefits from research on poisonous plants include the development of animal models for the study of human diseases, new techniques and technologies for diagnosis and treatment of livestock poisoning, development of antibody-based diagnostic tools (ELISAs), novel treatments (chemotherapeutic agents), the discovery of new bioactive compounds, and improved livestock management strategies to enhance animal and human health.

2.5 REFERENCES

Blackwell, W.H. (1990). *Poisonous and medicinal plants*. Prentice Hall, Englewood Cliffs, New Jersey.

Beasley, V. (1997). *A systems affected approach to veterinary toxicology*. Reference Notes for Toxicology, University of Illinois.

Beier, R.C. and Norman, J.O. (1990). The toxic factor in white snakeroot: Identity, analysis and prevention, *Hum. Vet. Toxicol.*, 32, 81–88.

Binns, W., Shupe, J.L., Keeler, R.F. and James, L.F. (1965). Chronological evaluation of teratogenicity in sheep fed *Veratrum californicum*, *J. Am. Vet. Med. Assoc.*, 147, 839–842.

Botha, C.J., Van der Lugt, J.J., Erasmus, G.L., Kellerman, T.S., Schultz, R.A. and Vleggaar, R. (1998). Krimpsiekte, a paretic condition of small stock poisoned by bufadienolide-containing plants of the Crassulaceae in South Africa, in Garland, T. and Barr, A.C., Eds., *Toxic plants and other natural toxicants*, CAB International, Wallingford, pp. 407–412.

Burrows, G.E. and Tyrl, R.J. (2001). *Toxic plants of North America*, Iowa State Press, Ames.

Carey, D.B. and Wink, M. (1994). Elevational variation of quinolizidine alkaloid contents in a lupine (*Lupinus argenteus*) of the Rocky Mountains, *J. Chem. Ecol.*, 20, 849–857.

Cheeke, P.R., ed., (1989). *Toxicants of plant origin*, Vol. I. Alkaloids, Vol. II. Glycosides, Vol. III. Proteins and Amino Acids, Vol. IV. Phenolics, CRC Press, Boca Raton.

Cheeke, P.R. (1998). *Natural toxicants in feeds, forages, and poisonous plants.* Interstate Publishers Inc., Danville.

Colegate, S.M., Dorling, P.R. and Huxtable, C.R. (1979). A spectroscopic investigation of swainsonine: an α-mannosidase inhibitor isolated from *Swainsona canescens*. *Aust. J. Chem.*, 32, 2257–2264.

Cronin, E.H. and Nielsen, D.B. (1979). *The ecology and control of rangeland larkspurs*, UT Agri. Exp. Sta. Bull., 499, Utah State University, Logan.

Crosby, D.G. and Aharonson, N. (1967). The stucture of carotatoxin, a natural toxicant from carrot, *Tetrahedron*, 23, 465–472.

Daugherty, C.G. (1995). The death of Socrates and the toxicology of hemlock, *J. Med. Biography* 3, 178–182.

Davis, A.M. and Stout, D.M. (1986). Anagyrine in western American lupines, *J. Range Manage.*, 39, 29–30.

de Balogh, K.K.I.M., Dimande, A.P., vander Lugt, J.J., Molyneux, R.J., Naude, T.W. and Welmans, W.G. (1999). A lysosomal storage disease induced by *Ipomoea carnea* in goats in Mozambique, *J. Vet. Diagn. Invest.*, 11, 266–273.

Dennis, J.W., White, S.L., Freer, A.M. and Dime, D. (1993). Carbonoyloxy analogs of the anitmetastatic drug swainsonine. Activation in tumor cells by esterases, *Biochem. Pharmacol.*, 46, 1459–1466.

Dobelis, P., Madl, J.E., Pfister, J.A., Manners, G.D. and Walrond, J.P. (1999). Effects of Delphinium alkaloids on neuromuscular transmission, *J. Pharmacol. Exp. Ther.*, 291, 538–546.

Dorling, P.R., Huxtable, C.R. and Vogel, P. (1978). Lysosomal storage in *Swainsona* spp. toxicosis: An induced mannosidosis, *Neuropathol. Appl. Neurobiol.*, 4, 285–295.

Edgar, J.A. and Smith, L.W. (2000). Transfer of pyrrolizidine alkaloids into eggs: Food safety implications, in Tu, A.T. and Gaffield W., Eds., *Natural and selected synthetic toxins: biological implications*, American Chemical Society, Washington, pp. 118–128.

Fodor, G.B. and Colasanti, B. (1985). The pyridine and piperidine alkaloids: chemistry and pharmacology, in Pelletier S., Ed., *Alkaloids: chemical and biological perspectives*, Vol. 3, John Wiley and Sons, New York, pp. 3–91.

France, B. (1997). Personal Communication.

Frank, B.S., Michelson, W.B., Panter, K.E. and Gardner, D.R. (1995). Ingestion of poison-hemlock (*Conium maculatum*), *West. J. Med.*, 163, 573–574.

Frandsen, E. and Boe, D. (1991). Economics of noxious weeds and poisonous plants, in James, L.F., Evans, J.O., Ralphs, M.H. and Child, R.D, Eds., *Noxious range weeds,* Westview Press, Boulder, pp. 442–458.

Gaffield, W. (2000). The *Veratrum* alkaloids: Natural tools for studying embryonic development, in Atta-ur-Rahman, Ed., *Studies in natural products chemistry* 23, Elsevier Science, Amsterdam, pp. 563–589.

Gaffield, W., Incardona, J.P., Kapur, R.P. and Roelink, H. (2000). Mechanistic investigation of Veratrum alkaloid-induced mammalian teratogenesis, in Tu, A.T. and Gaffield W., Eds., *Natural and selected synthetic toxins: biological implications*, American Chemical Society, Washington, pp. 173–187.

Gaffield, W. and Keeler, R.F. (1994). Structure–activity relations of teratogenic natural products, *Pure and Appl. Chem.*, 66, 2407–2410.

Gaffield, W. and Keeler, R.F. (1996). Steroidal alkaloid teratogens: molecular probes for investigation of craniofacial malformations, *J. Toxicol. Toxin Rev.*, 15, 303–326.

Gardner, D.R. and James, L.F. (1999). Pine needle abortion in cattle: Analysis of isocupressic acid in North American Gymnosperms, *Phytochem. Anal.*, 10, 1–5.

Gardner, D.R., Molyneux, R.J., James, L.F., Panter, K.E. and Stegelmeier, B.L. (1994). Ponderosa pine needle-induced abortion in beef cattle: Identification of isocupressic acid as the principal active compound, *J. Agric. Food Chem.*, 42, 756–761.

Gardner, D.R. and Panter, K.E. (1993). Comparison of blood plasma alkaloid levels in cattle, sheep and goats fed *Lupinus caudatus*, *J. Nat. Toxins*, 2, 1–11.

Gardner, D.R., Panter, K.E., James, L.F. and Stegelmeier, B.L. (1998). Abortifacient effects of lodgepole pine (*Pinus contorta*) and common juniper (*Juniperus communis*) on cattle, *Vet. Human Toxicol.*, 40, 260–263.

Habermehl, G.G., Martz, W., Tokarnia, C.H., Dobereiner, J. and Mendez, M.C. (1988). Livestock poisoning in South America by species of the *Senecio* plant, *Toxicon*, 26, 275–286.

Hall, J. (2003). Unpublished Data.

Hammerschmidt, M., Brook, A. and McMahon, A.P. (1997). The world according to hedgehog, *Trends Genet.*, 13, 14–21.

Harborne, J.B. (1988). *Introduction to ecological biochemistry*, 3rd ed., Academic Press, London.

Harborne, J.B. (1993). *Introduction to ecological biochemistry*, 4th ed., Academic Press, London.

Harborne, J.B. and Baxter, H. (1996). *Dictionary of plant toxins*, John Wiley and Sons, New York.

Hegarty, M.P. (1978). Toxic amino acids of plant origin, in Keeler, R.F., VanKampen, K.R. and James, L.F., Eds. *Effects of poisonous plants on livestock*, Academic Press, New York, pp. 575–585.

Huxtable, R.J. and Cooper, R.A. (2000). Pyrrolizidine alkaloids: physicochemical correlates of metabolism and toxicity, in Tu, A.T. and Gaffield W., Eds., *Natural and selected synthetic toxins: biological implications*, American Chemical Society, Washington, D.C., pp. 100–117.

James, L.F. (1978). Oxalate poisoning in livestock, in Keeler, R.F., Van Kampen, K.R. and James, L.F., Eds., *Effects of poisonous plants on livestock*, Academic Press, New York, NY, pp. 139–145.

James, L.F. (1999). Teratological research at the USDA-ARS Poisonous Plant Research Laboratory, *J. Nat. Toxins*, 8, 63–80.

James, L.F. and Hartley, W.J. (1977). Effects of milk from animals fed locoweed in kittens, calves, and lambs, *Amer. J. Vet. Res.*, 38, 1263–1265.

James, L.F., Hartley, W.J. and Van Kampen, K.R. (1981). Syndromes of *Astragalus* poisoning in livestock, *J. Amer. Vet. Med. Assoc.*, 178, 146–150.

James, L.F., Panter, K.E., Gaffield, W. and Molyneux, R.J. (2004). Biomedical applications of poisonous plant research, *J. Agric. Food Chem.*, submitted 2003.

James, L.F., Short, R.E., Panter, K.E., Molyneux, R.J., Stuart, L.D. and Bellows, R.A. (1989). A review and report of 1973–1984 research, *Cornell Vet.*, 79, 39–52.

Keeler, R.F. (1986). Teratology of steroidal alkaloids, in Pelletier, S.W., Ed., *Alkaloids: chemical and biological perspectives*, John Wiley and Sons, New York, pp. 389–425.

Keeler, R.F. 1989. Quinolizidine alkaloids in range and grain lupins, in Cheeke, P.R., Ed., *Toxicants of plant origin*, Vol. I: Alkaloids, CRC Press, Boca Raton, pp. 133–168.

Keeler, R.F. and Balls, L.D. (1978). Teratogenic effects in cattle of *Conium maculatum* and conium alkaloids and analogs,. *Clin. Toxicol.*, 12, 49–64.

Keeler, R.F. and Crowe, M.W. (1984). Teratogenicity and toxicity of wild tree tobacco, *Nicotiana glauca* in sheep, *Cornell Vet.*, 74, 50–59.

Keeler, R.F. and Panter, K.E. (1989). Piperidine alkaloid composition and relation to crooked calf disease-inducing potential of *Lupinus formosus*, *Teratology*, 40, 423–432.

Keeler, R.F. and Young, S. (1986). When ewes ingest poisonous plants: The teratogenic effects. *Veterinary Medicine, Food Animal Practice*, May, 449–454.

Kellerman, T.S., Coetzer, J.A.W. and Naude, T.W. (1988). *Plant poisonings and mycotoxicoses of livestock in southern Africa*. Oxford University Press, Cape Town.

Kim, I.H., Choi, K.C., An, B.S., Choi, I.G., Kim, B.K., Oh, Y.K. and Jeung, E.B. (2003). Effect on abortion of feeding Korean pine needles to pregnant Korean native cows, *Can. J. Vet. Res.*, 67, 194–197.

Kim, S.K. and Melton, D.A. (1998). Pancreas development is promoted by cyclopamine, a hedgehog signaling inhibitor, *Proc. Natl. Acad. Sci.*, 95, 13,036–13,041.

King, L.A., Lewis, M.J., Parry, D., Twitchett, P.J. and Kilner, E.A. (1985). Identification of oenanthotoxin and related compounds in hemlock water dropwort poisoning, *Hum. Toxicol.*, 4, 355–364.

Kinghorn, A.D. and Balandrin, M.F. (1984). Quinolizidine alkaloids of the Leguminosae: Structural types, analysis, chemotaxonomy and biological activities, in Pelletier, S.W., Ed., *Alkaloids: chemical and biological perspectives*, John Wiley and Sons, New York, pp. 105–148.

Kingsbury, J.M. (1964). *Poisonous plants of the United States and Canada*. Prentice Hall, Englewood Cliffs.

Knight, A.P. and Walter, R.G. (2001). *A guide to plant poisoning of animals in North America*. Teton NewMedia, Jackson.

Landenburg, H. (1886). Research with the synthesis of coniine, *Chem. Ber.*, 19, 439–441.

Lavie, Y., Harel-Orbital, T., Gaffield, W. and Liscovitch, M. (2001). Inhibitory effect of steroidal alkaloids on drug transport and multidrug resistance in human breast cancer cells, *Anticancer Res.*, 21, 1189–1194.

Majak, W., Mcdiarmid, R.E., Hall, J.W. and Willms, W. (2000). Alkaloid levels of a tall larkspur species in southwestern Alberta, *J. Range Manage.*, 53, 207–210.

Majak, W. and Pass, M.A. (1989). Aliphatic nitrocompounds, in Cheeke, P.R., Ed., *Toxicants of plant origin*, Vol. II: Glycosides, CRC Press, Boca Raton, pp. 143–159.

Marsh, C.D. (1909). *The Loco-Weed Disease of the Plains*, Bulletin 112, U.S. Dept. Agri., Bureau of Animal Industry, Washington.

Matsunaga, E. and Shiota, K. (1977). Holoprosencephaly in human embryos: Epidemiologic studies of 150 cases, *Teratology*, 16, 261–272.

Molyneux, R.J., Gardner, D.R., James, L.F. and Colegate, S.M. (2002). Polyhydroxy alkaloids: Chromatographic analysis, *J. Chromatogr. Anal.*, 967, 57–74.

Molyneux, R.J. and James, L.F. (1982). Loco Intoxication: indolizidine alkaloids of spotted locoweed (*Astragalus lentiginosus*), *Science*, 216, 190–191.

Molyneux, R.J., James, L.F., Panter, K.E. and Ralphs, M.H. (1991b). Analysis and distribution of swainsonine and related polyhydroxyindolizidine alkaloids by thin layer chromatography, *Phytochem. Anal.*, 2, 125–129.

Molyneux, R.J., James, L.F., Ralphs, M.H., Pfister, J.A., Panter, K.E. and Nash, R.J. (1994). Polyhydroxy alkaloid glycosidase inhibitors from poisonous plants of global distibution: Analysis and identification, in Colegate, S.M. and Dorling, P.R., Eds., *Plant-associated toxins: agricultural, phytochemical and ecological aspects*, CAB International, Wallingford, pp. 107–112.

Molyneux, R.J., Johnson, A.E., Olsen, J.D. and Baker, D.C. (1991a). Toxicity of pyrrolizidine alkaloids from riddell groundsel (*Senecio riddellii*). to cattle, *Am. J. Vet. Res.*, 52, 146–151.

Molyneux, R.J., McKenzie, R.A., O'Sullivan, B.M. and Elbein, A.D. (1995). Identification of the glycosidase inhibitors swainsonine and calystegine B_2 in Weir vine (*Ipomoea* sp. Q6 [aff. calobra]) and correlation with toxicity, *J. Nat. Prod.*, 58, 878–886.

Molyneux, R.J., Pan, Y.T., Goldmann, A., Tepfer, D.A. and Elbein, A.D. (1993). Calystegins, a novel class of alkaloid glycosidase inhibitors, *Arch Biochem Biophys.*, 304, 81–88.

Nielsen, D.B. and James, L.F. (1992). The economic impacts of livestock poisonings by plants, in James, L.F., Keeler, R.F., Bailey Jr., E.M, Cheeke, P.R. and Hegarty, M.P., Eds, *The ecology and economic impact of poisonous plants on livestock production*, Iowa State University Press, Ames, pp. 3–10.

Nielsen, D.B. and Ralphs, M.H. (1987). Larkspur economic considerations, in James, L.F., Ralphs, M.H. and Nielsen, D.B., Eds., *Ecology and economic considerations of poisonous plants*, Westview Press, Boulder, pp. 119–129.

Panter, K.E., Baker, D.C. and Kechele, P.O. (1996). Water hemlock (*Cicuta douglasii*). toxicosis in sheep: Pathologic description and prevention of lesions and death, *J. Vet. Diagn. Invest.*, 8, 474–480.

Panter, K.E., Bunch, T.D., Keeler, R.F., Sisson, D.V. and Callan, R.J. (1990). Multiple congenital contractures (MCC). and cleft palate induced in goats by ingestion of piperidine alkaloid-containing plants: Reduction in fetal movement as the probable cause, *Clin. Toxicol.*, 28, 69–83.

Panter, K.E., Gardner, D.R., James, L.F., Stegelmeier, B.L. and Molyneux, R.J. (2000a). Natural toxins from poisonous plants affecting reproductive function in livestock, in Tu, A.T. and Gaffield, W., Eds., *Natural and selected synthetic toxins: biological implications*, ACS Symposium Series 745, American Chemical Society, Washington, pp.154–172.

Panter, K.E., Gardner, D.R. and Molyneux, R.J. (1994). Comparison of toxic and teratogenic effects of *Lupinus formosus*, *L. arbustus* and *L. caudatus* in goats, *J. Nat. Toxins*, 3, 83–93.

Panter, K.E., Gardner, D.R. and Molyneux, R.J. (1998a). Teratogenic and fetotoxic effects of two piperidine alkaloid-containing lupines (*L. formosus* and *L. arbustus*) in cows, *J. Nat. Toxins*, 7, 131–140.

Panter, K.E., Gardner, D.R. and Molyneux, R.J. (1998b). Toxic and teratogenic piperidine alkaloids from *Lupinus*, *Conium* and *Nicotiana* species, in Garland, T.

and Barr, A.C., Eds., *Toxic plants and other natural toxicants*, CAB International, Wallingford, pp. 345–350.

Panter, K.E., James, L.F. and Gardner, D.R. (1999). Lupines, poison-hemlock and *Nicotiana* spp: Toxicity and teratogenicity in livestock, *J. Nat. Toxins*, 8, 117–134.

Panter, K.E. and Keeler, R.F. (1992). Induction of cleft palate in goats by *Nicotiana glauca* during a narrow gestational period and the relation to reduction in fetal movement, *J. Nat. Toxins*, 1, 25–32.

Panter, K.E. and Keeler, R.F. (1989). Piperidine alkaloids of poison hemlock (*Conium maculatum*), in Cheeke, P.R., Ed., *Toxicants of plant origin*, Vol. I: Alkaloids, CRC Press, Boca Raton, pp. 109–132.

Panter, K.E., Manners, G.D., Stegelmeier, B.L., Lee, S.T., Gardner, D.R., Ralphs, M.H., Pfister, J.A. and James, L.F. (2002). Larkspur poisoning: Toxicology and alkaloid structure-activity relationships, *Biochem. Systematics Ecol.*, 30, 113–128.

Panter, K.E., Ralphs, M.H., Smart, R.A. and Duelke, B. (1987). Death camas poisoning in sheep: A case report, *Vet. Human Toxicol.*, 29, 45–48.

Panter, K.E., Weinzweig, J., Gardner, D.R., Stegelmeier, B.L. and James, L.F. (2000b). Comparison of cleft palate induction by *Nicotiana glauca* in goats and sheep, *Teratology*, 61, 203–210.

Pelletier, S.W. (1983). The nature and definition of an alkaloid, in Pelletier, S.W., Ed., *Alkaloids: Chemical and biological perspectives*, Vol. 1, Wiley, New York, pp. 1–31.

Pfister, J.A. (2003). Personal Communication.

Pfister, J.A. and Adams, D.C. (1993). Factors influencing consumption of ponderosa pine needles by grazing cattle during winter, *J. Range Manage.*, 46, 394–398.

Pfister, J.A., Ralphs, M.H., Gardner, D.R., Stegelmeier, B.L., Manners, G.D., Panter, K.E. and Lee, S.T. (2002). Management of three toxic *Delphinium* species based on alkaloid concentrations, *Biochem. Systematics Ecol.*, 30, 129–138.

Powell, M.J. (1990). Poisonous and medicinal fungi, in Blackwell, W.H., Ed., *Poisonous and medicinal plants*, Prentice Hall, Englewood Cliffs, pp. 71–110.

Ralphs, M.H., James, L.F., Nielsen, D.B. and Panter, K.E. (1984). Management practices reduce cattle loss to locoweed on high mountain range, *Rangelands*, 6, 175–177.

Ralphs, M.H., Manners, G.D., Pfister, J.A., Gardner, D.R. and James, L.F. (1997). Toxic alkaloid concentration in tall larkspur species in the western United States, *J. Range Manage.*, 50, 497–502.

Ralphs, M.H. (2003). Unpublished Data.

Roberts, M.F. and Wink, M. (1998). *Alkaloids: Biochemistry, ecology, and medicinal applications.* Plenum Press, New York.

Roitman, J.N. and Panter, K.E. 1995. Livestock poisoning caused by plant alkaloids, in Blum, M.S., Ed., *The toxic action of marine and terrestrial alkaloids.* Alaken Inc., Fort Collins, pp. 53–124.

Sharma, R.P. and Salunkhe, D.K. (1989). Solanum glycoalkaloids, in Cheeke, P.R., Ed., *Toxicants of plant origin*, Vol. I Alkaloids, CRC Press, Boca Raton, pp. 179–236.

Smetzer, D.L., Coppock, R.W. and Ely, R.W. (1983). Cardiac effects of white snakeroot intoxication in horses, *Equine Practice*, 5, 26–32.

Smith, L.W. and Culvenor, C.C.J. (1981). Plant sources of hepatotoxic pyrrolizidine alkaloids, *J. Nat. Prod.*, 44, 129–152.

Stegelmeier, B.L., Gardner, D.R., James, L.F., Panter, K.E. and Molyneux, R.J. (1996). The toxic and abortifacient effects of Ponderosa pine, *Vet. Pathol.*, 33, 22–28.

Stegelmeier, B.L., James, L.F., Panter, K.E., Ralphs, M.H., Gardner, D.R., Molyneux, R.J. and Pfister, J.A. (1999). The pathogenesis and toxicokinetics of locoweed (*Astragalus* and *Oxytropis* spp.) poisoning in livestock, *J. Nat. Toxins*, 8, 35–45.

Stegelmeier, B.L., Panter, K.E., Pfister, J.A., James, L.F., Manners, G.D., Gardner, D.R., Ralphs, M.H. and Olsen, J.D. (1998). Experimental modification of larkspur (*Delphinium* spp.) toxicity, in Garlandand, T. and Barr, A.C., Eds., *Toxic plants and other natural toxicants*, CAB International, New York, pp. 205–210.

Taipale, J., Chen, J.K., Cooper, M.K., Wang, B., Mann, R.K., Milenkovic, L., Scott, M. and Beachy, P.A. (2000). Effects of oncogenic mutations in Smoothened and Patched can be reversed by cyclopamine, *Nature*, 406, 1005–1009.

Weinzweig, J., Panter, K.E., Pantaloni, M., Spangenberger, A., Harper, J.S., Lui, F., Gardner, D.R. and Wierenga, T.L. (1999a). The fetal cleft palate: I. Characterization of a congenital model, *Plastic and Reconstr. Surg.*, 103, 419–428.

Weinzweig, J., Panter, K.E., Pantaloni, M., Spangenberger, A., Harper, J.S., Lui, F., James, L.F. and Edstrom, L.E. (1999b). The fetal cleft palate: II. Scarless healing after *in utero* repair of a congenital model, *Plastic and Reconstr. Surg.*, 104, 1356–1364.

Weinzweig, J., Panter, K.E., Spangenberger, A., Harper, J.S., McRae, R. and Edstrom, L.E. (2002). The fetal cleft palate: III. Ultrastructural and functional analysis of palatal development following *in utero* repair of the congenital model, *Plastic and Reconstr. Surg.*, 104, 2355–2362.

Wiley, R.G. (2000). Molecular neurosurgery: using plant toxins to make highly selective neural lesions, in Tu, A.T. and Gaffield, W., Eds., *Natural and selected synthetic toxins: Biological implications*, American Chemical Society, Washington, pp. 194–203.

Wink, M. (1999). *Functions of secondary metabolites and their exploitation in biotechnology: Annual plant reviews*, Vol. 3, CRC Press, Boca Raton.

Wink, M. and Carey, D.B. (1994). Variability of quinolizidine alkaloid profiles of *Lupinus argenteus* (Fabaceae) from North America, *Biochem. Systematics Ecol.*, 22, 663–669.

Wink, M., Hofer, M.A., Bilfinger, M., Englert, E., Martin, M. and Schneider, D. (1993). Geese and plant dietary allelochemicals- food palatability and geophagy, *Chemoecology*, 4, 93–107.

Wink, M., Meibner, C. and Witte, L. (1995). Patterns of quinolizidine alkaloids in 56 species of the genus Lupinus, *Phytochemistry*, 38, 139–153.

Young, J.A., Martinelli, P.C., Eckert, R.E. and Evans, R.A. (1999). *Halogeton: A history of mid-20th Century range conservation in the Intermountain Area.* USDA-ARS Publication Number 1553.

Yu, F., Barry, T.N., Moughan, P.J. and Wilson, G.F. (1993). Condensed tannin and gossypol concentrations in cottonseed and in processed cottonseed meal, *J. Sci. Food Agric.*, 63, 7–15.

Zhang, Y. and Talalay, P. (1998). Mechanism of differential potencies of isothiocyanates as inducers of anticarcinogenic phase 2 enzymes, *Cancer Res.*, 58, 4632–4639.

3

Mushroom Toxins

Heinz Faulstich

CONTENTS

3.1 INTRODUCTION

This chapter provides an overview of our present knowledge on mushroom toxins, and discusses the toxins in order of importance. The chapter includes: information on the mushroom species producing the toxin; chemistry and detection of the toxin; and the medical impact of the toxin, i.e., the symptoms produced, and the appropriate treatment of the poisoning. The information is based on several reviews (Spoerke and Rumack, 1994; Faulstich and Wieland, 1992; Wieland and Faulstich, 1983), which may be consulted for more details, as well as on data taken from the current literature.

3.2 AMATOXINS

3.2.1 MUSHROOMS PRODUCING AMATOXINS

By far the largest number of fatalities due to ingestion of mushrooms are caused by amatoxins. At the top of the list of amatoxin-containing mushrooms is the green death cap, *Amanita phalloides*, because of its wide distribution and the high content of amatoxins (5 to 8 mg per 25 g fresh tissue, corresponding to 2.5 to 4.0 mg/g dry weight). This mushroom is common all over Europe and also increasingly found in North America. Given the estimated lethal dose for humans (0.1 mg/kg body weight), a full-grown mushroom (25 g) will be sufficient to kill a human. The olive green cap of this mushroom may appear as pale or even white, prompting the classification as a separate species, *A. verna*, which, however, is nowadays regarded as a subspecies, *A. phalloides var. verna*. In the few specimens of this subspecies tested so far, the amatoxin content was lower than in *A. phalloides* (1 to 6 mg per 25 g fresh tissue). The white species, *A. virosa*, the destroying angel, is easily distinguished from this subspecies by its cone-shaped cap and by a differing toxin pattern. The overall concentration of amatoxins in *A. virosa* is 1 to 5 mg per 25 g fresh tissue, composed of α-amanitin, or amaninamide, with no acidic amatoxins present. Fatal cases reported for *A. virosa* come from areas with mild climate, such as Virginia, central France, or southern Sweden. More recently, however, there have been reports of casualties caused by *A. virosa* from Mexico (Perez-Moreno et al., 1994), Thailand (Chaiear et al., 1999), and Korea (Lim et al., 2000). Another white species, *A. bisporigera,* seems to be identical to *A. virosa.* In particular, the white-coloured species of the deadly *Amanitas* may be mistaken for edible species of *Macrolepiota* or *Agaricus.*

Amatoxins have also been found in genera other than *Amanita,* for example in *Galerina* and *Lepiota.* Galerinas (*G. marginata, G. autumnalis*) are little, brown mushrooms (LBM), with brown spores. Some grow on earth, others on rotting wood. They contain less amatoxins (0.5 to 2.4 mg per 25 g fresh tissue) than the Amanitas, but nonetheless have been reported as the cause of amatoxin poisoning in humans; a recent poisoning by *G. fasciculata* was reported from Japan (Kaneko et al., 2001). Small *Lepiota* mushrooms (*L. helveola, L. brunneoincarnata, L. josserandii,*) contain amatoxins in concentrations comparable with those in the Galerinas (up to 2.6 mg per 25 g fresh tissue) and are increasingly responsible for fatal cases of amatoxin poisoning in France (Ramirez et al., 1994; Meunier et al., 1995), Spain (Puig Hernandez et al., 2001), and Turkey (Paydas et al., 1990).

3.2.2 CHEMISTRY AND ACTION

Amatoxins are a family of cyclic peptides, with α-amanitin and β-amanitin (Figure 3.1) accounting for $>90\%$ of the total amatoxins. In *A. virosa,* mushrooms collected in Virginia α-amanitin found to be completely replaced by amaninamide (Figure 3.1). The peptides are not destroyed by cooking and

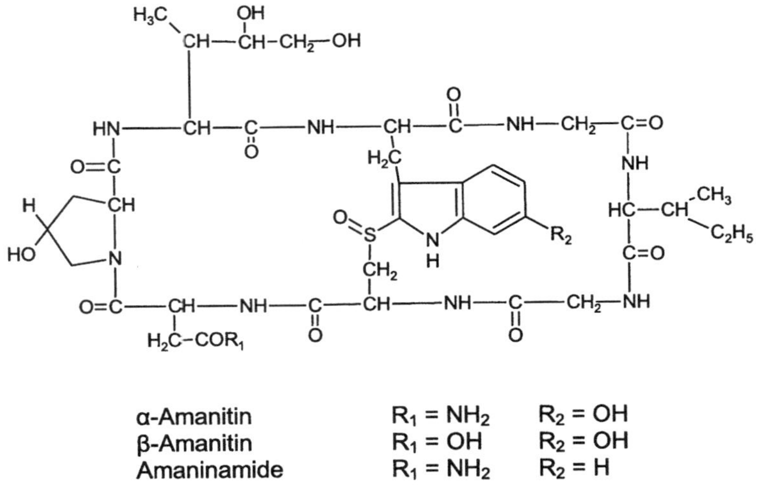

α-Amanitin	$R_1 = NH_2$	$R_2 = OH$
β-Amanitin	$R_1 = OH$	$R_2 = OH$
Amaninamide	$R_1 = NH_2$	$R_2 = H$

FIGURE 3.1 Structures of the main amatoxins α-amanitin, β-amanitin, and amaninamide.

can be kept for years if dried, but will decompose slowly when exposed to ultraviolet (UV) light for several months. No protease known would cleave the peptide bonds in the cyclic peptide. Amatoxins inhibit protein biosynthesis at the transcriptional level. There was virtually no difference found in the toxic activities of α-amanitin, β-amanitin, and amaninamide. By tightly binding to the enzyme transcribing DNA into mRNA, the toxins inhibit the synthesis of the templates required for proteins to be synthesized in the cell. If transcription is not restored within a certain period of time, cells poisoned by amatoxins die from programmed cell death (apoptosis). Amatoxins have a poor rate of penetration through cell membranes and therefore preferentially enter cells possessing an amanitin-transporting system, as is present in cells of the intestinal mucosa and in hepatocytes.

3.2.3 SYMPTOMS

The specificity of amatoxins for cells in the gastrointestinal (GI) tract and in the liver explains the symptoms of amatoxin poisoning. Onset of symptoms occurs at the earliest six hours, in most cases eight to twelve hours, after the mushroom meal, with vomiting, diarrhea, abdominal cramps, and nausea, known as the GI phase. A plausible explanation for the long latent period is that poisoned cells can live on their stock of mRNA for some hours until the RNAs are degraded, according to their specific life time. The latent period is so characteristic that it represents an important diagnostic tool for amanitin poisoning. After the GI phase (days one to two), patients experience a treacherous phase of recovery, but may suffer from the first coagulation disorders, such as decrease in prothrombin time. The hepatic phase (days three to four) develops with an increase of liver transaminases in serum, LDH, and bilirubin. In severe cases, acute hepatic failure will develop, associated with severe coagulation disorders and encephalopathy. Acute renal failure may occur at this stage, indicating a poor prognosis due to heavy toxin exposure. Patients eventually die after six to sixteen days, exceptionally as late as twenty days after ingestion.

3.2.4 TREATMENT

There is no specific therapy for amatoxin poisoning. Intense supportive care, including rehydration, balance of electrolyte loss, substitution of blood glucose, administration of activated charcoal, and, if necessary, enhanced diuresis, should be started as soon as possible. Extracorporal purification procedures, such as hemodialysis, hemoperfusion, or plasmapheresis, are no longer recommended because of the low plasma concentration of amatoxins at the time of hopitalization; however, infusion of charcoal slurry may prevent residual amatoxins, or amatoxins excreted in bile, from being (re)absorbed. Kidney function should be controlled carefully, and slightly enhanced diuresis seems important (100 to 200 ml/h). Silymarin (silibinin), and, less efficiently, penicillin, have been proved in experimental animals to intercept reabsorption of amanitin excreted by the liver due to enterohepatic circulation. If very high doses of amanitin were ingested, a fatal outcome seems avoidable only by liver transplantation, which has recently been performed successfully. Mortality rates were 30% in former decades but have now dropped to around 11%, mainly due to intense supportive care. Such values are ambiguous, however, given the lack of an obligatory classification system of severity. (For recent reviews on the management of amatoxin poisoning, see: Faulstich and Zilker, 1994; Enjalbert et al., 2002; Persson and Karlson-Stiber, in press).

3.2.5 DETECTION OF AMATOXINS

It is possible to use the newspaper test to detect amatoxins in a drop of mushroom juice. In this test, amatoxins develop a purple-brownish color when concentrated hydrochloric acid is added to the dried spot due to the lignin present in the newspaper. However, several mushroom species that contain no amatoxins will give a false-positive result with this test (Seeger, 1984). Analytical procedures with much higher sensitivity for detecting amatoxins include high performance liquid chromatography (HPLC) and various radioimmunoassays. These are suited also for detecting amanitin in urine samples of patients, with a limit of detection of ca. 10 ng/ml. In the past, two amatoxin-specific radioimmunoassays were brought to market, one from the author's laboratory, the other from a Swiss group. However, interest in the analysis of urine samples has since declined because general agreement was reached that amatoxin concentration in urine is of no prognostic value for the course of an individual intoxication. Radioimmunoassays and HPLC analysis work for serum samples also, but in most cases the serum of patients is free of amatoxins at the time of hospitalization. However, such analytical procedures may still be useful for analysing mushroom remains.

3.2.6 OTHER TOXINS IN AMANITA MUSHROOMS

Beside amatoxins, *A. phalloides* and *A. virosa* contain a second family of toxic, cyclic peptides, the phallotoxins, with phalloidin and phallacidin being the main components. There is convincing evidence that phallotoxins do not contribute to human mushroom poisoning. The same is true for the virotoxins, a family of cyclic peptides structurally related to the phallotoxins and found exclusively in *A. virosa*. Phallotoxins and virotoxins share the target protein polymeric actin, in non-muscle cells, preferentially in hepatocytes. Several species of *Amanita*, among them *A. phalloides* and *A. virosa*, but also edible species of this genus such as *A. rubescens*, contain so-called hemolysins, proteins with very potent cytolytic activity. These proteins are destroyed during cooking (temperature $> 65°C$), and hence do not contribute to human poisoning.

3.3 ORELLANINE

3.3.1 MUSHROOMS PRODUCING ORELLANINE

Orellanine is exclusively found in mushrooms of the genus *Cortinarius* (*C. orellanus, C. speciocissimus*). Orellanine is absent from *C. splendens*, although in a few cases of intoxication from this mushroom the symptoms developed were typical for orellanine poisoning (renal failure). The content of orellanine was determined as ca. 14 mg/g dry weight in *C. orellanus*, and 9 mg/g dry weight in *C. speciocissimus*. Toxicity of the medium-sized, fox-colored *Cortinarius* mushrooms remained undetected until 1952, when in Bydgosz (Poland) 102 persons fell ill after ingestion of *C. orellanus*, with 11 of them dying from renal failure 4 to 16 days after the meal (Grzymala, 1965). Remarkably, a similar collective poisoning with *C. orellanus* was reported from France, with 26 persons involved but no fatalities (due to timely intermittent dialysis) (Bouget et al., 1990). Lethal doses of orellanine are known for the mouse only, corresponding to 15 to 20 mg/kg body weight for intraperitoneal, and 33 to 90 mg/kg body weight for oral administration. Recently, three cases of suspected *Cortinarius* intoxication were reported from Australia (Mount et al., 2002).

3.3.2 CHEMISTRY AND ACTION

Orellanine is a hydroxylated bipyridyl-N,N'-dioxide (Figure 3.2a), associated in the mushroom with the corresponding monoxide, orellinine (Figure 3.2b). Under UV light, orellanine and orellinine stepwise lose the N-oxides, leading to orelline (Figure 3.2c) as the stable, but non-toxic, end product. Orellinine is less toxic than orellanine, and there is evidence that the species with toxic activity is not orellanine itself but an oxidation product, the semiquinone (Figure 3.2d), produced in cells by a peroxidase reaction (Oubrahim, et al., 1998). The semiquinone is a radical that probably causes intracellular depletion of glutathione and ascorbate as the toxic event. Toxicity mainly develops in the

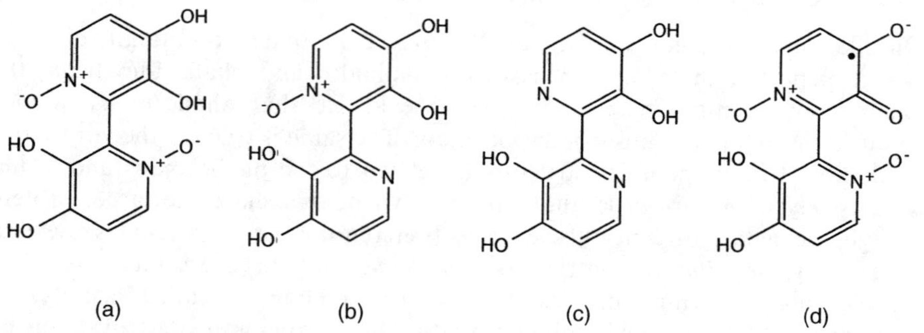

(a)   (b)   (c)   (d)

FIGURE 3.2 Structures of (a) orellanine, (b) orellinine, (c) orilline, and (d) the radical semiquinone of orellanine, suggested as the toxic species.

kidney, leading to renal failure. No toxic effects were found in the liver. On the molecular level, orellanine was shown to be an inhibitor of alkaline phosphatase (Ruedl et al., 1989).

3.3.3 SYMPTOMS AND TREATMENT

Symptoms of orellanine poisoning are typical of renal damage, developing two to four days, in some cases up to fourteen days, after the mushroom meal. During the latent period, patients have mild GI symptoms which may be overlooked. Accordingly, patients present themselves at hospital only at the stage when renal failure has developed. At that stage, patients suffer from abdominal or lumbar pain, headache, muscular pain, and fatigue, and present laboratory values showing leukocyturia, hematuria, and increased serum values of creatinine and potassium. Out of a group of 22 patients treated in Sweden in the years 1979 to 1993, nine patients developed chronic renal failure requiring dialysis or transplantation.

As with amatoxin poisoning, attempts to remove the toxin from plasma by extra-corporal purification methods at the time of hospitalization do not seem promising because of the long latent period. However, beside supportive care, hemodialysis is the option during the clinical course. For a recent review on *Corinarius* spp. poisoning, see Danel et al. (2001). A renal transplantation should not be carried out too early; the mean time for a transplant among the cases published so far was 6 to 30 months.

A method for estimating the prognosis in individual cases was recently proposed by Holmendahl; the Cortinarius Nephro Toxicity (CNT) Prognosis Index. This test is based on the serum creatinine level before treatment (y) and the number of days elapsed (X):

$$\text{CNT} = (y + 316)/X \times 10^2$$

where CNT < 1.1 indicates a good prognosis; CNT $= 1.1$–2.2 indicates a probable chronic failure; and CNT > 2.1 suggests a poor outcome requiring renal replacement therapy (Persson and Karlson-Stiber, in press).

3.3.4 DETECTION

The toxins are easily detected, after separation of the compounds from plasma and renal tissue on silica thin layers, by their fluorescence in UV light: orellanine is visible as navy blue, orellinine as dark blue, and orelline as light blue (Horn et al., 1997). Beside thin-layer chromatography (TLC), use of HPLC for the analysis of orellanine, e.g., in mushroom extracts, has also been reported. Quantitative analysis of orellanine in plasma samples, or in (rat) urine samples, was performed by extraction of orellanine on XAD-4 resin, two-dimensional TLC on cellulose, and spectrophotometric evaluation of the orelline produced on the TLC plates after UV-induced decomposition of the orellanine.

3.4 GYROMETRIN

3.4.1 MUSHROOMS PRODUCING GYROMETRIN

Gyrometrin toxin is produced by the false morel (*Gyromitra esculenta*), a short-stalked mushroom with a brain-like cap of dark brown color. Fruiting bodies of this mushroom appear mostly in spring and are valued as edible, even as delicacies. While many people consume the mushroom without any troubles, others become ill, some of them severely. It has been shown that the toxin content may vary with growth conditions, such as altitude and temperature. More probably, however, the variation is caused by differences in handling or cooking as the toxic components are volatile. The toxin has been detected in cooked, frozen, and dried specimens.

3.4.2 CHEMISTRY AND ACTION

Gyrometrin is the formyl-methylhydrazone of acetaldehyde (Figure 3.3a), a volatile and unstable compound. By hydrolysis, which occurs in the cooking process as well as in the GI tract, gyrometrin is cleaved into formyl-methylhydrazine (Figure 3.3b), and further into monomethylhydrazine, MMH (Figure 3.3c), representing the real poison. Both reaction products are volatile, therefore intoxications may also occur by inhalation of the fumes emitted during cooking. However, insufficient cooking, or cooking in a covered pot, may increase toxicity by leaving too much of the toxin in the meal. Fresh mushrooms contain 0 to 1.5 mg/g of the poison. The estimated lethal dose for humans has been estimated as 20 to 50 mg/kg body weight, less for children, i.e., 10 to 30 mg/kg body weight. Formyl-methylhydrazine and methylhydrazine are reported to be cancerogenic, possibly by methylating guanine moieties in DNA (Bergman and Hellenas, 1992).

3.4.3 SYMPTOMS AND TREATMENT

After a latency period of six to twenty hours a GI phase develops, with vomiting, abdominal pain, headache, and nausea. In the majority of cases neurological symptoms prevail, such as incoordination, vertigo, seizures, and coma. In severe cases a hepato-renal phase can follow with elevated liver

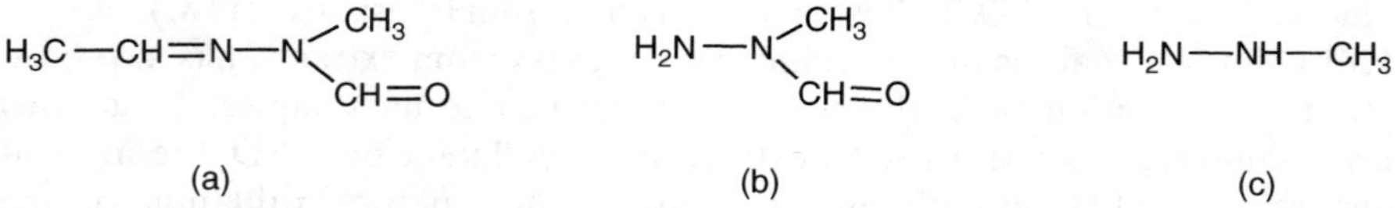

$$H_3C-CH=N-N\begin{array}{c}CH_3\\CH=O\end{array} \qquad H_2N-N\begin{array}{c}CH_3\\CH=O\end{array} \qquad H_2N-NH-CH_3$$

| (a) | (b) | (c) |

FIGURE 3.3 Structures of (a) gyrometrin, (b) formyl-methylhydrazine, and (c) methylhydrazine.

enzymes, jaundice and, finally, liver injury. However, life-threatening poisonings, or even fatalities, are nowadays rare.

After decontamination by emesis or lavage, patients should be carefully monitored for alterations in liver and kidney function, and treated symptomatically if necesseray. Seizures can be treated with anti-convulsant drugs. Because the toxin produces a deficiency of γ-amino-butyric acid (GABA), specific treatment with pyridoxine (vitamin B_6) has been recommended.

3.4.4 Detection

There is evidence that gyrometrin does not exist in the free state in the mushroom, but rather is bound to an unknown high-molecular component. Therefore, fruiting bodies have to be heated with water in a closed tube at 120°C for several hours before methylhydrazine can be extracted with chloroform under an atmosphere of nitrogen. Gas chromotography and TLC have been used for its identification.

3.5 COPRIN

3.5.1 Mushrooms Producing Coprine

During autumn (fall), mushrooms with egg-shaped, grey-white fruiting bodies occasionally appear, very often on road-sides, which after a few days deliquesce into an ink-colored liquid. The mushroom, *Coprinus atramentarius*, or inky cap, is edible when young, but can cause alcohol incompatability when consumed before, or together with, ethanol.

3.5.2 Chemistry and Action

The offending toxin is a conjugate of cyclopropanone and glutamine, called coprin (Figure 3.4a). In the liver, the amidohemiketal is cleaved into glutamine and cyclopropanone (Figure 3.4b), regarded as the toxic species. Its activity is understood as blocking the enzyme acetaldehyde dehydrogenase by reacting with the essential SH-group in the enzyme with formation of a hemi-thioketal (Figure 3.4c). As a consequence, acetaldehyde, the toxic metabolite of alcohol, will accumulate in the body.

3.5.3 Symptoms and Treatment

The symptoms are described as similar to those observed after application of disulfiram (Antabus), a drug used to discourage alcoholics from drinking. Typical symptoms include flashes, mydriasis, paraesthesia, tachycardia, and sweating, beside nausea and occasionally vomiting. This syndrome is brief in duration and will usually disappear after three to four hours, but may linger up to twenty-four hours.

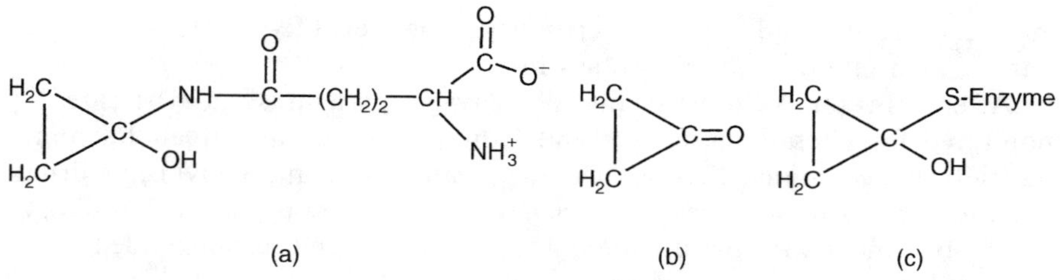

(a)   (b)   (c)

FIGURE 3.4 Structures of (a) coprin, (b) cyclopropanone, and (c) the thio-hemiketal of cyclopropanone formed at the essential SH-group of acetaldehyde dehydrogenase that blocks the activity of the enzyme.

The majority of reported cases have shown relatively mild and short-lived toxicity; therefore, in general, supportive care is regarded as the adequate treatment.

3.6 PSILOCYBIN AND PSILOCIN

3.6.1 MUSHROOMS PRODUCING PSILOCYBIN AND PSILOCIN

Mushrooms containing hallucinogenic indole derivatives (for a recent review see Wurst et al., 2002) were known in the 16th Century in the Mayan culture of ancient Mexico (teonanacatel). They comprise mainly four genera, *Psilocybe, Conocybe, Panaeolus*, and *Gymnopilus*. Most common are *Psilocybe semilanceata* (liberty cap), and *Psilocybe cubensis* (golden tops), small brown and cone-shaped mushrooms with slender stalks. They contain psilocybin, the main hallucinogenic component, in amounts of 2 to 16 mg/g dry weight, and a second hallucinogenic component, psilocin, in amounts of 0 to 10 mg/g dry weight. In dry form, but also as a supplement in honey (Bogusz et al., 1998), the mushrooms are available on the black market, particularly in England, the U.S., and the Netherlands. According to recent reports, use of *Psilocybe* is increasing in France (Pierrot et al., 2000), Denmark (Lassen et al., 1990), Japan (Musha et al., 1986), and in Thailand (where the mushrooms are consumed in omelettes by natives and tourists) (Gartz et al., 1994).

The quantity of toxins in the mushrooms can vary widely. In an analytical study on material confiscated by local authorities in Germany, *P. cyanescens* had the highest toxin content (Musshoff et al., 2000). As a species that always contains psilocin, *P. cyanescens* shows bluing. Species that do not always contain psilocin sometimes do not. The reason for this is that the blue color is caused by an oxidation product of psilocin. Both psilocibin and psilocin are temperature-sensitive; mushrooms in the freeze-dried state have been reported to retain activity for over two years when kept at −5°C.

3.6.2 Chemistry and Action

Psilocybin (Figure 3.5a) and psilocin (Figure 3.5b) are indole derivatives substituted in position 4 by a hydroxyl group, where psilocybin is phosphorylated. Due to its ionic properties, psilocybin is soluble in water. In addition, phosphorylation protects psilocybin from oxidative degradation. Both compounds are found to affect laboratory animals, but there is evidence that only the dephosphorylated form, psilocin, is the active species. In their structure the toxins resemble serotonine, a biogenic amine known to be a neurotransmitter.

3.6.3 Symptoms and Treatment

The toxins affect the central nervous system (CNS). Symptoms start within twenty minutes and may last for two to four hours, but peak hallucinogenic activity rarely lasts for more than one hour. Symptoms include anxiety and tension, visual effects such as blurring, euphoria, increased color perception with closed eyes, but also headache and fatigue. The overall sensation is usually described as pleasant.

Treatment is infrequently required. Severe agitation, anxiety, and aggressive behavior respond to diazepam, for example. Rest in a dark, quiet room is sufficient for the majority of the cases.

3.6.4 Detection

The toxins can be separated by TLC on silica and detected with Ehrlich reagent, dimethyl-aminobenzaldehyde, or, for higher sensitivity, with dimethyl-aminocinnamic aldehyde, yielding spots of violet or blue color. As a field test, lignine in newspapers can be used, as described for amatoxins (Section 3.2.5). For quantitation, gas chromatography in combination with mass spectrometry (Keller et al., 1999), HPLC and capillary-zone electrophoresis (Pedersen-Bjergaard et al., 1997), and even a DNA based test (Lee et al., 2000) have been used successfully. For the analysis of urine samples it must be considered that psilocin is excreted as glucuronide (Sticht and Käferstein, 2000).

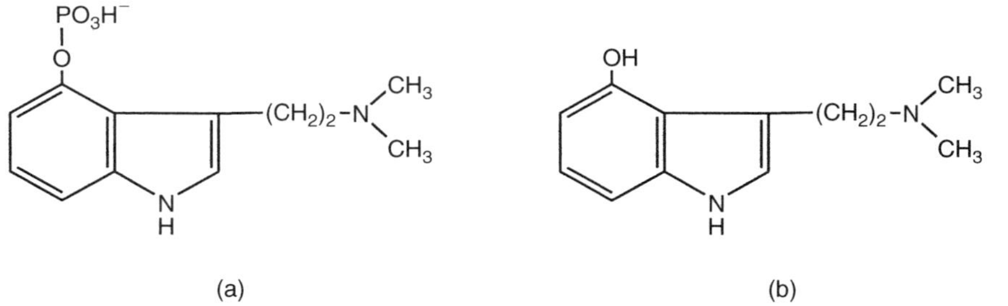

(a)   (b)

FIGURE 3.5 Structures of (a) psilocybin, and (b) psilocin.

3.7 IBOTENIC ACID AND MUSCIMOL

3.7.1 MUSHROOMS PRODUCING IBOTENIC ACID AND MUSCIMOL

These toxins, which target the CNS, are mainly found in two *Amanita* species, *A. muscaria* and *A. pantherina*, and to a lesser extent in *A. gemmata* and some other Amanitas. The fly agaric (*A. muscaria*) is frequent in coniferous and deciduous forests, growing singly or in groups. With its bright red cap (which, however, may also be orange or yellow) and the white warts, it is one of the most impressive forest mushrooms. *A. pantherina* has a greyish-brown cap with creamy-white warts and is frequently found under fir trees in autumn (fall). Toxic doses of ibotenic acid (30 to 60 mg) and muscimol (6 mg) can be found in single specimens of *A. muscaria*; other authors estimated the total amount of the two toxins in dry mushroom tissue of *A. muscaria* and *A. pantherina* as 2 and 4 mg/g, respectively. Commonly, two to four mushrooms of *A. muscaria* are ingested to produce mind-altering effects.

3.7.2 CHEMISTRY AND ACTION

Both toxins are isoxazole derivatives. In the mushroom, as well as in the eater, ibotenic acid (Figure 3.6a) is decarboxylated to muscimol (Figure 3.6b), which seems to be the active species. Muscimol is an agonist of GABA, and acts on the CNS in a way similar to diazepam. In animal experiments, both ibotenic acid and muscimol caused a decrease in muscle tone and motor activity, and an increase in brain levels of serotonine, but did not affect the cerebellar content of GABA. For a recent review on ibotenic acid and muscimol see Michelot and Melendez-Howell (2003).

3.7.3 SYMPTOMS AND TREATMENT

Patients may appear to be intoxicated, presenting nausea, vomiting, and diarrhea. They have color hallucinations, slow pulse, hypotension, irritability, and incoordination. Children may develop fever and seizures. Death from *A. muscaria* is rare, usually occurring only in severely poisoned young children, older patients, or persons with serious chronic illnesses. *A. pantherina* caused

(a)   (b)

FIGURE 3.6 Structures of (a) ibotenic acid, and (b) muscimol.

only one death out of 24 mushroom poisoning fatalities recorded in the literature before 1961.

There is no specific treatment for ingestion of ibotenic acid or muscimol; rather, treatment is symptomatic and supportive. Anxiety, hysteria, or convulsions can be treated with sedatives, such as diazepam. This should be done cautiously, however, and with the lowest effective dose because animal studies revealed that respiratory arrest may occur. In severe cases, with prolonged nausea, vomiting, or diarrhea, monitoring of fluid and electrolyte status may be required. Recent cases of muscarine poisonings were reported by Benjamin (1992), and Tupalska-Wilczynska et al. (1997).

3.7.4 DETECTION

Separation and quantitation of the toxic components of *A. muscaria* and related mushrooms can be achieved by HPLC, or by TLC using ninhydrine and heating for detection. With ninhydrine, muscimol develops a yellow spot and has a limit of detection of 0.1 µg.

3.8 MUSCARINE

3.8.1 MUSHROOMS PRODUCING MUSCARINE

Muscarine is found in mushrooms of the genera *Inocybe* and *Clitocybe* (*I. patouillardi, I. fastigiata, I. geophylla,* and *C. dealbata*), in which it accounts for 1 to 3 mg/g of dry weight. Both genera occur commonly and have a worldwide distribution. While *Inocybe* mushrooms are mycorrhizal on conifers or broad-leafed trees, *Clitocybe* mushrooms are saprophytic and grow on forest litter or grassland humus. Confusion with edible mushrooms most commonly occurs with the species growing on grassland.

Muscarine is found in tiny amounts, usually under 20 µg/g, in other agaric genera, too, such as *Amanita, Boletus, Hygrocybe, Lactarius, Mycena,* and *Russula*. It was by the small amounts of muscarine present in *A. muscaria,* 90 µg/g, that the toxin was detected and identified (and got its name); but muscarine in *A. muscaria* usually does not account for the symptoms that occur after ingestion of this fungus, which are produced by muscimol and its precursor ibotenic acid.

3.8.2 CHEMISTRY AND ACTION

Muscarine is a tetrahydrofuran derivative with the structure shown in Figure 3.7a. Because of the three chirality centers present in the molecule, muscarine exists in eight isomers, of which only one, L-(+)-muscarine, is active. The remaining isomers also have been detected in toxic fungi, but because of their low biological activity and low concentration they do not contribute to toxicity.

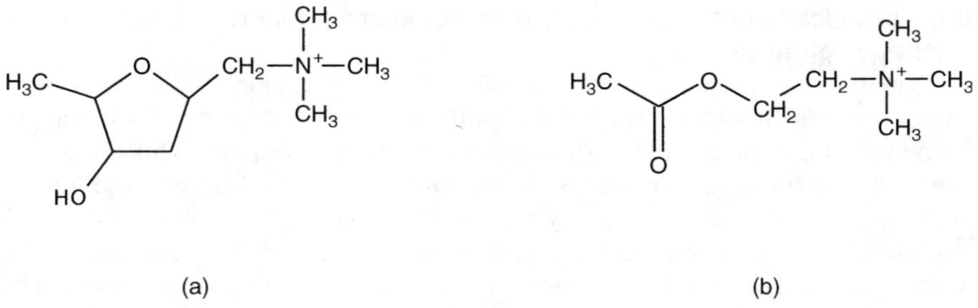

(a)   (b)

FIGURE 3.7 Structures of (a) muscarine, and (b) the neurotransmitter acetylcholine

Through its structural similarity to acetylcholine (Figure 3.7b), muscarine binds to the acetylcholine receptor on the synapses of nerve endings of smooth muscles and endocrine glands, causing the well-known parasympaticomimetic effects. Because muscarine is not an ester like acetylcholine, and hence resists esterase activity, it is not degraded and so can cause continuous stimulation of the affected neurons.

3.8.3 SYMPTOMS AND TREATMENT

Muscarine poisoning is characterized by profuse perspiration, salivation, and lachrymation. The constriction of the pupils is a typical syndrome and can strengthen diagnosis. Vomiting may occur. Symptoms typically appear within thirty minutes and can last for up to two hours, in severe cases up to six to twenty four hours.

Where muscarinic symptoms are mild, supportive therapy may be sufficient. Severe cases will require intramuscular or intravenous administration of atropin.

From recent literature it must be concluded that mushrooms of the genera *Inocybe* and *Clitocybe* contain toxic components that are different from muscarine. The severe symptoms reported of an Israeli child poisoned with *I. tristis* therefore departed from what is known of muscarine poisoning (Amitai et al., 1982). The toxic activities of *C. acromelalga* and *C. amoenolens*, two *Clitocybe* species containing clitidine and acromelic acid A, respectively, were studied in rats (Fukuwatari et al., 2001; Saviuc et al., 2003).

3.8.4 DETECTION

Muscarine is detected by high-performance thin-layer chromatography (HPTLC), with a limit of detection of 50 ng (Stijve, 1981). Using Dragendorff reagent, muscarine appears as an orange spot.

3.9 MUSHROOMS CAUSING GASTROINTESTINAL DISORDERS

This large group of mushrooms accounts by far for the largest number of mushroom poisonings, but fatalities are very rare, possibly absent. In the great majority of cases the toxins involved remain unidentified, and may differ from species to species.

3.9.1 *CHLOROPHYLLUM MOLYBDITIS*

This mushroom was originally classified in the genus *Lepiota*, and is also known as *Lepiota morgani* or *Lepiota molybditis* (false parasol). It is a species often involved in poisonings in the U.S. and throughout the world, but apparently not in Europe. The attractive mushroom grows in grassland and can be distinguished from edible lepiotas by its greenish spores and greenish gills. The toxin was suggested to be a protein of high molecular weight, composed of monomers of 40 to 60 kDa. Symptoms typically start within one to two hours after ingestion, with profuse vomiting and nausea, followed by diarrhea, intestinal cramps, and sweating. In severe cases symptoms may last up to two to three days. Vomiting and diarrhea can cause significant fluid and electrolyte depletion, which must be balanced. No hepatic or renal sequelae are known. (For a review see Augenstein, 1994.)

3.9.2 *ENTOLOMA SINUATUM* (OR *LIVIDUM*)

This mushroom is responsible for a significant number of mushroom poisonings in Europe. Symptoms such as vomiting, abdominal pain, and diarrhea may be seen between thirty minutes and two hours after ingestion. No *Entoloma* poisonings have been fatal and symptoms disappear within a day or two.

3.9.3 *TRICHOLOMA PERDIDUM*

Of all mushroom poisonings in two Swiss studies, 20 to 50% were due to this mushroom. One to two hours postingestion the patient may experience abdominal pain, violent vomiting, sweating, diarrhea, and cramping in the calf muscles. Symptoms usually last for two to six hours, but full recovery may take three to six days.

3.9.4 *AGARICUS XANTHODERMUS*

GI reactions have occurred from ingestion of yellow-staining *Agaricus* species. *Agaricus xanthodermus* has a strong phenol-like odor and taste, and phenol has indeed been discovered in it and in a number of other *Agaricus* mushrooms. It is unclear, however, whether phenol or another agent is responsible for the GI upset.

3.9.5 *OMPHALOTUS OLEARIUS* (OR *ILLUDENS*)

This mushroom known as Jack O'Lantern, can cause severe gastroenteritis after a latent period of one to three hours, with headache, nausea, sweating, vomiting, abdominal pain, sometimes associated with bitter taste, and a feeling of coldness. It has been argued that these effects may be due to a muscarine-like reaction, but no muscarine has been identified. A sesquiterpene, illudin S, is believed to be at least one of the toxic components.

3.9.6 *LACTARIUS HELVUS*

Lactarius species are 'milk'-containing mushrooms. Poisonous *Lactarius* are generally found in species with white latex. After eating large quantities of these mushrooms, symptoms such as vomiting, profuse diarrhea, and sweating will occur fifteen minutes to one hour after the meal. The nature of the toxin is unknown.

3.9.7 *RAMARIA* (OR *CLAVARIA*) *PALLIDA*

This mushroom has been known to produce gastroenteritis and profuse diarrhea. The toxin responsible has not been identified.

3.9.8 *BOLETUS CALOPUS*, *B. SANTANAS*

GI irritants are the most common toxins in Boletes, particularly in red-spored and yellow-spored species. Muscarine is present in a few species, but too low to be significant. Symptoms are nausea, vomiting, and diarrhea. In more severe cases there may be muscle cramps and circulatory disturbance. Treatment is largely symptomatic, and recovery is usually complete one to two days after ingestion.

3.9.9 *PAXILLUS INVOLUTUS*

Paxillus syndrome is a food allergy, not a true poisoning. As a consequence, some who eat the mushrooms will not develop symptoms. Symptoms may include colic, vomiting, diarrhea, oliguria or anuria, kidney pain, hemoglobinuria, and renal failure. A hemagglutination test has been used for confirmation (Bresinsky and Besl, 1990).

3.10 CONCLUSION

Fortunately, of the vast number of mushroom species that exists, only a few produce secondary metabolites that cause fatal poisonings. If toxins causing benign symptoms, such as abdominal pain and diarrhea, hallucinations, or alcohol incompatibility, are disregarded, the most significant mushroom toxins are the extremely hazardous compounds of amatoxins, orellanine, and, to a lesser extent, methylhydrazine and its derivatives. Consequently, there is only a handful of mushroom species that one should strictly keep away from, or at least avoid ingesting. Studying to identify these few species seems more profitable than learning to identify all the edible mushrooms, of which there are so many. Moreover, considering that more than 90% of all fatal cases of mushroom poisoning in Europe are due solely to *Amanita phalloides,* the abilility to discern *Amanita phalloides* infallably in all its varieties and stages of development would save nine lives of ten otherwise lost by mushroom poisoning.

3.11 REFERENCES

Amitai, I., Peleg O., Ariel, I. and Binjamini, N. (1982). Severe poisoning of a child by the mushroom *Inocybe tristis,* Malencon and Bertault, *Isr. J. Med. Sci.,* 18, 798–801.

Augenstein, W.L. (1994), Chlorophyllum Molybditis, in Spoerke, D.G. and Rumack, B.H., Eds., *Handbook of mushroom poisoning,* CRC Press, Boca Raton, chap. 17.

Benjamin, D.R. (1992). Mushroom poisoning in infants and children: The Amanita pantherina/muscaria group, *J. Toxicol. Clin. Toxicol.,* 30, 13–22.

Bergman, K. and Hellenas, K.E. (1992). Methylation of rat DNA by the mushroom poison gyrometrin and its metabolite monomethylhydrazine, *Cancer Lett.,* 61, 165–170.

Bogusz, M.J., Maier, R.D., Schafer, A.D. and Erkens, M. (1998). Honey with Psilocybe mushrooms: a revival of a very old preparation on the drug market?, *Int. J. Legal Med.,* 111, 147–150.

Bouget, J., Bousser, J., Pats, B., Ramee, M.P., Chevet, D., Rifle, G., Giudicelli, C.P. and Thomas, R. (1990). Acute renal failure following collective intoxication by *Cortinarius orellanus, Intensive Care Med.,* 16, 506–510.

Bresinsky, A. and Besl, H. (1990). *A colour atlas of fungi,* Wolfe Publishing Ltd, London.

Buck, R.W. (1961). Mushroom Toxins – a brief review of the literature, *N. Engl. J. Med.,* 265, 681–689.

Chaiear, K., Limpaiboon, R., Meechai, C. and Poovorawan, Y. (1999). Fatal mushroom poisoning caused by *Amanita virosa* in Thailand, *Southeast Asian J. Trop. Med. Public Health,* 30, 157–160.

Danel, V.C., Saviuc, P.F. and Garon, D. (2001). Main features of *Cortinarius* ssp. poisoning: a literature review, *Toxicon,* 39, 1053–1060.

Enjalbert, F., Rapior, S., Nougier-Soule, J. Guillon, S., Amouroux, N. and Cabot, C. (2002). Treatment of amatoxin poisoning: 20-year retrospective analysis, *J. Toxicol. Clin. Toxicol.,* 40, 715–757.

Faulstich H. and Wieland, T. (1992). Mushroom Poisons, in Tu, A.T., Ed., *Food poisoning,* Marcel Dekker, New York.

Faulstich, H. and Zilker, T.R. (1994). Amatoxins, in Spoerke, D.G. and Rumack, B.H., eds., *Handbook of mushroom poisoning,* CRC Press, Boca Raton, Chap. 10.

Fukawatari, T., Suigimoto, E. and Shibata, K. (2001). Effect of feeding with a poisonous mushroom *Clitocybe acromelalga* on the metabolism of tryptophan-niacin in rats. *Shokuhin Eiseigaku Zasshi,* 42, 190–196.

Gartz, J., Allen, J.W. and Merlin, M.D. (1994). Ethnomycology, biochemistry, and cultivation of *Psilocybe samuensis* Guzman, Bandala and Allen, a new psychoactive fungus from Koh Samui, Thailand, *J. Ethnopharmacol.*, 43, 73–80.

Grzymala, S. (1965). Etude clinique des intoxications par les champignons du genre *Cortinarius orellanus* Fr. *Bull. Med. Leg., Toxicol. Med.*, 8, 60–70.

Horn S., Horina, J.H., Krejs G.J., Holzer, H. and Ratschek, M. (1997). Endstage renal failure from mushroom poisoning with *Cortinarius orellanus*: report of four cases and review of literature, *Am. J. Kidney Dis.*, 30, 282–286.

Kaneko, H., Tomomasa, T., Inuoe, Y., Kunimoto, F., Fukusato, T., Muraoka, S., Gonmori, K., Matsumoto, T. and Morikawa, A. (2001). Amatoxin poisoning from ingestion of Japanese Galerina mushrooms, *J. Toxicol. Clin. Toxicol.*, 39, 413–416.

Keller, T., Schneider, A., Regenscheit, P., Dirnhofer, R., Rucker, T., Jaspers, J. and Kisser, W. (1999). Analysis of psilocybin and psilocin *Psilocybe subcubensis* Guzman by ion mobility spectrometry and gas chromatography-mass spectrometry, *Forensic Sci. Int.*, 99, 93–105.

Lassen, J.F., Ravn, H.B. and Lassen, S.F. (1990). Hallucinogenic psilocybin containing mushrooms. Toxins contained in Danish wild mushrooms, *Ugeskr Laeger.*, 152, 314–317.

Lee, J.C., Cole, M. and Linacre, A. (2000). Identification of members of the genera *Panaeolus* and *Psilocybe* by a DNA test. A preliminary test for hallucinogenic fungi, *Forensic Sci. Int.*, 112, 123–133.

Lim, J.G., Kim, J.H., Lee, C.Y., Lee, S.I. and Kim, Y.S. (2000). *Amanita virosa* induced toxic hepatitis: report of three cases, *Yonsei Med. J.*, 41, 416–421.

Meunier, B.C., Camus, C.M., Houssin, D.P., Messner, M.J., Gerault, A.M. and Launois, B.G. (1995). Liver transplantation after severe poisoning due to amatoxin-containing *Lepiota* – report of three cases, *J. Toxicol. Clin. Toxicol.*, 33, 165–171.

Michelot, D. and Melendez-Howell, L.M. (2003), *Amanita muscaria*: chemistry, biology, toxicology and ethnomycology, *Mycol. Res.*, 107, 231–246.

Mount, P., Harris, G., Sinclair. R., Finlay, M. and Becker, G.J. (2002). Acute renal failure following ingestion of wild mushrooms, *Int. Med. J.*, 32, 187–190.

Musha, M., Ishii, A., Tanaka, F. and Kusano, G. (1986). Poisoning by hallucinogenic mushroom higakeshibiritake (*Psilocybe argentipes* K. Yokohama) indigenous to Japan, *Tohoku J. Exp. Med.*, 148, 73–78.

Musshoff, F., Madea, B. and Beike, J. (2000). Hallucinogenic mushrooms on the German market – simple instructions for examination and identification, *Forensic Sci. Int.*, 113, 389–395.

Oubrahim, H., Richard, J.M., Cantin-Esnault, D. (1998). Peroxidase-mediated oxidation, a possible pathway for activation of the fungal nephrotoxin orellanine and related compounds. ESR and spin-trapping studies, *Free Radic. Res.*, 28, 497–505.

Paydas, S., Kocak, R., Erturk, F., Erken, E., Zaksu, H.S. and Gurcay, A. (1990). Poisoning due to amatoxin-containing *Lepiota* species, *Br. J. Clin. Pract.*, 44, 450–453.

Pedersen-Bjergaard, S., Sannes, E. Rasmussen, K.E. and Tonnesen F. (1997). Determination of psilocybin in *Psilocybe semilanceata* by capillary zone electrophoresis, *J. Chromatogr. B Biomed Sci.* Appl., 694, 375–381.

Perez-Moreno, J., Perez-Moreno, A. and Ferrera-Cerrato, R. (1994). Multiple fatal mycetism caused by *Amanita virosa* in Mexico, *Mycopathologia*, 125, 3–5.

Persson H. and Karlson-Stiber, C. Cytotoxic fungi – an overview, *Toxicon*, in press.

Pierrot, M., Josse, P., Raspiller, M.F., Goulmy, M., Rambourg, M.O., Manel, J. and Lambert, H. (2000). Intoxication by hallucinogenic mushrooms, *Ann. Med. Interne* (Paris), 151, Suppl. B:B16–19.

Puig Hernandez, A., Chumillas Cordoba, C., Camprodon Calveras, J., de Francisco Enciso, E.F., Marco, M.P. and Ferran Martinez, G. (2001). *Lepiota brunneoincarnata* fatal intoxication, *An. Med. Interna*, 18, 481–482.

Ramirez, P., Parrilla, P., Sanchez Bueno, F., Robles, R., Pons, J.A., Bixquert, V., Nicolas, S., Nunez, R., Alegria, M. S. and Miras, M. (1994). Fulminant hepatic failure after *Lepiota* poisoning, *J. Hepatol.*, 19, 51–54.

Ruedl, C., Gstrauntaler, G. and Moser, M. (1989). Differential inhibitory activity of the fungal toxin orellanine on alkaline phosphatase isoenzymes, *Biochim. Biophys. Acta*, 991, 280–283.

Saviuc, P., Dematteis, M., Mezin, P., Danel, V. and Mallaret, M. (2003). Toxicity of the *Clitocybe amoenolens* mushroom in rat, *Vet. Hum. Toxicol*, 45, 180–182.

Seeger, R. (1984). Zeitungspapiertest für Amanitine – falsch-positive Ergebnisse, *Z. Mykol.*, 50, 353–359.

Spoerke, D.G. and Rumack, B.H., Eds. (1994). *Handbook of mushroom poisoning, diagnosis and treatment*. CRC Press, Boca Raton.

Sticht, G. and Käferstein, H. (2000). Detection of psilocin in body fluids, *Forensic Sci. Int.*, 113, 403–407.

Stijve, T. (1981). High performance thin-layer chromatographic determination of the toxic principles of some poisonous mushrooms, *Mitt. Geb. Lebensmittelunters. Hyg.*, 72, 2432–2436.

Tupalska-Wilczynska, K., Ignatowicz, R., Poziemski, A., Wojcik, H. and Wilczynski, G. (1997). *Amanita pantherina* and *Amanita muscaria* poisonings – pathogenesis, symptoms and treatment, *Pol. Merkuriusz Lek.*, 3, 30–32.

Wieland, T. and Faulstich, H. (1983). Peptide Toxins from Amanita, in Keeler, R.F. and Tu, A.T., Eds., *Handbook of natural toxins*, Marcel Dekker, New York, Chap. 18.

Wurst, M., Kysilka, R. and Flieger, M. (2002). Psychoactive tryptamines from basidiomycetes, *Folia Microbiol.* (Praha), 47, 3–27.

4

Phytoestrogens in Food Plants

Paola Albertazzi

Contents

4.1 INTRODUCTION

Phytoestrogens are a group of plant-derived molecules (Figure 4.1) that are so named because they possess an estrogen-like activity. In 1949, adverse effects on fertility were observed in animals that had been grazing on phytoestrogen-rich plants (Shutt, 1976). In the early 1980s it became clear that phytoestrogens could produce biological effects in humans, but it was not until the early 1990s that interest around these compounds really soared. What caused such a stir was the observation of a lower incidence of hot flushes in Japanese menopausal women compared with their Western counterparts (Lock, 1993). Japanese women also appeared to have a lower incidence of breast cancer, cardiovascular disease, and osteoporosis. In addition, Japanese men have a low incidence of prostate cancer. The low incidence of these conditions appeared

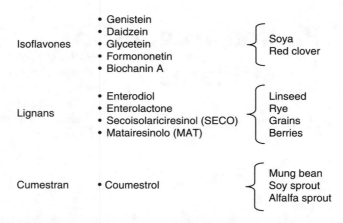

FIGURE 4.1 Different types of phytoestrogen and food where they can typically be found.

to be strictly correlated with the consumption of the traditional diet (Nagata et al., 2002).

The Japanese diet differs in many aspects from its Western counterpart, not only in consumption of soy but also of fish. To date, however, soy alone appears to have attracted the attention of researchers. The structural similarity between the isoflavones contained in soy and estrogen has perhaps made it conceptually easier to associate soy consumption and the low incidence of hot flushes in Japanese women. This may prove to be too simplistic as it is highly likely that a combination of nutrients, rather than just one compound, may determine the favorable health effects of the diet.

Although the issue is still unresolved, postmenopausal women all over the Western world have caught onto the idea that phytoestrogens may be beneficial to their health. In 2000, the value of the European market for phytoestrogens was estimated to be €106 million. Dietary supplements containing isoflavones are an expanding market and presently represent 9% of the phytonutrient market value. Research from market analysis predicts that the combined phytonutrient market will increase to an estimated €163 million by 2008 (Frost & Sullivan, 2002). This growth is due to several reasons, however the main one is that ageing women are the largest consumers of food supplements (Mintel, 2001) and they are the fastest growing segment of the population in the Western world.

4.2 SOURCES OF PHYTOESTROGEN AND ESTROGENIC EFFECTS

Phytoestrogens are a diverse group of polyphenolic non-steroidal plant compounds that bind to human estrogen receptors (Cos et al., 2003). The best studied of these compounds are the isoflavones, the phytoestrogens present in soy and red clover.

Phytoestrogens *in vitro* bind to and stimulate the activity of both estrogen receptors (ERs), α and β, but have a stronger affinity for the latter (Kuiper et al., 1998). The distribution of ERα and ERβ in different tissues has been used to explain the tissue selectivity of phytoestrogens, as well as other pharmacological compounds. But this is most certainly not the whole story. Different phytoestrogens have different affinities for binding to the ERs, in the order: 17-β-estradiol > coumestrol > genistein > equol > daidzein > biochanin A. The ER binding affinity, however, cannot distinguish between agonistic and antagonistic activity (Diel et al., 1999).

There are several *in vitro* test systems, including cell-proliferation assays and reporter gene assays, that are used to evaluate the estrogenic activity of natural compounds. The cell-proliferation assay, also called the 'E-screen,' measures the ability of a compound to stimulate the proliferation of human estrogen dependent breast cancer cell lines, such as MCF-7 and T47-D. The reporter gene assay is used to check the capability of a compound to activate the transcription of an estrogen-sensitive promoter. Application of these tests to phytoestrogens has clearly demonstrated that coumestrol is the most active of the phytoestrogens and binds as strongly as 17-β-estradiol to both ERs. Differences in estrogen-binding affinity have suggested that phytoestrogens, and in particular the isoflavones, are weakly estrogenic but induce distinct patterns of ER agonist or antagonist activities that are cell context- and promoter-dependent, suggesting that these compounds may induce tissue-specific effects similar to those observed for a class of compound called selective estrogen receptor modulators (SERM) (Diel et al., 2001; Setchell, 2001)

4.3 PHYTOESTROGEN METABOLISM

The isoflavones that occur naturally in most soy foods are conjugated almost exclusively to sugars, called the glycoside forms. Bioavailability of isoflavone glycosides, and the mechanism of intestinal absorption of isoflavones in humans, are unclear. Evidence from intestinal perfusion and *in vitro* cell-culture studies indicates that isoflavone glycosides are poorly absorbed and their bioavailability requires initial hydrolysis of the sugar moiety by intestinal β-glucosidases for uptake to the peripheral circulation. (Setchell et al., 2002a). It is possible that products that contain mostly isoflavones in the glycoside state, such as soy and red clover, may be less effective as they may be less absorbed or more susceptible to the variability of individual metabolisms.

The glycosides forms of the isoflavones have a weaker estrogenic action compared with their aglycone counterparts. In fact, they bind weakly to both ERα and ERβ and the receptor-dependent transcriptional expression is poor. Once the glucose molecule is removed, the isoflavones bind more strongly to the estrogen receptor (Morito et al., 2001).

Equol [7-hydroxy-3-(4'-hydroxyphenyl)-chroman] is a nonsteroidal estrogen of the isoflavone class. It is exclusively a product of intestinal bacterial metabolism of dietary isoflavones and possesses estrogenic activity, having affinity for both ERα and ERβ. Equol appears to be superior to all other isoflavones for antioxidant activity. It is the end product of the biotransformation of the phytoestrogen daidzein, one of the two main isoflavones found in abundance in soybeans and most soy foods. Once formed, equol is relatively stable; however, it is not produced in all healthy adults in response to dietary challenge with soy or daidzein. Several recent dietary intervention studies examining the health effects of soy isoflavones allude to the potential importance of equol for obtaining maximal clinical responses to soy protein diets (Setchell et al., 2002b).

4.4   EFFECT OF PROCESSING PHYTOESTROGENS AND THEIR ACTIVITY

The bulk of data available about the processing of phytoestrogens again reflects the primary interest in the isoflavones subclass of phytoestrogen.

Before 1990 the composition of isoflavones in soy foods was thought to be largely determined by whether the food had been fermented. Fermented foods (e.g., miso and tempeh) contain the unconjugated isoflavones agycones, while non-fermented food (e.g., tofu, soy flower, and soy milk) contain the conjugated glucoside. Subsequent experiments have demonstrated that fermentation of soy decreased the isoflavone content of the food product, but increased the urinary isoflavonoid recovery, suggesting that fermentation increases availability of isoflavones in soy (Slavin et al., 1998).

The principal chemical forms of isoflavones in soybean are their 6″-O-malonyl-β-glucoside (6OMalGlc) conjugates. Hot alcohol extraction of ground soybean yields deesterified 6OMalGlc conjugates. Although room temperature extraction slows the conversion, extraction at 4°C for 2 to 4 hours led to the highest yield of 6OMalGlc conjugates and the lowest proportion of β-glucoside conjugates. Analysis of soy food products by reversed-phase high performance liquid chromatography (HPLC)-mass spectrometry reveals that defatted soy flour that had not been heat treated consisted mostly of 6OMalGlc conjugates; in contrast, toasted soy flour contained large amounts of 6″-O-acetyl-β-glucoside conjugates, formed by heat-induced decarboxylation of the malonate group to acetate. Soymilk and tofu consist almost entirely of β-glucoside conjugates; low-fat versions of these products were markedly depleted in isoflavones. Alcohol-washed soy-protein concentrate contains few isoflavones. Isolated soy protein and textured vegetable protein consisted of a mixture of all three types of isoflavone conjugates. Baking or frying of textured vegetable protein at 190°C and baking of soy flour in cookies does not appear to alter total isoflavone content, but produces a steady increase in β-glucoside conjugates at the expense of 6OMalGlc conjugates (Coward et al., 1998).

4.5 BENEFICIAL AND ADVERSE EFFECTS OF PHYTOESTROGENS IN HUMANS

4.5.1 INTRODUCTION

The bulk of the available data on the effects of phytoestrogen on humans is mostly from postmenopausal women, and in particular on the effects on hot flushes. Data are beginning to emerge on the effect of phytoestrogens in bone, but very little is known about the effects of these compounds on the uterus and breast. This information is urgently required to allow evaluation of long-term safety of these compounds, particularly in view of long-term treatment of postmenopausal women for the prevention of osteoporosis. Very little is known about the therapeutic potential of phytoestrogen in men.

4.5.2 EFFECTS OF SOY OR RED CLOVER DERIVED PHYTOESTROGEN ON CLIMACTERIC SYMPTOMS

To date, six randomized studies (Murkies et al., 1995; Albertazzi et al., 1998; Washburn et al., 1999; St Germain et al., 2001; Kotsopoulos et al., 2000; Knight et al., 2001) have investigated the effect of soy or other pulses on incidence and severity of hot flushes in perimenopausal and postmenopausal women (Table 4.1). Some of the studies utilized soy as whole grains, some in flour form. Other studies have utilized isolated soy protein that is a soy-derived powder containing over 90% protein and a high concentration of isoflavones. This is possibly a more physiological diet-like way of administering isoflavones as it maintains intact the original food matrix, which may be of importance for absorption and clinical efficacy.

The results of studies on the effects of soy on hot flushes are quite contradictory. Three studies have failed to observe any effects (St Germain et al., 2001; Kotsopoulos et al., 2000; Knight et al., 2001), while others have observed some benefit. Soy preparations appear, at best, to only halve the incidence of hot flushes (Albertazzi et al., 1998), which is somewhat in contrast with a complete lack of hot flushes observed in Japanese women (Lock, 1993).

One could argue that efficacy may be improved by extracting and concentrating in tablets the compound considered to be the active principal of soy. This should also, at least theoretically, improve compliance. Western women, in general, do not find the traditional Japanese diet easy to follow, hence, isolated isoflavones in tablet form have been used.

Four studies (Scambia et al., 2000; Upmalis et al., 2000; Han et al., 2002; Faure et al., 2002) using isolated isoflavones in tablet form have been performed to date (Table 4.2). Doses ranging from 50 to 100 mg per day were used. Again, at best, number of hot flushes was halved. This is not an obvious improvement in the treatment effects over those achieved with whole soy and suggests that the effect of these compounds is small. It will be necessary to use a large population size with a high number of severe symptoms to obtain an effect that is statistically significant.

Table 4.1
Randomized placebo-controlled studies performed with soy and other grains.

Trial reference	Phytoestrogen source	n	Trial type and duration	Hot flushes
Murkies et al. (1995). *Maturitas*, 21, 189–195.	45 g soy flour, 45 g wheat flour	58	Wheat as placebo, parallel, 12 weeks	↓40%, $p. < .001$ ↓25%, $p. < .001$
Albertazzi et al. (1998). *Obstet. Gyncecol.*, 91, 6–11.	60 g soy protein, 76 mg isoflavones, aglycone	104	Parallel, 12 weeks	↓45%, $p. < .001$
Washburn et al. (1998). *Menopause*, 6, 7–13.	20 g soy protein containing 34 mg of phytoestrogen	51	Cross-over, 6 weeks	↓ severity
Germain et al . (2001). *Menopause*, 8, 17–26.	Soy protein containing 4.4 mg isoflavones, 80 mg aglicone	69	Parallel, 6 months	↓ severity
Kotsopoulos et al. (2000). *Climacteric*, 31, 161–167.	Soy protein containing 118 mg of phytoestrogen	95	Parallel, 3 months	↓ severity
Knight et al. (2001). *Climacteric*, 4, 13–18.	60 g Take Care®, 77 mg aglycone	24	Parallel, 12 weeks	↓ severity

Red clover is a plant that contains isoflavones in a slightly different composition compared with soy. Red clover contains formononetin and biochanin A, which are not present in soy and may thus have additional biological activity. So far, four studies (Barber et al., 1999; Knight et al., 1999; van de Weijer, 2002; Tice et al., 2003) have been performed using isoflavones derived from red clover (Table 4.3). These have used doses of isoflavones ranging from 40 to 160 mg. Three out of four of these studies did not show any effects, even in spite of a very large sample size (Tice et al., 2003). Only one study showed a reduction in the number of hot flushes. The reduction, however, was small (van de Weijer and Barentsen, 2002). Red clover therefore does not appear to have much of an effect on the reduction of hot flushes.

Two studies have been performed so far on women with breast cancer complaining of hot flushes – neither showed an improvement (Table 4.4). Quella et al. (2000) did not show any reduction in hot flushes in breast cancer survivors using 150 mg of phytoestrogen in tablets. The study was a cross-over design and had two phases lasting only four weeks, which were not separated by a wash-out period thus a carry-over effect cannot be excluded.

Table 4.2
Effects of soy-derived isolated isoflavones.

Trial reference	Phytoestrogen source	n	Trial type and duration	Hot flushes
Scambia et al. (2000). *Menopause*, 7, 105–111.	50 mg isoflavones glycone û ~ 31 mg aglycone	39	Parallel, 6 weeks	↓45%, $p. < .001$
Upmalis et al. (2000). *Menopause*, 7, 236–242.	50 mg isoflavones	177	Parallel, 12 weeks	↓28%, $p. < .078$
Han et al. (2002). *Obstet. Gynecol.*, 99, 389–94.	100 mg	82	Parallel, 4 months	↓ Kupperman index
Faure et al. (2002). *Menopause*, 9, 329–334.	70 mg isoflavones	75	Parallel, 4 months	ITT ↓51%, $p. = .01$

Table 4.3
Effects of isolated isoflavones derived from red clover.

Trial reference	Phytoestrogen	n	Trial type and duration	Hot flushes
Barber et al. (1999). *Climacteric*, 2, 85–92.	40 mg	51	Cross-over, 12 weeks	NS
Knight et al. (1999). *Climacteric*, 2, 79–84.	40 mg, 160 mg	37	Parallel, 12 weeks	NS
Van de Weijer and Barentsen (2002). *Maturitas.*, 42, 187–193.	80 mg	30	Parallel, 12 weeks	↓44%, $p. < .01$
Tice et al. (2003). *JAMA*, 290, 207–214.	82 mg, 57 mg	252	Parallel, 12 weeks	NS

Table 4.4
Effects of phytoestrogen on hot flushes in patients with breast cancer.

Trial reference	Phytoestrogen	n	Trial type and duration	Hot flushes
Quella et al. (2000). *J. Clin. Oncol.*, 18, 1068–1074.	150 mg	177	Cross-over, 4 weeks	NS
Van Patten et al. (2002). *J. Clin. Oncol.*, 20, 1436–1438.	90 mg isoflavones in 500 ml soy beverage	123	Parallel, 12 weeks	NS

Van Patten et al. (2002), in a very well conducted randomized study, divided 157 women into two groups: 500 ml soy beverage containing 90 mg of isoflavones versus a rice beverage for 12 weeks. No improvement in the number of hot flushes was found in the population taking soy compared with the placebo. Tamoxifen was used on 68% of women on the Quella et al. trial and in 24% in the van Patten trial. In spite of differences in the phytoestrogen preparation tested and prevalence of tamoxifen usage, the outcome was similarly negative.

4.5.3 EFFECTS OF PHYTOESTROGENS ON BONE

Four short-term (six months) human studies have been performed on the effects of different isoflavone preparations on bone mineral density (Alekel et al., 2000; Potter et al., 1998,; Clifton-Bligh et al., 2001; Hsu et al., 2001) and one on bone markers (Wagen et al., 2000).

One of the studies, that by Potter et al. (1998), was double blind and placebo-controlled, involving 66 postmenopausal women, but only lasted six months. A dose of 40 mg per day of isolated soy protein containing 90 mg of isoflavones resulted in a 2.2% increase in bone mineral density at the lumbar spine compared with the baseline. This difference was statistically significant. A second similar study, by Alekel et al. (2000), was performed in 69 perimenopausal women. A dose of 80 mg of phytoestrogen in the daily diet prevented lumbar spine bone loss, while a 1.28% loss was observed in the placebo group. Clifton-Bligh et al. (2001) performed a double-blind six months study in postmenopausal women. Two daily doses (57 and 85 mg) of isolated isoflavones derived from red clover determined a non-dose-dependent increase of mineral density of 3 to 4% at proximal radius and ulna. Unfortunately, given the precision of forearm densitometry, 24 weeks is probably too short a time to observe conclusive changes in bone mineral. Hsu et al. (2001) performed an uncontrolled study on 37 postmenopausal women using 150 mg per day of isoflavone from a non-specified source for six months. The study was looking for changes in calcaneal bone mineral density. However, again, the calcaneous is a site not particularly sensitive to modification of bone density over such a short period. Not surprisingly, no-changes were observed after six months of treatment compared with the baseline.

Three cohort studies have been performed, one in European women, and two in oriental women eating a traditional soy-based diet. The study in European women, performed by Kardinaal et al. (1998), failed to show a correlation between change in forearm bone mineral density and urinary excretion of isoflavonoids. Excretion of enterolactone, a marker of intake of grain and berries, was found to correlate positively with bone mineral density. This may be explained with the difficulty of correlating bone mineral density – a multifactorial variable, influenced by diet only on long-term basis – with excretion of phytoestrogens that only quantify the last 24 to 48 hours of phytoestrogen intake.

A well-conducted interventional study, which was undertaken using 54 mg per day of pure genistein in the aglycone form, was recently published (Morabito et al., 2002). A statistically highly significant increase of over 3% in bone mineral density of both the spine and the femoral neck was observed. The increase was similar to that observed with hormonal replacement therapy. This is the first suggestion that pure isoflavones in the aglycone form may have a role in the treatment of osteoporosis.

4.5.4 EFFECTS OF PHYTOESTROGENS ON THE UTERUS

Increasing doses of genistein have been found to be a stimulatory effect on the uterus in ovariectomized mice (Ishimi et al., 2000). In humans, different isoflavone preparations have not, so far, produced any increase in endometrial thickness (Barber et al., 1999; Scambia et al., 2000; Han et al., 2002; Morabito et al., 2002) or changes in uterine histology (Balk et al., 2002). However, these human studies have been all of short duration and not large enough to observe incidence of endometrial hyperplasia. It is thus important to obtain long-term data on the effects of different doses of phytoestrogen on uterine safety. There is, in fact, at least one report in the literature that suggests a link between massive consumption of phytoestrogen supplement and endometrial cancer in a postmenopausal woman (Johnson et al., 2001).

4.5.5 EFFECTS OF PHYTOESTROGENS ON THE BREAST

Asians consume high amounts of phytoestrogens and have a low incidence of breast cancer. High excretion of phytoestrogens in plasma and urine, indicating high intake, has been connected with a low incidence of breast cancer in two Australian case-control studies (Ingram et al., 1997; Murkies, 2000). The time of life during which exposure to phytoestrogens occurs may actually determine whether the effects on carcinogenesis are beneficial. The greatest cancer preventive effects occur in animals exposed during breast development (Murrill et al., 1996; Hilakivi-Clarke et al., 1999), most likely as a result of enhanced mammary-gland development with growth of fewer terminal end buds (the mammary structure most vulnerable to carcinogenesis). Consistent with this observation are data from an epidemiological study performed in China in which a retrospective evaluation of early food intake shows that soy food intake by adolescents is inversely associated with adult breast-cancer risk, with an odds ratio of 0.5 at the highest quintile of intake. (Shu et al., 2001). Results are significant for both pre- and postmenopausal women.

Only two short-term prospective studies on the effect of soy on the breast have been performed to date. The first reported the effects of two weeks of soy supplementation on the breast of women who were due to have surgery for either benign or malignant breast disease (Hargreaves, 1999). Soy had no adverse effects on any histological index of proliferation. However, a rise of pS2 protein and lowering of apolipoprotein D was observed in the nipple aspirate of women taking soy compared with controls. (A similar effect has been observed *in vitro* when breast cells are challenged with estrogen (Brown et al., 1984; Harding et al., 1996). This latter result has been interpreted as possible evidence of an estrogenic effect of soy on the breast epithelium, although it is not known whether it corresponds with *in vivo* effects on breast histology.) The second study showed an increased secretion from the nipple in premenopausal but not postmenopausal women taking soy for six months (Petrakis et al., 1996). This might suggest a slight stimulatory effect of soy in premenopausal women, although continued stimulation of the breast alone, necessary to produce the nipple aspirate, might have also explained this finding.

In vitro and animal studies of the effects of phytoestrogens on established tumors have raised some concerns that may be relevant to women at high risk of breast cancer. Although some studies have shown inhibitory effects of phytoestrogens (e.g., Hawrylewicz et al., 1995), others have reported increased carcinogenesis in rodents (e.g., Ju et al., 2001). Of particular concern is a recent report that dietary genistein negates the inhibitory effect of tamoxifen in the athymic nude mouse model (Ju et al., 2002).

4.5.6 EFFECTS OF PHYTOESTROGENS ON HEART DISEASE

In 1999, the Food and Drug Administration approved a health claim relating to soy protein and cholesterol lowering, stating "diets low in saturated fat and cholesterol that include 25 g of soy protein/day may reduce the risk of heart disease" (Food and Drug Administration, 1999). This followed several reports that linked the dietary intake of soy-based foods with a reduction of coronary heart disease (CHD) (Beaglehole et al., 1990; Thom et al., 1992). Intact soy protein appears to be effective, in both animal and humans, in lowering plasma total cholesterol, LDH cholesterol and triacylglycerols. The magnitude of LDL cholesterol improvement in humans is directly related to the initial cholesterol concentration. The benefit is also proportional to amount of soy intake (Anderson et al., 1995). Improvement of HDL cholesterol is also directly proportional to the initial plasma HDL cholesterol concentration (Sirtori et al., 1998) and to gender (Baum et al., 1998).

A greater effect is apparent in postmenopausal women compared with men. The protein component seems to play a crucial role in the cardio-protective effect of soy. When soy-extracted phytoestrogens are added to animal-derived protein (casein), no effects on lipids are observed (Greaves et al., 1999). It is therefore clear that both the proteins from soy and the phytoestrogens need to be present to have a beneficial effect on lipid. In the presence of soy protein, the lipid-lowering effect is dose dependent on the phytoestrogen present (Crouse et al., 1999).

Isolated soy protein, rich in phytoestrogen, enhances vascular reactivity in female monkeys with atherosclerosis, an effect similar to that observed with estrogen replacement therapy. The effect appears dependent on the phytoestrogen content of soy and is not observed when animals are fed soy protein devoid of its phytoestrogen content (Honore' et al., 1997). One *in vitro* study performed on rabbit coronary arteries has demonstrated that the effect is likely due to a calcium channel blocking mechanism (Figtree et al., 2000), although an ERβ-mediated action cannot be excluded (Makela et al., 1999). Supplementation with purified genistein, one of the isoflavones present in soy, has been shown to reduce the extension of ischaemic lesions in murine models of stroke (Trieu and Utckum, 1999) and mycardial infarction (Deodato et al., 1999). This protective effect of genistein on ischaemia appears to be mediated by its antioxidant effect. In humans, a similar mechanism has been used to describe the reduced susceptibility of LDL to oxidation observed in both normal (Tikkanen et al., 1998) and hypercholesterolemic (Jenkins et al., 2000) individuals fed a soy or phytoestrogen diet. Both the antioxidant effect and the enhancement of vascular reactivity may further contribute to the cardiovascular disease protection of soy.

Red clover contains isoflavones in high concentrations, but in a rather different composition compared with soy. Clover has an high concentration of formononetine and biochanin A compared with soy. For reasons still unknown, concentrated phytoestrogens derived from red clover do not appear to be effective in improving the lipid profile in either normal or hypercholestolemic subjects (Nestel et al., 1999; Howes et al., 2000). The only potentially useful finding obtained so far with these compounds has been the improvement of ultrasound-measured arterial compliance in postmenopausal women. This was defined as the increase in volumetric blood flow in both thoracic aorta and right carotid artery.

4.5.7 PHYTOESTROGENS IN MEN

There has been some concern that the recently observed decline in sperm quality may be related to exposure to environmental estrogens (Sharpe and Skakkebaek, 1993) and at the same time there has been speculation that these estrogenic compounds may exert inhibitory effects against prostate cancer (Kurzer, 2002). Theoretically, exposure to high levels of dietary estrogens could alter the hypothalamic-pituitary-gonadal axis in men, but dietary studies to date have not shown such an hormonal effects.

One study directly evaluated semen and testicular endpoints in men consuming soy phytoestrogens. Mitchell et al. (2001) reported a study of 14 young men (18 to 35 years old) who consumed 40 mg per day of soy isoflavones (in a tablet form) for two months. The subjects were followed for two months before and three months after taking the supplement. The isoflavone supplement did not change testicular or ejaculate volume, or sperm concentration, count, or motility.

Three dietary intervention studies reported the effects of soy or soy phytoestrogen consumption on reproductive hormones in men and very modest alterations of doubtful clinical significance were found (Habito et al., 2000; Nagata et al., 2001). None of these studies evaluated the prostate itself, and it is possible that soy consumption alters local hormone metabolism and action within the gland.

4.5.8 Toxicity of Phytoestrogen

In the mid-1940s it was reported that ewes grazing on subterranean clover in western Australia become sterile (Bennetts et al., 1946). This effect has not been observed for other species being fed isoflavones and or in humans on high-soy diets (Munro et al., 2003).

Administration of single oral or subcutaneous doses of up to 10,000 mg soy daidzein per kg body weight did not produce toxic effects in mice or rats (Takeda Chemical Industries Ltd, 1984). No adverse effects were reported in rats or dogs following oral administration of genistein and daidzein for a period of three months (National Cancer Institute, 1996). Chronic feeding studies in rats, ranging from eight to twenty-two months in duration, were also shown not to produce toxicity following oral exposure to soy isoflavone concentrates at concentrations of up to 39 mg/kg body weight per day (Rackis et al., 1979).

Decreased prostatic lobe weights have been demonstrated in mice exposed via subcutaneous injection, but not in rats exposed orally to soy isoflavones at doses of 2.5 to 500 mg/kg body weight per day during neonatal or perinatal periods (Strauss et al., 1998). Increased mean sexually dimorphic nucleus volume and decreased pituitary responsiveness to gonadotrophin releasing hormone in female rats that were administered genistein neonatally via subcutaneous injection were studied by Faber and Hughes (1993), and increased central nucleus volume of the medial preoptic area in male rats exposed pre- and postnatally to genistein through diet was reported by Slikker et al. (2001). Sexually dimorphic differences in behavior in pups following prenatal exposure were not seen. Male reproductive development and mating were shown in rats to be adversely affected by dietary soy isoflavone exposure (Atanassova et al., 2000); however, these effects were not observed consistently throughout the study, and the proportion of animals assessed for mating was small.

4.5.9 Carcinogeneticity Studies

Subcutaneous administration of genistein to neonatal mice produced significant inductions in uterine weight at postnatal day five, and, after eighteen months, abnormal proliferations in the oviduct were seen, and corpora lutea were absent (Newbold et al., 2001). Atypical hyperplasia, squamous metaplasia, and uterine adenocarcinoma also were reported in genistein-treated mice compared with a control group; however, the relevance of the route of administration (subcutaneous injection) and the high dose (50 mg/kg body weight) to possible effects from dietary exposure is unclear.

4.5.10 Possible Adverse Effects on Infant Development and Thyroid Gland

Infants that are fed soy-based formula experience one of the highest exposures to phytoestrogen and during a stage of development at which permanent effects are theoretically possible. The concerns expressed about possible detrimental effects have so far proven to have had no factual support (Strom et al., 2001).

There have been occasional case-reports of infants with goiter and hypothyroidism associated with soy-based infant formula consumption (Tuohy, 2003). There has been one case control study, by Fort et al. (1990), which suggested a higher prevalence of soy-based formula feeding in infants with subsequent autoimmune thyroid disease. However, an alternative explanation may be a greater tendency for atopic infants (who may be more likely to be fed soy-based infant formulas) to have such antibodies.

Early studies suggested that the goitrogenic effect of soy was related to reduced enterohepatic recirculation of thyroid hormones following their secretion in bile into the intestine (Van Middlesworth, 1957). However, it has been shown that genistein and daidzein in aglycone (unconjugated) form can inhibit thyroid peroxidase reactions by a competitive substrate mechanism (Divi et al., 1997), although the doses required for inhibition were significantly higher than those reported in infants fed soy-based formula. Recent studies in rats fed high doses of genistein indicated that despite clear evidence of biochemical changes in the thyroid there was no clinical evidence of alteration in thyroid function (Chang and Doerge, 2000), and suggested that in rats, iodine deficiency contributed to the peripheral goitrogenic effect of soy (Doerge and Chang, 2002).

4.6 METHODOLOGY FOR THE DETECTION OF PHYTOESTROGENS

In 1987, Ken Setchell first described the method for the isolation of phytoestrogen in soy (Setchell et al., 1987). The phytoestrogens daidzein, genistein, coumestrol, formononetin, and biochanin-A were separated on a C18 reversed-phase column (Hypersil ODS) with methanol-0.1 M ammonium acetate buffer, pH 4.6 (60:40 v/v), as eluent. The retention and resolution were affected by buffer concentrations, pH type, and proportion of organic solvent in the mobile phase. Detection in the low picograms range was achieved with an electrochemical detector, and the compounds were positively identified by HPLC-thermospray mass spectrometry.

An assay has been produced for three isoflavones (daidzein, genistein, and glycitein), two metabolites of daidzein (O-desmethylangolensin and equol), and two lignans (enterodiol and enterolactone) in human serum using electrospray ionization liquid chromatography/mass spectrometry (LC/MS) with selective reaction monitoring. A simple, highly-automated sample preparation procedure requires only 200 µl of sample and utilizes one solid-phase extraction stage. Limits of detection are in the region of 10 pg/ml for all analytes, except equol, which had a limit of detection of approximately 100 pg/ml. The method developed is suitable for measuring the concentrations of phytoestrogens in blood samples collected from large epidemiological studies (Grace et al., 2003).

4.7 CONCLUSIONS

Isoflavones do appear to exert some health benefits. The majority of data available relate to their effects on menopausal symptoms. Consumption of as little as 30 mg of soy isoflavones, in soy protein or as an extract, reduces vasomotor menopausal symptoms by approximately 30 to 50%, including the placebo effect, or approximately 10 to 20% after subtracting the placebo effect. Soy protein and isoflavones work together to lower LDL cholesterol and increase HDL cholesterol. Benefits to bone health are less certain, although some data suggest that they may prevent bone loss over the short term. Effects on breast cancer risk are complex. Isoflavones are likely to be cancer preventive when consumed early in life, but a few animal studies that show stimulation of breast cancer cell growth raise sufficient concerns that phytoestrogen supplements should not be recommended for women at high risk of breast cancer.

Numerous questions concerning the effects of phytoestrogen supplements for women remain unanswered. Further studies should be performed to clarify the effects of isoflavone extracts, their optimal doses, the significance of individual variation in phytoestrogen metabolism and long-term effects, particularly on men. Risk, benefits, and interactions between phytoestrogens and drugs also need to be carefully evaluated.

4.8 REFERENCES

Albertazzi, P., Pansini, F., Bonaccorsi, G., Zanotti, L., Forini, E. and De Aloysio, D. (1998). The effects of soy supplementation on hot flushes, *Obstet. Gynecol.*, 91, 6–11.

Alekel, D.L., Germain, A.S., Peterson, C.T., Hanson, K.B., Steward, J.W. and Toda, T. (2000). Isoflavone-rich soy protein isolate attenuate bone loss in the lumbar spine of perimenopausal women, *Am. J. Clin. Nutr.*, 72, 844–852.

Anderson, J.W., Johnstone, B.M. and Cook-Newell, M.E. (1995). Meta-analysis of the effects of soy protein intake on serum lipids, *N. Engl. J. Med.*, 333, 276–282.

Atanassova, N., McKinnell, C., Turner, K.J., et al. (2000). Comparative effects of neonatal exposure of male rats to potent and weak (environmental) estrogens on spermatogenesis at puberty and the relationship to adult testis size and fertility: evidence for stimulatory effects of low estrogen levels, *Endocrinology*, 141, 3898–3907.

Baber, R.J., Templeman, C., Morton, T., Kelly, G.E. and West, L. (1999). Randomised placebo-controlled trial of an isoflavone supplement and menopausal symptom in women, *Climacteric*, 2, 85–92.

Balk, J.L., Whiteside, D.A., Naus, G., DeFerrari, E. and Roberts, J.M. (2002). A pilot study of the effects of phytoestrogen supplementation on postmenopausal endometrium, *Soc. Gynecol. Investig.*, 9, 238–242.

Baum, J.A., Teng, H., Erdman, J.W., et al. (1998). Long-term intake of soy protein improves blood lipids profiles and increases mononuclear cell LDL receptor mRNA in hypocholesterolemic postmenopausal women, *Am. J. Clin. Nutr.*, 68, 545–551.

Beaglehole, R. (1990). International trends in coronary heart disease mortality, morbidity and risk factors, *Epidemiol Review*, 12, 1–15.

Bennetts, H.W., Underwood, E.J. and Sheir, F.L. (1946). A specific breeding problem of sheep on subterranean clover pastures in Western Australia, *Austr. Vet. J.*, 22, 2–12.

Brown, A.M.C., Jeltsch, J.M., Roberts, M. and Chambon, P. (1984). Activation of the PS2 gene transcription is a primary response to estrogen in human breast cancer cell line MCF-7, *Proc. Natl. Acad. Sci. U.S.A.*, 81, 6344–6348.

Chang, H.C. and Doerge, D.R. (2000). Dietary genistein inactivates rat thyroid peroxidase *in vivo* without an apparent hypothyroid effect, *Toxicol. Appl. Pharmacol.*, 168, 244–252.

Clifton-Bligh, P.B., Barber, R.J., Fulcher, G.R., Nery, M.L. and Moreton, T. (2001). The effect of isoflavones extracted from red clover (rimostril) on lipid and bone metabolism, *Menopause*, 8, 259–265.

Cos, P., De Bruyne, T., Apers, S., Vanden Berghe, D., Pieters, L. and Vlietinck, A.J. (2003). Phytoestrogens: recent developments, *Planta Med.*, Jul, 69, 7, 589–599.

Coward, L., Smith, M., Kirk, M. and Barnes, S. (1998). Chemical modification of isoflavones in soyfoods during cooking and processing, *Am. J. Clin. Nutr.*, Dec, 68, 6 (Suppl.), 1486S–1491S.

Crouse, J.R., Morgan, T., Terry, J.G., Ellis, J., Vitolins, M. and Burke, G.L. (1999). A randomized trial comparing the effect of caseine with that of soy protein containing varying amount of isoflavones on plasma concentration of lipids and lipoproteins, *Arch. Intern. Med.*, 159, 2070–2076.

Deodato, B., Altavilla, D., Squadrito, G., et al. (1999). Cardioprotection by the phytoestrogen genistein in experimental ishaemia-reperfusion injury, *Br. J. Pharmacol.*, 128, 1683–1690.

Diel, P., Olff, S., Schmidt, S. and Michna, H. (2001). Molecular identification of potential selective estrogen receptor modulator (SERM) like properties of phytoestrogens in the human breast cancer cell line MCF-7, *Planta Med.*, Aug, 67, 6, 510–514.

Diel, P., Smolnikar, K. and Michna, H. (1999). In vitro test systems for the evaluation of the estrogenic activity of natural products, *Planta Med.*, Apr, 65, 3, 197–203.

Divi, R.L., Chang, H.C. and Doerge, D.R. (1997). Anti-thyroid isoflavones from soybean, *Biochem. Pharmacol.*, 54, 1087–1096.

Doerge, D.R. and Chang, H.C. (2002). Inactivation of thyroid peroxidase by soy isoflavones, *in vitro* and *in vivo*. *J. Chromotogr. B*, 777, 269–279.

Faber, K.A. and Hughes Jr, C.L. (1993). Dose-response characteristics of neonatal exposure to genistein on pituitary responsiveness to gonadotropin releasing hormone and volume of the sexually dimorphic nucleus of the preoptic area (SDN-POA) in postpubertal castrated female rats, *Reprod. Toxicol.*, 7, 35–39.

Faure, E.D., Chantre, P. and Mares, P. (2002). Effects of a standardized soy extract on hot flushes: a multicenter, double-blind, randomized, placebo-controlled study, *Menopause*, 9, 329–334.

Figtree, G.A., Griffiths, H., Lu, Y.Q., Webb, C.M., MacLeod, K. and Collins, P. (2000). Plant-derived estrogen relax coronary artery *in vitro* by a calcium antagonist mechanism, *Am. J. Coll. Cardiol.*, 35, 1977–1985.

Food and Drug Administration (1999). Food labeling: health claims; soy protein and coronary heart disease, *Fed. Regist.*, 64, 57700–57733.

Fort, P., Moses, N., Fasano, M., Goldberg, T. and Lifshitz, F. (1990). Breast and soy-formula feedings in early infancy and the prevalence of autoimmune thyroid disease in children, *J. Am. Coll. Nutr.*, 9, 164–167.

Frost & Sullivan (2002). *The European phytonutrients*, Frost & Sullivan Market Analysis Report, 1.1-1.

Grace, P.B., Taylor, J.I., Botting, N.P., et al. (2003). Quantification of isoflavones and lignans in serum using isotope dilution liquid chromatography/tandem mass spectrometry, *Rapid Commun. Mass Spectrom.*, 17, 1350–1357.

Greaves, K.A., Parks, J.S., Williams, J.K. and Wagner, J.D. (1999). Intact dietary soy protein, but not adding an isoflavone-rich soy extract to casein, improves plasma lipids in ovariectomized cunomologus monkeys, *J. Nutr.*, 129, 1585–1592.

Habito, R.C., Montalto, J., Leslie, E. and Ball, M.J. (2000). Effects of replacing meat with soyabean in the diet on sex hormone concentrations in healthy adult males, *Br. J. Nutr.*, 84, 557–563

Han, K.K., Soares Jr, J.M., Haidar, M.A., de Lima, G.R. and Baracat, E.C. (2002). Benefits of soy isoflavone therapeutic regimen on menopausal symptoms, *Obstet Gynecol.*, 99, 389–94.

Harding, C., Osudenko, O., Tetlow, L., Howell, A. and Bundred, N.J. (1996). Non invasive measurement of anti-oestrogen activity in the breast, *Eur. J. Cancer.*, 32A, 13.

Hargreaves, D.F., Potten, C.S., Harding, C., et al. (1999). Two-week dietary soy supplementation has an estrogenic effect on normal premenopausal breast, *J. Clin. Endocrinol. Metab.*, 84, 4017–4024.

Hawrylewicz, E.J., Zapata, J.J. and Blair, W.H. (1995). Soy and experimental cancer: animal studies, *J. Nutr.*, 125, 698S–708S.

Hilakivi-Clarke, L., Onojafe, I., Raygada, M., Cho, E., Skaar, T., Russo, I. and Clarke, R. (1999). Prepubertal exposure to zearalenone or genistein reduces mammary carcinogenesis, *Br. J. Cancer.*, 80, 1682–1688.

Ho, S.C., Chan, S.G., Yi, Q., Wong, E. and Leung, P.C. (2001). Soy intake and the maintenance of peak bone mass in Hong Kong Chinese women, *J. Bone. Miner. Res.*, 16, 1363–1369.

Honore', E.K., Williams, J.K., Antony, M.S. and Clarkson, T.B. (1997). Soy isoflavones enhance coronary vascular reactivity in atherosclerotic female macaques, *Fertil. Steril.*, 67, 148–154.

Howes, J.B., Sullivan, D., Lai, N., Nestel, P., Pomeroy, S., West, L., Eden, J.A. and Howes, L.G. (2000). The effects of dietary supplementation with isoflavones from red clover on the lipoprotein profiles of post menopausal women with mild to moderate hypercholesterolaemia, *Atherosclerosis*, 152, 143–147.

Hsu, C.-S., Shen, W.W., Hsueh, Y.M. and Yeh, S.L. (2001). Soy Isoflavone supplementation in postmenopausal women, *J. Reprod. Med.*, 42, 221–226.

Ingram, D., Sanders, K., Kolybaba, M. and Lopez, D. (1997). Case control study of phytoestrogens and breast cancer, *Lancet*, 350, 990–994.

Ishimi, Y., Arai, N., Wang, X., et al. (2000). Difference in effective dosage of genistein on bone and uterus in ovariectomized mice, *Biochem. Biophys. Res. Commun.*, 274, 697–701.

Jenkins, D.J.A., Kendall, C.W.C., Garsetti, M., et al. (2000). Effects of soy protein food on low density lipoprotein oxidation and *ex vivo* sex hormone receptor activity – a controlled cross over trial, *Metabolism*, 49, 537–543.

Johnson, E.B., Muto, M.G., Yanushpolsky, E.H. and Mutter, G.L. (2001). Phytoestrogen supplementation and endometrial cancer, *Obstet. Gynecol.*, 98, 947–955.

Ju, Y.H., Allred, C.D., Allred, K.F., Karko, K.L., Doerge, D.R. and Helferich, W.G. (2001). Physiological concentrations of dietary genistein dose-dependently stimulate growth of estrogen-dependent human breast cancer (MCF-7) tumors implanted in athymic nude mice, *J. Nutr.*, 131, 2957–2962.

Ju, Y.H., Doerge, D.R., Allred, K.F., Allred, C.D. and Helferich, W.G. (2002). Dietary genistein negates the inhibitory effect of tamoxifen on growth of estrogen-dependent human breast cancer (MCF-7) cells implanted in athymic mice, *Cancer Res.*, 62, 2474–2477.

Kardinaal, A.F.M., Morton, M.S., Bruggermann-Rotgans, I.E.M. and van Beresteijn, E.C.H. (1998). Phytoestrogen excretion and rate of bone loss in postmenopausal women, *Europ. J. Clin. Nutr.*, 52, 850–855.

Kuiper, G.G., Lemmen, J.G., Carlsson, B., Corton, J.C., Safe, S.H., van der Saag, P.T., van der Burg, B. and Gustafsson, J.A. (1998). Interaction of estrogenic chemicals and phytoestrogens with estrogen receptor beta, *Endocrinology*, Oct, 139, 10, 4252–4263.

Knight, D.C., Howes, J.B. and Eden, J.A. (1999). The effects of Promensil[TM] an isoflavone extract on menopausal symptoms, *Climacteric*, 2, 79–84.

Knight, D.C., Howes, J.B., Eden, J.A. and Howes, L.G. (2001). Effects on menopausal symptoms and acceptability of isoflavones-containing soy powder dietary supplementation, *Climacteric*, 4, 13–18.

Kotsopoulos, D., Dalais, F.S., Liang, Y.L., McGrath, P.B. and Teede, H.J. (2000). The effects of soy protein containing phytoestrogens on menopausal symptoms on postmenopausal women, *Climacteric*, 316, 161–167.

Kurzer, M.S. (2002). Hormonal effects of soy in premenopausal women and men, *J. Nutr.*, Mar, 132, 3, 570S–573S.

Lock, M. (1993). *Encounters with ageing. Mythology of menopause in Japan and North America*. University of California Press Ltd.

Makela, S., Savolainen, H., Aavik, E., et al. (1999). Differentiation between vasculoprotective and uterotrophic effects of ligands with different binding affinities to estrogen α and β, *Proc. Natl. Acad. Sci. U.S.A.*, 96, 7077–7082.

Mintel (2001). *Vitamins and supplements*, Mintel Market Research, Mintel UK, May 2001, 1–37.

Mitchell, J.H., Cawood, E., Kinniburgh, D., Provan, A., Collins, A.R. and Irvine, D.S. (2001). Effect of a phytoestrogen food supplement on reproductive health in normal males, *Clin. Sci.*, 100, 613–618.

Morabito, N., Crisafulli, A., Vergara C., et al. (2002). Effects of genistein and hormone-replacement therapy on bone loss in early postmenopausal women: a randomized double-blind placebo-controlled study, *J. Bone Miner. Res.*, 10, 1904-1912.

Morito, K., Hirose, T., Kinjo, J., et al. (2001). Interaction of phytoestrogens with estrogen receptors alpha and beta, *Biol. Pharm. Bull.*, 4, 351–356.

Munro, I.C., Harwood, M., Hlywka, J.J., Stephen, A.M., Doull, J., Flamm, W.G. and Adlercreutz, H. (2003). Soy isoflavones: a safety review, *Nutr. Rev.*, Jan, 61, 1, 1–33.

Murkies, A., Dalais, F.S., Briganti, E.M., Burger, H.G., Healy, D.L., Wahlqvist, M.L. and Davis, S.R. (2000). Phytoestrogen and breast cancer in postmenopausal women: a case control study, *Menopause*, 7, 289–296.

Murkies, A.L., Lombard, C., Strauss, B.J.G., Wilkox, G., Burger, H.G. and Morton, M.S. (1995). Dietary flower supplementation decreases post-menopausal hot flushes: effect of soy and wheat, *Maturitas*, 21, 189–195.

Murrill, W.B., Brown, N.M., Zhang, J.X., Manzolillo, P.A., Barnes, S.A. and Lamartiniere, C.A. (1996). Prepubertal genistein exposure suppresses mammary cancer and enhances gland differentiation in rats, *Carcinogenesis*, 17, 1451–1457.

Nagata, C., Takatsuka, N. and Shimizu, H. (2002). Soy and fish oil intake and mortality in a Japanese community, *Am. J. Epidemiol.*, 156, 824–831.

Nagata, C., Takatsuka, N., Shimizu, H., Hayashi, H., Akamatsu, T. and Murase, K. (2001). Effect of soymilk consumption on serum estrogen and androgen concentrations in Japanese men, *Cancer Epidemiol. Biomarkers Prev.*, 10, 179–184.

National Cancer Institute, Chemoprevention Branch and Agent Development Committee (1996). Clinical development plan: genistein, *J. Cell Biochem.*, 26S, 114–126.

Nestel, P.J., Pomeroy, S., Kay, S., Komesaroff, P., Behrsing, J., Cameron, J.D. and West, L. (1999). Isoflavones from red clover improve systemic arterial compliance but not plasma lipids in menopausal women, *J. Clin. Endocrinol. Metab.*, 84, 895–898.

Newbold, R.R., Banks, E.P., Bullock, B. and Jefferson, W.N. (2001). Uterine adenocarcinoma in mice treated neonatally with genistein, *Cancer Res.*, 61, 4325–4328.

Petrakis, N.L., Barnes, S., King, E.B., et al. (1996). Stimulatory influence of soy protein isolate on breast secretion in pre- and post menopausal women, *Cancer Epidemiol Biomark and Prevention*, 5, 785–794.

Potter, S.M., Baum, J.A., Teng, H., Stillman, R.J., Shay, N.F. and Erdman, J.W. (1998). Soy protein and isoflavones: effects on blood lipids and bone density in postmenopausal women, *Am. J. Clin. Nutr.*, 68, 1375S–1379S.

Quella, S.K., Loprinzi, C.L., Barton, D.L., et al. (2000). Evaluation of soy phytoestrogens for the treatment of hot flushes in breast cancer survivors: A North Central Cancer Treatment Group trial, *J. Clin. Oncol.*, 5, 1068–1074.

Rackis, J.J., McGee, J.E., Gumbmann, M.R. and Booth, A.N. (1979). Effect of soy protein containing trypsin inhibitors in long term feeding studies in rats, *J. Am. Oil. Chem. Soc.*, 56, 162–1628.

Scambia, G., Mango, D., Signorile, P.G., et al. (2000). Clinical effects of a standardized soy extract in postmenopasual women: a pilot study, *Menopause*, 2, 150–111.

Setchell, K.D. (2001). Soy isoflavones – benefits and risks from nature's selective estrogen receptor modulators (SERMs), *J. Am. Coll. Nutr.*, Oct, 20, 5 Suppl, 354S–362S, discussion 381S.

Setchell, K.D., Brown, N.M., Zimmer-Nechemias, L., et al. (2002a). Evidence for lack of absorption of soy isoflavone glycosides in humans, supporting the crucial role of intestinal metabolism for bioavailability, *Am. J. Clin. Nutr.*, 2, 447–53.

Setchell, K.D., Brown, N.M., and Lydeking-Olsen, E. (2002b). The clinical importance of the metabolite equol-a clue to the effectiveness of soy and its isoflavones, *J. Nutr.*, Dec, 132, 12, 3577–3584.

Setchell, K.D., Welsh, M.B., and Lim, C.K. (1987). High-performance liquid chromatographic analysis of phytoestrogens in soy protein preparations with ultraviolet, electrochemical and thermospray mass spectrometric detection, *J. Chromatogr.*, Jan, 16, 386, 315–323.

Sharpe, R.M. and Skakkebaek, N.E. (1993). Are oestrogens involved in falling sperm counts and disorders of the male reproductive tract? *Lancet*, 341, 1392–1395.

Shu, X.O., Jin, F., Dai, Q., Wen, W., Potter, J.D., Kushi, L.H., Ruan, Z., Gao, Y.-T. and Zheng, W. (2001). Soyfood intake during adolescence and subsequent risk of breast cancer among Chinese women, *Cancer Epidemiol. Biomarkers Prev.*, 10, 483–488.

Shutt, D.A. (1976). The effects of plant oestrogens of dietary origin, *Endevour*, 35, 110–113.

Sirtori, C.R., Galli, G., Lovati, M.R., CXarrara, P., Bosisio, E. and Kienle, M.G. (1998). Effects of dietary proteins on regulation of liver lipoprotein receptors in rats, *J. Clin. Nutr.*, 114, 1493–1500.

Slavin, J.L., Karr, S.C., Hutchins, A.M. and Lampe, J.W. (1998). Influence of soybean processing, habitual diet, and soy dose on urinary isoflavonoid excretion, *Am. J. Clin. Nutr.*, Dec, 8, 6 Suppl., 1492S–1495S.

Slikker Jr, W., Scallet, A.C., Doerge, D.R. and Ferguson, S.A. (2001). Gender-based differences in rats after chronic dietary exposure to genistein, *Int. J. Toxicol.*, 20, 175–179.

Somekawa, Y., Chguchi, M., Ishibashi, T. and Aso, T. (2001). Soy intake related to menopausal symptoms, serum lipids and bone mineral density in postmeno-pausal Japanese women, *Obstet. Gynecol.*, 97, 109–115.

St Germain, A., Peterson, C.T., Robinson, J.G. and Alekel, D.L. (2001). Isoflavone-rich or isoflavones-poor soy protein does not reduce menopausal symptoms during 24 weeks of treatment, *Menopause*, 8, 17–26.

Strauss, L., Makela, S., Joshi, S., Huhtaniemi, I. and Santti, R. (1998). Genistein exerts estrogen-like effects in male mouse reproductive tract, *Mol. Cell Endocrinol.*, 144, 83–93.

Strom, B.L., Schinnar, R., Ziegler, E.E., et al. (2001). Exposure to soy-based formula in infancy and endocrinological and reproductive outcomes in young adulthood, *JAMA*. 286, 807–814.

Takeda Chemical Industries Ltd (1984). EP 0135172. *Method for treating osteoporosis*, European Patent Application.

Thom, T.J., Epstein, F.H., Feldman, J.J., Leaveton, P.E. and Wolz, M. (1992). *Total mortality from heart disease, cancer and stroke from 1950 to 1987 in 27 Countries.* National Institutes of Health publication no. 02-3088. National Institutes of Health, National Heart, Lung and Blood Institute, Bethesda.

Tice, J.A., Ettinger, B., Ensrud, K., Wallace, E.R., Blackwell, T. and Cummings, R.S. (2003). Phytoestrogen supplements for the treatment of hot flushes: The Isoflavone Clover Extract (ICE) Study: A randomized controlled trial, *JAMA*, 290, 207–214.

Tikkanen, M.J., Whahala, K., Ojala, S., Vihma, V. and Adlercreutz, H. (1998). Effects of phytoestrogen intake on low density lipoprotein oxidation resistance, *Proc. Natl. Acad. Sci. U.S.A.*, 95, 3106–3110.

Trieu, V.N. and Utckun, F.M. (1999). Genistein is neuroprotective in murine models of familiar amyotrophys lateral sclerosis and stroke, *Biochem. and Biophys. Res. Comun.*, 258, 685–688.

Tuohy, P.G. (2003). Soy infant formula and phytoestrogens, *J. Paediatr. Child Health*, 39, 401–405.

Upmalis, D.H., Lobo, R., Bradley, L., Warren, M., Cone, F.C. and Lamia, C.A. (2000). Vasomotor symptoms relief by soy isoflavone extract tablets in postmenopausal women; a multicenter, double-blind, randomized, placebo-controlled study, *Menopause*, 7, 236–242.

van de Weijer, P.H. and Barentsen, R. (2002). Isoflavones from red clover (Promensil) significantly reduce menopausal hot flush symptoms compared with placebo, *Maturitas*, 42, 187–193.

Van Middlesworth, L. (1957). Thyroxine excretion, possible cause of goiter, *Endocrinology*, 61, 570–573.

Van Patten, C.L., Olivotto, I.A., Chambers, G.K., et al. (2002). Effect of soy phytoestrogens on hot flushes in postmenopausal women with breast cancer: a randomized, controlled clinical trial, *J. Clin. Oncol.*, 20, 1449–1455.

Wagen, K.E., Dunkan, A.M., Merz-Demlow, B.E., et al. (2000). Effects of soy isoflavones on markers of bone turnover in premenopausal and postmenopausal women, *J. Clin. Endocrinol. Metab.*, 85, 3043–3048.

Washburn, S., Burke, G.L., Morgan, T. and Antony, M. (1999). Effect of soy protein supplementation on serum lipoproteins, blood pressure, and menopausal symptoms in perimenopausal women, *Menopause*, 6, 7–13.

5

Food Allergies and Food Intolerance

Elżbieta Kucharska

Contents

5.1   WHAT IS AN ALLERGY?

The European Academy of Allergology and Clinical Immunology (EAACI) defines a food allergy in the following way (Johansson, 2002):

> We propose that an adverse reaction to food should be called food hypersensitivity. When immunologic mechanisms have been demonstrated, the appropriate term is food allergy, and, if the role of IgE [Immunoglobulin E] is highlighted, the term is IgE-mediated food allergy. All other reactions, previously sometimes referred to as "food intolerance," should be referred to as nonallergic food hypersensitivity. Severe, generalized allergic reactions to food can be classified as anaphylaxis.

The EAACI also defines atopy:

> Atopy is inborn and characterized by genetic markers and increased IgE-antibody concentration. The increased concentration must be accompanied by clinical symptoms of a disease. If only the level of IgE is exceeded, it is not a sign of a disease, however it may forecast developing of the allergy in the future.

5.2   INFLUENCE OF GENETIC FACTORS

Until now the reasons for why allergies affect only some patients and not others are not evident. It is also not known what causes an allergy to a specific allergen. A positive correlation between the rate of occurrence of major histocompatibility complex (MHC) genes (especially DR locus) and the frequency of allergies to specific allergens is being verified.

An allergy is a multi-gene syndrome and its inheritance pattern causes additional hindrances to analyzing a genetic background of an atopy. The identical phenotypic set of symptoms, e.g., gastrointestinal (GI) disorders, may be determined by various gene mosaics in different people. Therefore, understanding the mutual connections between a genetic make-up and its phenotypic expression remains problematic. To reveal such links, the characteristic phenotypes are determined among related people and confirmed by a probability analysis of a relatedness of polymorphic DNA markers. Markers are not specific or characteristic for a disease gene, but include numerous alleles accumulated throughout generations.

If the connection between genotype and phenotype is confirmed, the next steps include sequencing and gene mapping. Generally, genes are classified as (Marsh, 1994):

- disease-specific genes
- genes determining immunological response
- regulatory genes for an IgE synthesis

Results of population studies carried out in atopy-affected families revealed that an increased IgE concentration in blood serum observed among tested individuals was inherited and that the 5q31.1 gene was responsible for this phenomenon. In addition, the chromosome 5 contains genes for colony stimulating factor (CSF) 2 encoding granulocyte-macrophage (GM) CSF genes for interleukin (IL) 13, IL 5, IL 4, IL 3 and interferon regulatory factor (IRF) 1, cell division cycle (CDC) 25C, IL 9, epidermal growth factor (EGF 1), lymphocyte-specific transcription factor (TCF) 7 (Marsh et al., 1995). A tendency to excessive antibody synthesis is connected with chromosome 11q. The presence of a gene encoding β-chain of a receptor characterized by a high affinity to IgE was detected on the same chromosome (Sandford et al., 1993). Similarly, a genetic linkage between the TcR lymphocyte complex Tγ/δ, chromosome 14, and the synthesis of specific IgE antibodies was reported (Moffat et al., 1994). Genes encoding IFNγ and STAT6 proteins (which transmit a critical signal for growth of helper Th2 cells) are located on chromosome 12q14.3-q24.1. Additionally, chromosomes 3q21 and 16q21 containing a gene for the IL 4 receptor may be also considered as atopy markers (Marsh et al., 1995).

The risk of acquiring an allergy is higher for people who have cases allergy in their family medical histories. If one parent manifests allergy symptoms, the probability of having a child affected by atopy is 40%. If both parents suffer from allergy, the probability may reach 60%. Atopy is inherited on the distaff side. It affects boys 1.5 times more frequently than girls.

5.3 INFLUENCE OF ENVIRONMENTAL FACTORS

The influence of environmental factors has been established, but remains controversial. The strategy of strict avoidance of exposure to bacteria, viruses, and allergens until sensitization diminishes belongs to the canons of prophylaxis and treatment of choice of atopic diseases. For years, elimination of allergens from the environment of potentially-affected patients was not undermined as the method for preventing allergy. According to medical instructions, children with an atopy in their case history should have stayed in virtually sterile conditions.

Some years ago, however, the first reports against this opinion appeared. It was observed that children living in urban areas who did not experience an 'immunological training' through a moderate exposure to infections were more prone to diseases than children in rural areas having more contact with allergens and bacterial endotoxins (Braun-Fahrländer et al., 1999; von Mutius, 2002). Th 1 cells are responsible for this phenomenon. The contrary dependence was also observed, between the frequency of disease occurrence and positive tuberculin-test reactions (Shirakawa, 1997). Similar effects were also reported by Matricardi et al. (2000). The percentage of children suffering from allergy of the upper respiratory tracts and having raised IgE concentration was lower if children had recovered from hepatitis A, *Toxoplasma gondii*, *Helicobacter pylorii* or orofecal infections. Gereda et al. (2000) highlighted the value of Th1 lymphocyte stimulation with endotoxins. Saito et al. (2003) presented a very interesting hypothesis according to which toll-like receptors (TLR) are molecules responsible for an hereditary and acquired immunogenicity because they recognize molecules present on the surface of microorganisms – the Cpg motif (Akira et al., 2001).

During the era of an increase in GI allergy diseases, probiotics seem to play a more significant role (Kirjavainen et al., 1999) in preventing against allergies by their immunoregulatory effects on immunity (TLR ligands) and Th1 lymphocyte stimulation (Lignau et al.,1995). The occurrence of food allergy among children is linked to:

- low acidity of gastric juices
- physiological condition of mucus, which is permeable for allergens during the first months of a child life
- leakiness of mucus caused by a chronic inflammation, as a result of introducing various foods to an infant's diet too early and the effect of iatrogenic factors

5.4 FOOD ALLERGENS

5.4.1 INTRODUCTION

Food allergens are substances of a plant or animal origin; the most common are the glycoprotein antigens, the least common are the haptens. The difference in allergenicity depends on the number of IgE-binding determinants, although the structure of a molecule also plays a significant role.

Allergens with linear epitopes are resistant to denaturation, whereas in the case of conformational epitopes high temperatures will easily destroy the ability to cause allergy. Therefore, fruit and vegetable allergens are sensitive to denaturation, while nut, soy, egg, and milk proteins are resistant to heat. Based on their allergenicity potential, allergens are divided into major and minor allergens. Major allergens are defined as affecting over 50% of patients in a particular group, e.g., among persons allergic to birch pollens. Major allergens are indicated with the number 1, minor allergens are indicated by succeeding Roman numbers.

Many attempts have been made to classify allergens rationally. The result has been the following factors for classification of allergens (Steinman and Lee, 2003):

- denaturating and non-denaturating under the influence of physico-chemical conditions
- soluble and insoluble in water
- identical and present in many plant species botanically related
- identical and present in many unrelated plant species, etc.

In practice, a useful classification scheme is that based on revealing a common antigen in a maximally large number of foods – the term 'panantigen' was used by Valenta et al. in 1992 for profilins (Valenta et al., 1992). If a cause of allergy is correctly diagnosed, a patient may be immediately informed about other food components that may cause allergy symptoms. Another useful classification is a 'technological' one, which enables prediction of the decrease in food allergenicity, e.g., due to thermal processes, enzymatic and chemical hydrolysis, and sometimes also due to the fermentation processes.

Unfortunately, patients do not acquire allergies according to allergen classifications. Most frequently they are allergic to many various substances, triggering compatible (but different if a pathomechanism is considered) crossreactions. Moreover, allergy symptoms are intensified by food components that provoke non-immunological hypersensitivity (formerly called a pseudoallergy). The ubiquity of panallergens does not facilitate their elimination, either for patients or doctors.

5.4.2 PANALLERGENS

5.4.2.1 Introduction

Panallergens are proteins present in plant pollens, fruit, and vegetables. They cause symptoms of a crossreactivity (i.e., simultaneous hypersensitivity to food, or to inhaled or contact allergens) in the same person.

The degree of allergen similarity may differ, resulting in different allergic reactions. If a food allergen is identical with an inhaled one, the symptoms of asthma may be caused by a smell of food or food ingestion. If the allergens are only similar, the symptoms from upper respiratory and GI tracts may not manifest at the same time, an asthmatic dyspnoea may occur within a few hours after food consumption. If only some epitopes are similar, the respiratory symptoms may be less advanced. An oral allergy syndrome (OAS) is a frequently diagnosed disease caused by panallergens.

The categories of panallergens, which are described in the following sections, comprise the following:

- Bet v 1-homologues
- profilins
- chitinases
- lipid transfer proteins
- tropomyosin
- isoflavone reductase

- 2S albumins
- thaumatin-like proteins

5.4.2.2 Bet v 1-Homologues

Bet v 1-homologues are the allergens found in birch pollens. They are crossreactivate with allergens of apples, apricot, chamomile, celery, carrot, cherry, European chestnut tree, mango, pear, poppy seed, timothy grass, etc. (Hoffman-Sommergruber et al., 1999a and 1999b; Ebner et al., 2001; Karamloo et al., 2001).

5.4.2.3 Profilins

Profilins are proteins first detected in 1977 and present in eucaryotic cells. They control actin binding in cells or participate in the cell fertilization process. Profilins are present both in plants and in fruits. The profilins from plants and fruits are structurally very similar; IgE created against plant allergens may react with fruit allergens. This is an example of a co-sensitization phenomenon.

Profilins may also cause the allergy to latex. If present in plant pollens or in food products, they may trigger food allergy or respiratory symptoms in patients allergic to latex (Scheurer et al., 1999).

5.4.2.4 Chitinases

Chitinases belong to a group of enzymes that decompose chitin, such as that present in insect carapaces and cell walls of fungi. They are stress proteins inactivated during heating, and are found in cereals, tomatoes, kiwi, avocado, bananas, green bean, and cherimoya. Chitinases may also cause disease symptoms in patients allergic to latex (Diaz-Perales et al., 1999; Sanchez-Monge et al., 1999; Posch et al., 2003). The quantity of enzymes found in fruit is increased if the fruit has been stimulated into ripening by using ethylene oxide.

5.4.2.5 Lipid Transfer Proteins

Lipid transfer proteins (LTPs) are widely distributed in the plant environment, and are small, highly-conservative proteins involved in non-specific lipid transportation throughout cell membranes. They are often present in the surface parts of plants, e.g., in peels, and the quantity present increases during fruit ripening. LTPs are resistant to pepsin digestion. There is a cross-consistency between LTP, birch allergens (Bet v 1 and Bet v 2) and apple profilins. LTPs are found in apples, peaches, cherries, plums, apricots, tomatoes, soybean, parsley, carrot, celery, broccoli, cabbage, peanuts, sunflower seeds, almonds, and grapevine pollens (Salcedo et al., 1999; Pastorello et al., 2000).

5.4.2.6 Tropomyosin

Tropomyosin is a protein found in vertebrates and invertebrates, but only the protein from invertebrates has allergic properties. It is frequently found in sea foods, such as shrimps, crabs, American lobsters, Pacific flying squids, and also in some species of cockroaches (*Blattela germanica, Periplaneta americana*), moths, spiders, and house dust mites (*Dermatophagoides pteronyssinus, Dermatophagoides farinae*) (Witteman et al., 1994).

5.4.2.7 Isoflavone Reductase

Isoflavone reductase is a substance that belongs to the group of stress proteins formed during ultraviolet (UV)-C irradiation in plants, e.g., pineapples, and prevents molding caused by *Penicillium digitatum*. Isoflavone reductase is also a minor birch allergen (Bet v 5). Patients allergic to birch pollens may suffer from OAS after consuming bananas, carrots, chickpeas, maize, pears, peas, or oranges. Isoflavone reductase is also found in alfalfa and tobacco (Karamloo et al.,1999).

5.4.2.8 2S Albumins

2S albumins are highly allergic, small molecule 'storage proteins' present in many seeds, such as sesame, castor bean, sunflower, oriental and yellow mustard, as well as in Brazil nuts and walnuts (Pastorello et al., 2001).

5.4.2.9 Thaumatin-Like Proteins

Thaumatin-like proteins provide a sweet taste in food. They may display antifungal activity and are treated as potential allergens. These proteins are found in strawberries, apples, bell peppers, and cherries (Scheurer et al., 1999; Aalberse et al., 2001).

5.4.3 SPECIFIC ALLERGENS

5.4.3.1 Introduction

While many allergens are present in a variety of foods, specific allergens are found only in particular products. Most have a low molecular weight, except for immunoglobulins 9S, Ig M class, from milk.

5.4.3.2 Cows' Milk Proteins

Cows' milk contains five protein fractions, α-lactoalbumin, β-lactoglobulin, α-casein, and immunoglobulins. (Their homologues are present in goats' milk.) Homogenization of milk may increase its allergenicity by reducing the size of the lipid molecules and opsonizing proteins, which consequently facilitates the transmission of micellae throughout the intestine wall.

Heat processes reduce the allergic properties of milk, as temperature and exposure time increase. A similar effect is produced by fermentation carried out by *Lactobacillus* sp. (Wróblewska and Jędrychowski, 1994; van Beresteijn et al., 1995). Moreover, the allergenicity of milk may be also reduced by chemical modifications and application of high pressure (Nakamura, 1993; Nakamura et al., 1993).

5.4.3.3 Egg Proteins

Egg proteins contain many fractions, of which ovoalbumin, ovomucoid, and livetin (an egg-yolk allergen) are the strongest allergens. They are resistant to digestion, thermal denaturation and low pH (for example the allergic properties of ovoalbumin can still be observed at pH 3.0).

The major causes of food allergies diagnosed in children in the U.S., Germany, Spain, Switzerland, Israel, and Japan were eggs, followed by cows' milk. As allergies to eggs, milk, and wheat caused 60% of allergy cases among children in Japan, the Japanese Ministry of Health and Social Welfare has since 1999 required that all food products are labeled with their actual contents of nine major allergens responsible for increased frequency of food allergy cases (Ebisawa et al., 2003). The increased frequency of food allergy in Japan is explained by the wider availability of foods that were not processed, handled or prepared in the traditional ways.

5.4.3.4 Wheat Proteins

Wheat proteins are polypeptide glutens, and include gliadin (responsible for a celiac disease), globulins, albumins, and α-amylase inhibitor (which causes asthma among bakers or elevator workers [Baur and Posch, 1998]). 'Hypoallergenic' flour is a result of interactions among different enzymes: actinase, collagenase, and transglutaminase (Watanabe, 1994).

5.4.3.5 Seafood

Cod meat contains allergen M – a sarcoplasmic protein – and parvalbumens crossreactivate with proteins from other fish (Pascual et al., 1992). Allergy symptoms may be caused not only by the consumption of fish meat, but also by to the smell of fish meat. However, in most cases, non-immunological hypersensitivity is the cause of GI disorders that develop after ingestion of fish meat, e.g., tuna or mackerel, containing biogenic amines.

5.4.4 INFLUENCE OF SOME TECHNOLOGICAL PROCESSES

It has been shown that new technological processes applied in food production, such as ethylene oxide sterilization, UV-C irradiation, or prolonged storage, may promote formation of new allergens (Sanchez-Monge et al., 1999).

The new processes may lead to increased allergenicity of protein-like contamination, such as casein, gliadin, soy protein, and lysosyme (Zitouni et al., 1999). Residues of plant proteins in oils (Moneret-Vautrin et al., 2002) and allergens created by gene transfer into genetically modified plants and animals may reveal allergic properties (Taylor and Hefle, 2001). Moreover, food contaminants, e.g., antibacterial substances (such as salicylic acid) and residues of antibiotics, herbicides, and pesticides, may become allergens (van der Klauw et al., 1996; Lieberman, 2002; Franck et al., 2002). Emerging sources of allergens also include imported food, and cuisine traditionally not consumed in a given country.

The IgE-mediated food allergy is one of the main atopic diseases. Its symptoms, especially among children, are not disease-characteristic. GI symptoms observed after an ingestion of particular food are commonly thought to be the result of previously diagnosed respiratory or skin disorders, thus food allergy may remain misdiagnosed if it coexists with asthma or atopic eczema/dermatitis.

5.5 PATOMECHANISM OF FOOD ALLERGY

5.5.1 INTRODUCTION

A repeated contact with an allergen that leads to a secondary immunological response that is disproportionate to the allergen exposure is a condition to develop allergy. According to the internationally recognized system of Gell and Coombs, there are four basic types of allergy, Type I to Type IV, which develop through various immunological mechanisms.

5.5.2 ALLERGY TYPE I

This is the most frequently diagnosed type of allergy. It is an immediate, IgE-mediated hypersensitivity that is caused by attachment of specific IgE (which is increasingly released after repeated exposure to allergens) to mastocyte surfaces. The number of mastocyte receptors varies between individuals. Repeated exposure to allergens leads to gradual binding of receptors with specific IgE, and induces cross-linking of IgE-antibody by specific allergen. It is followed by mastocyte degranulation and a release of preformed or generated mediators, e.g., biogenic amines, leukotriens, prostaglandins, lipotoxins, tromboxans, and many others. These mediators cause an increased permeability of capillaries, contraction of smooth muscles, increased mucus secretion, irritation of nerves endings, and increased permeability of epithelium. Between six and eight hours after contact with an allergen, a migration of eosinophils, neutrophils and a few lymphocytes is observed (late phase of early allergic reaction).

5.5.3 ALLERGY TYPE II

According to the Gell and Coombs classification, allergy Type II is called 'antibody-mediated cytotoxicity'. It is triggered by excessive destruction of hapten-binding cells, which become antigens and induce the production of IgM and IgG class antibodies. Attachment of antibodies to haptens on the cells membranes activates complement proteins and results in cell lysis.

An alternative mechanism is based on non-complement dependent cytotoxicity, e.g., food allergen stimulation of mechanisms of antibody dependent cellular cytotoxicity (ADCC), cytotoxicity of natural killer cells or macrophages. The contribution of ADCC in gastroenteropathy of children induced by cow's milk allergens was demonstrated by Owen et al. (1993).

5.5.4 ALLERGY TYPE III

According to Gell and Coombs classification, allergy Type III occurs when large numbers of antibody–antigen complexes accumulate in tissues. Complexes consist of IgM or IgG (IgG1 or IgG3) and an allergen. In the case of food allergy, antibody excess and mild antigen excess lead to the creation of complexes. They are localized to the site of introduction, activate complement, and trigger a process of infiltration with polymorphonuclear leucocytes. It results in acute inflammatory response and damage to cells with complexes attached. It is a probable mechanism of colitis ulcerosa, where high concentrations of antibodies against casein, lactoalbumin, and lactoglobulin are detected (Halstensen et al., 1990).

5.5.5 ALLERGY TYPE IV

According to the Gell and Coombs classification, allergy Type IV is a delayed hypersensitivity reaction. This type of allergy reaction occurs when an antigen interacts with antigen-specific lymphocyte, which releases inflammatory and toxic substances that attract other white blood cells and results in an inflammatory infiltration. This mechanism is part of those syndromes occurring as a reaction to cow's milk allergens (probably of colitis ulcerosa).

5.6 FOOD ALLERGY SYMPTOMS

Food allergy is a syndrome that affects 3 to 6% of the population in various countries. In early childhood it occurs as a result of contact with new food components and excessive permeability of GI mucous membranes. As the immunological systems develops, in most cases symptoms recede or food tolerance occurs – usually at the age of three. Studies carried out on a population of Japanese children revealed that the earliest remission occurs in case of allergy to soy, followed by allergy to egg yolk, egg white, wheat, and cows' milk (usually between the ages of two and three) (Ebisawa et al., 2003).

Allergic symptoms may be local or systemic and their manifestations may also vary. Local symptoms can manifest as a late phase reaction syndrome, which develops within 30 minutes (but may be delayed to six to eight hours). Changes characteristic for cell-mediated hypersensitivity, such as an inflammatory infiltration, may occur after 24 to 48 hours, e.g., enteritis granuloma. This is termed a 'late allergy'.

'Early allergy' (allergy Type I, II or III) may affect the mucous membrane of the oral cavity (OAS), the stomach (a surface or erosion-like mucous membrane inflammation), or the intestines (inflammatory changes of various degrees of intensity, from eosinophilic infiltration to ulceration or enteritis granuloma [Caffarelli et al., 1998]). Systemic manifestations may have a dramatic course, sometimes leading to death due to anaphylactic shock, which can develop in few minutes after food consumption. Early allergies may also affect internal organs, most frequently the upper respiratory tract (manifested as bronchial asthma). Delayed symptoms may affect the skin (nettle rash), joints (inflammations of single or numerous joints), muscles (myalgia), kidneys (nephrosis), and may also manifest as otitis media and recurrent pneumonia. They may also lead to changes in the central nervous system that cause character and mood changes, hypermotility or tiredness syndrome, headaches, 'chronic fatigue syndrome' (CSF), sleep disorders, and neurosis.

Despite medical progress, the diagnosis of food allergy remains difficult because the allergic symptoms are caused by a variety of different types of allergens, to which people may be simultaneously or successively exposed. Food allergy affects more and more people in the world, with many reported cases of deaths caused by anaphylaxis. To prevent such situations, many countries have changed their food laws, requiring prepackaging of processed foods which contain potential allergens and detailed labeling (Wütrich, 2003).

5.7 NON-ALLERGIC HYPERSENSITIVITY REACTION

5.7.1 INTRODUCTION

Non-allergic hypersensitivity reaction corresponds with the traditional term 'food intolerance'. It affects about 20% of patients, inducing symptoms similar to those observed during an allergy bout, however, it is triggered by non-immunological mechanisms.

5.7.2 DEGRANULATION OF MASTOCYTES

Degranulation of mastocytes is provoked by lectins, e.g., concanavalin A (Con A) found in nuts. Con A binds with Fc fragments of human IgE connected to a cell surface. Together with coexisting allergy to nuts, it may cause anaphylactic shock (Wütrich, 2003). Lectins are commonly present in bacteria and viruses, which may explain why allergy symptoms intensify during infection. Many microorganisms worsen allergy symptoms due to their direct lectin-way influence on mastocytes or cross-linking non specific to bacteria IgE on the cells surface. This may lead to increased levels of histamine and other preformed and generated substances in tissues and in the blood. (Norn, 1992; Kucharska, 1999). The release of granule contents does not increase in healthy individuals (Norn, 1992).

5.7.3 Effect of Some Medicines

Some medicines, such as non-steroid anti-inflammatory drugs, convertase inhibitors, and β-blockers, may intensify food allergy symptoms (Brooks et al., 1989; Meune et al., 2000; Tenenbaum et al., 2000).

5.7.4 A Direct Effect of Vasoactive Amines

A direct effect of vasoactive amines on the organism which are not degraded in GI tracts due to the lack of mono- and diaminooxidase (MAO and DAO) or their blockade by medicines or alcohol. This group of amines includes tyramine (in cheddar, emmental, roquefort cheeses, pickled fish, and walnuts), phenylethylamine (in chocolate), serotonin (in bananas), octopamine (in lemons), and histamine (in fermented foods, e.g., blue cheeses, but also in strawberries, tomatoes, wines, and in mackerel that have not been stored properly [scombrotoxin illness]).

5.7.5 Disorders of Nervous System Mediator Release

Disorders of nervous system mediator release may be caused by aspartame, monosodium glutamate (MSG) ('Chinese restaurant syndrome', 'Hot-dog headache,' or glutamate-induced asthma), and sulphites found in dried fruit, vegetables, pickled vegetables, and fruit juices.

5.7.6 Inborn or Acquired (Postinfection) Enzyme Deficiencies

Inborn or acquired (postinfection) enzyme deficiencies, e.g., deficiency of lactase, may lead to milk intolerance.

5.7.7 Psychological Problems

Psychological problems which inclines to 'alleged allergy' or generates an indirect reflex for a suggested allergen (Kallios and Kallos, 1980; Carter and Finch, 1993).

5.8 REFERENCES

Aalberse, R.C., Akkerdaas, J.H. and van Ree, R. (2001). Cross-reactivity of Ig E antibodies to allergens, *Allergy*, 56, 478–490.

Akira, S., Takeda, K. and Kaisho, T. (2001). Toll-like receptors: critical proteins linking innate and acquired immunity, *Nat. Immunol.*, 2, 675–680.

Baur, X. and Posch, A. (1998). Characterized allergens causing baker's asthma, *Allergy*, 53, 562–566.

van Beresteijn, E.C.H., Meijer, R.J.G.M. and Schmidt, D.G. (1995). Residual antigenicity of hypoallergenic infant formulas and the occurrence of milk-specific IgE antibodies in patients with clinical allergy, J. *Allergy. Clin. Immunol.*, 96, 365–374.

Braun-Fahrländer, C., Gassner, M. and Grize, L. (1999). Prevalence of hay fever and allergic sensitization in farmer's children and their peers living in the same rural community. SCARPOL team. Swiss Study on Childhood Allergy and Respiratory Symptoms with Respect to Air Pollution, *Clin. Exp. Allergy*, 32, 28–34.

Brooks, A.M., Burden, I.G. and Gilies, W.E. (1989). The significance of reactions to betaxolol reported by patients, *Aust. N.Z. J. Ophthalmol.*, 17, 353–355.

Caffarelli, C., et al. (1998). Clinical food hypersensitivity, the relevance of duodenal immunoglobulin E-positive cells, *Pediatr. Res.*, 44, 485–490.

Carter, C.M. and Finch, H.E. (1993). *Food intolerance*, in Macrae, E., Robinson, R.K. and Sadler, M.J., Eds., *Encyclopaedia of food science, food technology and nutrition*, Academic Press, London, pp. 1993–2011,

Diaz-Perales, A,. et al. (1999). Cross-reactions in the latex-fruit syndrome. A relevant role of chitinases but not of complex asparagines-linked glycans, *J. Allergy. Clin. Immunol.*, 104, 3, Part 1, 681–687.

Ebisawa, M., et al. (2003). Food allergy in Japan, *Allergy. Clin. Immunol. Int.*, 15, 214–217.

Ebner, C., Hoffman-Sommergruber, K. and Breitender, H. (2001). Plant food allergens homologous to pathogenesis-related protein, *Allergy*, 56, Suppl. 67, 43–44.

Franck P., et al. (2002). The allergenicity of soybean products is modified by food technologies, *Int. Arch. Allergy Immunol.*, 128, 212–219.

Gereda, J.E., Leung, D.Y.M. and Thatayatikom, A. (2000). Relation between house dust endotoxin exposure, type I T cell development, and allergen sensitization in infants at high risk of asthma, *Lancet*, 32, 1680–1683.

Halstensen, T.S., et al. (1990). Epithelial deposition of immunoglobulin G and activated complement (C3b and terminal complement complex) in ulcerative colitis, *Gastroenterology*, 98, 1264–1271.

Hoffmann-Sommergruber, K., et al. (1999a). Molecular characterization of Dau c 1, the Bet v 1 homologous protein from carrot and its cross-reactivity with Bet v 1 and Api g 1, *Clin. Exp. Allergy*, 29, 6, 840–847.

Hoffmann-Sommergruber, K,. et al. (1999b). IgE reactivity to Api g 1, a major celery allergen, in a Central European population is based on primary sensitization by Bet v 1, *J. Allergy. Clin. Immunol.*, 104, 2, Part 1, 478–484.

Johansson, S.G.O. (2002). A revised nomenclature for allergy. A condensed version of the EAACI position statement from the EAACI Nomenclature Task Force, *Allergy Clin. Immunol. Int.*, 14, 279–287.

Kallios, P. and Kallos, L. (1980). *Histamine and some other mediators of pseudoallergic reactions*, in, Dukor, P., Ed., *Pseudoallergic reactions: involvement of drug and chemicals*, Karger, Basel, 115–131.

Karamloo, F., et al.. (1999). Molecular cloning and characterization of a birch pollen minor allergen, Bet v 5, belonging to a family of isoflavone reductase-related proteins, *J. Allergy Clin. Immunol.*, 104, 991–999.

Karamloo, F., et al. (2001). Pyr c 1, the major allergen from pear (*Pyrus communis*), is a new member of the Bet v 1 allergen family, *J. Chromatogr. B. Biomed. Sci. Appl.*, 756, 1–2, 281–293.

Kirjavainen, P.V, et al. (1999). New aspects of probiotics – a novel approach in the management of food allergy, *Allergy*, 54, 909–915.

van der Klauw, M.M., Wilson, J.H.P. and Stricker, B.H.C. (1996). Drug associated anaphylaxis, 20 years reporting in the Netherlands (1974–1994). Review of the literature, *Clin. Exp. Allergy*, 26, 1355–1363.

Kucharska, E. (1999). The influence of bacteria and autovaccines on immunological parameters in obstructive inflammatory diseases of the airways, *Ann. Academiae Medicae Stetinensis*, 1–99.

Lieberman, P. (2002). Anaphylactic reactions during surgical and medical procedures, *J. Allergy Clin. Immunol.*, 110, 64–69.

Lingnau, K., et al. (1995). Il-4 in combination with TGF-β favours an alternative pathway of Th1 development independent of IL-12, *J. Immunol.*, 155, 3788–3792.

Marsh, D.G. (1994). *Genetics of asthma and atopy*, in Frank, M.M., Austen, K.F., Claman, H.N. and Unanue, E.R., Eds., *Samter's Immunological diseases*, 5th ed., Boston, Little, Brown, pp. 1257–1272.

Marsh, D.G., et al. (1995). Genetic basis of IgE responsiveness, relevance to the atopic diseases, *Int. Arch. Allergy Immunol.*, 107, 25–28.

Matricardi, P.M., et al. (2000). Exposure to foodborne and orofecal microbes versus airborne viruses in relation to atopy and allergic asthma, epidemiological study, *B.M.J.*, 320, 412–417.

Meune, C., et al. (2000). Interaction between angiotensin-converting enzyme inhibitors and aspirin, a review, *Eur. J. Clin. Pharmacol.*, 56, 609–620.

Moffatt, M., Mill, M. and Cornelis, F. (1994). Genetic linkage of T cell receptors and γ/δ complex to specific IgE response, *Lancet*, 343, 1997–2001.

Moneret-Vautrin, D.A., et al. (2002). Food allergy to peanuts in France. Evaluation of 142 observations, *Clin. Exp. Allergy*, 1998, 28, 1113–1119.

von Mutius, E. (2002). Environmental factors influencing the development and progression of pediatric asthma, *J. Allergy. Clin. Immunol.*, 109, S525–532.

Nakamura, T., (1993). Production of low antigenic whey protein hydrolysates by enzymatic hydrolysis and denaturation with high pressure, *Milchwiss.*, 48, 141–147.

Nakamura, T., et al. (1993). Enzymatic production of hypoallergenic peptides from casein, *Milchwiss.*, 11993, 48, 141–146.

Norn, S. (1992). Mediator release and its reinforcement, new aspects of microorganisms in asthma, *Pneumonol. Alergol. Pol.*, 60, Suppl. 2, 5–10.

Owen, M.J., et al. (1993). Relation of infant feeding practices cigarette smoke exposure and group children care to the onset and duration of otitis media with effusion in the first years of life, *J. Pediatric.*, 123, 702–710.

Pascual, C., Esteban, M. and Crespo, F. (1992). Fish allergy: Evaluation of the importance of cross-reactivity, *J. Pediatr.*, 121, 29–34.

Pastorello, E.A., et al. (2000). The maize major allergen, which is responsible food-induced allergic reactions, is a lipid transfer protein, *J. Allergy Clin. Immunol.*, 106, 4, 744–751.

Pastorello, E.A., et al. (2001). Lipid transfer proteins and 2S albumins as allergens, *Allergy*, 56, S67, 45–47.

Posch, A., et al. (1999). Class I endochitinase containing a hevein domain is the causative allergen in latex-associated avocado allergy, *Clin. Exp. Allergy*, 29, 5, 667–672.

Saito, H., Kato, A. and Matsumoto, K. (2003). Application of genomic science to clinical allergy, *Allergy Clin. Immunol. Int.*, 15, 218–222.

Salcedo, G., Diaz-Perales, A. and Sanchez-Monge, R. (1999). Fruit allergy: Plant defence proteins as novel potential panallergens, *Clin. Exp. Allergy*, 29, 9, 1158–1160.

Sanchez-Monge, R., et al. (1999). Isolation and characterization of major banana allergens, identification as fruit class I chitinases, *Clin. Exp. Allergy*, 29, 5, 673–680.

Sandford, A.O, Shirakawa, T.S and Moffat, M. (1993). Localisation of atopy and the β-subunit of the high affinity IgE receptor (FcεRI) on chromosome 11q, *Lancet*, 341, 332–334.

Scheurer, S., et al. (1999). Cross-reactivity and epitope analysis of Pru a 1, the major cherry allergen, *Mol. Immunol.*, 36, 155–167.

Shirakawa, T. (1997). The inverse association between tuberculin responses and atopic disorder, *Science*, 275, 77–79.

Steinman, H. and Lee, S. (2003). Concomitant clinical sensitivity (CCS) and cross-reactivity, *Allergy Clin. Immunol. Int.*, 15, 18–29.

Taylor, S. and Hefle, S. (2001). Will genetically modified foods be allergenic? *J. Allergy Clin. Immunol.*, 107, 765–771.

Tenenbaum, A., et al. (2000). Intermediate, but not low, doses of aspirin can suppress angiotensin-converting enzyme inhibitor-induced cough, *Am. J. Hypertens.*, 13, 776–782.

Valenta, R., et al. (1992). Profilins constitute a novel family of functional plant pan-allergens, *J. Exp. Med.*, 175, 377–385.

Watanabe, M. (1994). Controlled enzymatic treatment of wheat proteins for production of hypoallergenic flour, *Biosci. Biotech. Biochem.*, 58, 388–390.

Witteman, A.M., et al. (1994). Identification of a cross-reactive allergen (presumably tropomyosin) in shrimp, mite and insects, *Int. Arch. Allergy Immunol.*, 105, 1, 56–61.

Wróblewska, B. and Jędrychowski, L. (1994). The effect of selected microorganisms on the presence of immunoreactive fractions in cow and goat milks, *Pol. J. Food Nutr. Sci.*, 4/45, 3, 21–29.

Wütrich, B. (2003). Lethal or life-threatening food anaphylaxis. Notes from the lay press, *Allergy Clin. Immunol. Int.*, 15, 175–180.

Zitouni, N., et al. (1999). Influence of refining steps on trace allergenic protein content in sunflower oil, *J. Allergy Clin. Immunol.*, 104, 4, Part 1, 883–888.

6

Biogenic Amines in Foods

George J. Flick, Jr. and L. Ankenman Granata

Contents

6.1 INTRODUCTION

Different people display individual patterns of susceptibility to biogenic amines in foods. Clinical signs of histamine poisoning are more severe in people taking medications which inhibit enzymes that normally detoxify histamine in the intestines. Symptoms may be gastrointestinal (nausea, vomiting, diarrhea), circulatory (hypotension), or cutaneous (rash, urticaria, palpitations, tingling, flushing, burning, or itching). Antihistamines may be used effectively to treat the symptoms.

Histamine exerts its effects by binding to receptors on cellular membranes in the respiratory, cardiovascular, gastrointestinal, and hematological/immunological systems and the skin. The symptoms of histamine poisoning generally resemble those encountered with immunoglobulin E (IgE)-mediated food allergies (Taylor et al., 1989) and usually appear shortly after the food is ingested, with duration of up to 24 hours. Despite all uncertainties reported, histamine levels above 500 to 1000 mg per kg are considered potentially dangerous to human health, based on the concentrations found in food products involved in histamine poisoning (ten Brink et al., 1990). Even less is known about the toxic dose of other amines. Threshold values of 100 to 800 mg per kg for tyramine and 30 mg per kg for phenylethylamine have been reported (ten Brink et al., 1990). When estimating the toxic levels of biogenic amines, one should consider the amount of food consumed, the presence of other amines and dietary components in the food, and the use of alcohol and medicines. An additional concern, especially if nitrite were to be present, is that secondary amines, such as putrescine and cadaverine, can react with nitrate to form carcinogens (Hildrum et al., 1976; Taylor, 1986; ten Brink et al., 1990; Veciana-Nogues et al., 1997).

Cadaverine, putrescine, and histamine are diamines that may be produced postmortem from the decarboxylation of specific free amino acids (Table 6.1) in many foods (Silla Santos, 1996). The decarboxylation process can proceed through two biochemical pathways: endogenous decarboxylase enzymes naturally occurring in foods, or exogenous enzymes released by microorganisms associated with the product. Endogenous production of diamines is insignificant when compared with the exogenous pathway (Wendakoon et al., 1992A). The nature of the microflora and the composition of the product affect

Table 6.1
Biogenic amines and their chemical precursors.

Biogenic amine	Precursor
Histamine[a]	Histidine
Putrescine[b]	Ornithine
Cadaverine[b]	Lysine
Tyramine[c]	Tyrosine
Tryptamine[a]	Tryptophan
β-phenylethylamine[c]	Phenylalanine

[a] Heterocyclic amine.
[b] Alipathic amine.
[c] Aromatic amine.
Source: From Shalaby, A. (1996),
Food Res. Int., 29, 675.

the amount of decarboxylase a bacterial cell may release (Wendakoon et al., 1992A; Suzuki et al., 1990). In general, histamine, putrescine, cadaverine, tyramine, tryptamine, β-phenylethylamine, spermine, and spermidine are considered the most important biogenic amines in foods (Shalaby, 1996). However, β-phenylethylamine, spermine, and spermidine are not end products of bacterial decomposition in fishery products.

Some foods are naturally rich in free amino acids and the content may also increase postmortem. This is particularly true in muscle tissue due to the high content of proteolytic enzymes in the intestinal tract combined with a rapid autolytic process (Gildberg, 1978; Aksnes, 1988) and a high free amino acid content. Amino acid formation depends on such factors as the harvesting season, unit processing operation, ingredients, addition of certain microflora in a fermented food, and animal activity prior to slaughter. For example, large quantities of lysine and arginine are quickly liberated in fish harvested in summer or during feeding season (Aksnes et al., 1988).

The activity of amino acid decarboxylase depends on a range of factors, including availability of fermentable sugars, pH, and redox potential (Gale, 1946). The influence of microflora, decarboxylase activity, and intestinal tract content on biogenic amine formation may be major reasons for the discrepancies that have been reported in the literature concerning levels of biogenic amines in fresh and processed fish. Another reason for discrepancies that have been reported may be poor experimental design. Regardless of the discrepancies, it is clear that a high amino acid content and bacterial activity can rapidly result in an elevated concentration of biogenic amines if the proper controls are not in place (Table 6.2).

6.2 TOXICITY

6.2.1 HISTAMINE TOXICITY

Douglas (1970) reported that very large amounts of histamine could be given orally without causing adverse effects. He attributed this to the conversion of histamine to inactive N-acetylhistamine by intestinal microflora. Human subjects given up to 67.5 mg histamine orally, in a single dose, did not produce any subjective or objective symptoms of histamine poisoning (Granerus, 1968). Sjaastad (1966), however, administered 36 mg or more of histamine to subjects who subsequently developed symptoms associated with histamine toxicity. Symptoms appeared also with consumption of whole tuna sandwiches containing 100, 150, and 180 mg doses of histamine. It has been assumed that high histamine levels are able to cause a toxic response, but subsequent research has indicated that other factors may also be responsible. When Clifford et al. (1989) fed portions of spoiled mackerel containing 300 mg histamine and mackerel associated with an illness diagnosed as scombrotoxicosis to volunteers, there were no significant observable effects. A second study by Clifford et al. (1991) was conducted using mackerel fillets associated with an

Table 6.2
Production of biogenic amine by bacteria growing on media culture.

Histamine producers	Histamine concentration	Temperature and time	Reference
Morganella spp.	400 mg/100 g (max)	76 h	Aiso et al., 1958
Morganella spp.	100 mg/100 g 100 mg/100 g 0 mg/ 100g	25°C for 24 h 25°C for 19 h, followed by 5°C for 100 h	Klausen and Huss, 1987
Proteus spp.	Large	5°C for 100 h	Kimata et al., 1960
Proteus morganii	>200 nmol/ml Large	– 15, 30, 37°C for <24 h	Taylor et al., 1978 Behling and Taylor, 1982
Enterobacter aerogenes	>200 nmol/ml		Taylor et al., 1978
Klebsiella pneumoniae	Large	15, 30, 37°C or <24 h	Behling and Taylor, 1982
Hafnia alvei	Large	30, 37°C for >48 h	Behling and Taylor, 1982
Citrobacter freundii	Large	30, 37°C for > 48 h	Behling and Taylor, 1982
Escherichia coli	Large	30, 37°C for >48 h	Behling and Taylor, 1982
Lactobacillus (3 strains)	2.2 mg/ml		Masson et al., 1996
Proteus vulgaris (10 spp.)	3.03 to 4.80 g/l	25°C for 24 h	Bermejo et al., 2003
Proteus vulgaris (3 spp.)	2.04 to 6.35 g/l	5°C for 72 h	
Aeromonas hydrophila (6 spp.)	0.41 to 6.74 g/l	15°C for 24 h	Bermejo et al., 2003
Shingomonas paucimobilis (2 spp.)	2.45 to 2.54g/l	25°C for 24 h	Bermejo et al., 2003
Burkordelia cepacia (2 spp.)	1.61 to 3.35 g/l	25°C for 24 h	Bermejo et al., 2003
Photobacterium damsela (5 spp.)	1.02 to 2.26 g/l	25°C for 24 h	Bermejo et al., 2003
Pseudomonas putida (3 spp.)	1.57 to 2.26 g/l	5°C for 72 h	Bermejo et al., 2003

outbreak of scombrotoxicosis. Statistical analysis failed to detect any difference in the amine content between fillets shown to be scombrotoxic and those failing to induce nausea, vomiting, or diarrhea, and also failed to establish any significant relationship between the concentrations of six amines (including histamine, cadaverine, and putrescine) and the onset of scombrotoxic symptoms. Ienistea (1973) reported the deleterious effects in relation to the amount of histamine ingested at one meal as follows:

- 8 to 40 mg histamine – mild poisoning
- 70 to 1000 mg – histamine disorders of moderate intensity
- 1500 to 4000 mg – histamine severe incident

The role of saurine (implicated in histamine poisoning in Japan) as a compound able to act synergistically with histamine was reviewed by Arnold and Brown (1978), but it was later concluded that the compound in question was in fact histamine.

6.2.2 TOXICITY POTENTIATORS

Histamine appears not to be the sole factor in causing toxicity as cases of toxicity have also been observed where the histamine content has been low (Arnold and Brown, 1978; Murray et al., 1982; Taylor, 1986; Clifford et al., 1989; Soares and Gloria, 1994). Strong evidence exists that biogenic amines, such as putrescine, cadaverine, spermine, and spermidine, in fish tissue can potentiate the toxic effect of histamine by inhibiting intestinal histamine-metabolizing enzymes (such as diamine oxidase [Hungerford and Arefyev, 1992]), increasing histamine uptake, and liberating endogenous histamine in intestinal fluids (Chu and Bjeldanes, 1981; Hui and Taylor, 1983; Ibe et al., 1991; Halasz et al., 1994). It has been reported that fish implicated in a scombroid poisoning incident contained high levels of inhibitors that interfere with histamine metabolism. Monoamineoxidase inhibiting drugs used for the treatment of depression, hypertension, and tuberculosis have also been observed to potentiate the toxic effect of histamine (Maga, 1978; Taylor, 1986).

Studies have shown that the levels of cadaverine in toxic or decomposed fish are generally several times greater than the levels of putrescine. When cadaverine was administered through stomach catheters simultaneously with histamine, per oral toxicity was observed in the guinea pig (Bjeldanes et al., 1978). Klausen and Lund (1986) reported that at 10°C the high cadaverine content of mackerel in comparison with herring could be responsible for mackerel often being implicated in scombroid poisoning but not herring since histamine levels were similar in both. It has been suggested that cadaverine and putrescine, as well as other diamines, facilitate the transport of histamine through the intestinal wall and increase its toxicity (Fernandez-Salguero and Mackie, 1987).

Arnold and Brown (1978) reported on the possibility that bacterial endotoxins, which are widespread, could result in hypersensitivity to histamine. These compounds are complex, heat-stable, lipopolysaccharide materials produced primarily by Gram-negative bacteria. They also reported that endotoxin is known to be capable of inducing histamine release in animals (sometimes called endotoxin shock) similar to that seen in anaphylaxis. Baranowski et al. (1990), however, reported extremely low levels of endotoxin in both good tuna and tuna known to have caused illness in humans.

From these discussions, it is clear that the concentration of biogenic amines that produces observable toxicity may differ significantly, depending on a variety of circumstances. Furthermore, although a variety of histamine potentiators are known, there is no clear understanding of the level and the manner by which these synergistic effects occur.

6.3 BIOGENIC AMINES IN FISH

6.3.1 REGULATORY GUIDELINES FOR FISH

Fish is associated with biogenic amine poisoning more than any other food product. The fish most often associated with histamine poisoning are the scombroid fish, belonging to the families Scomberesocidae and Scombridae. Fish included in these families are the tunas, bonito, mackerels, bluefish, and saury. Tuna and mackerel are the fish most commonly connected with scombroid poisoning, but other fish are also linked with poisoning outbreaks. Examples include mahi-mahi, sardines, anchovies, herring, and marlin. The association of type of fish and biogenic amine poisoning may reflect differences in typical consumption of a specific fish.

Research by the Food and Drug Administrations (FDA) on the quantitative determination of histamine, cadaverine and putrescine in fishery products has resulted in the only two methods accepted by the Association of Official Analytical Chemists (AOAC) for regulatory purposes (Rogers and Staruszkiewicz, 1997). This research was the basis for the establishment of the defect action levels used in the FDA's regulatory programs. The FDA (21CFR123) recently established a guidance level for histamine of 5 mg per 100 g for assuring the safety of scombroid or scombroid-like fish and recommended the use of other data for judging the freshness of fish, such as the presence of other biogenic amines associated with fish decomposition (FDA, 1996). A maximum average histamine content of 10 mg per 100 g has been established in the European Community (EC) for acceptance of tuna and other species belonging to the Scomberesocidae and Scombridae families (Veciana-Nogues et al., 1997). The EC has suggested that in the future a maximum level of 30 mg per 100 g for total biogenic amines in fish and fish products may be an appropriate legal limit.

However, there may be a type of poisoning that does not arise from high levels of histamine, therefore a low histamine level may not be an absolute assurance of product safety. It may be more appropriate to state that the absence of decomposition in the fish renders it a safe product. As such, a safe product would have no evidence of spoilage, including odors of decomposition, high histamine levels, or other amines, e.g. cadaverine.

6.3.2 PREVALENCE IN FISH

The prevalence of biogenic amines in fish depends on several factors. In general, concentrations in newly caught fish are low. Mietz and Karmas (1978) found that cadaverine values ranged from 0.116 to 1.036 mg per 100 g in high-quality rockfish, salmon steaks, and shrimp and that putrescine levels were found to range from 0.136 to 0.63 mg per 100 g in high-quality lobster tail, salmon, and shrimp. A prior study by the investigators (Mietz and Karmas, 1977) reported that high-quality tuna contained cadaverine and putrescine in concentrations ranging from 0.024 to 0.532 and 0 to 0.184 mg per 100 g, respectively. There has, however, been some concern regarding the accuracy of the analytical methods used in these studies. Gloria et al. (1999) determined concentrations of biogenic amines in 102 samples of albacore tuna (*Thunnus alalunga*) harvested off the U.S. Northwest from 1994 to 1996. There were significant differences in the concentrations of amines detected (spermine, spermidine, putrescine, cadaverine, histamine, and tyramine), varying from 0.59 to 4.65 mg per 100 g. These levels were probably lower due to the fact that the samples were frozen on board, or chilled and immediately frozen after reaching the dock, and kept at −40°C until analysis. Spermine was present at the highest levels, followed by spermidine, putrescine, cadaverine, histamine, and tyramine.

6.3.3 MUSCLE TYPE

In the study by Gloria et al. (1999), no difference was observed in the amine levels of light upper- and lower-loin muscles, but dark muscles contained higher levels of spermidine. Intestinal wall samples contained high amine levels. Takagi et al. (1969) examined the amounts of histidine and histamine in 21 aquatic species during spoilage. Their conclusions were consistent with those of other researchers in that more histamine was produced in the red-muscled fish, such as tuna and mackerel, than in white-muscled species, such as rockfish. Within a given fish species, more histidine and histamine was found in white than in red muscle. In contrast to results reported by Wendakoon and Sakaguchi (1992A), they also reported that in the dark muscle, the amine levels were always much higher and the amine production was more rapid than in the white muscle.

6.3.4 MICROFLORA

A variety of microorganisms are able to produce biogenic amines. The production of cadaverine and putrescine by microorganisms is not surprising as the covalent linking of cadaverine and putrescine to peptidoglycan is necessary for normal microbial growth (Suzuki et al., 1988). Several inoculation studies, both on culture media and on fish, have demonstrated that *Morganella* spp., *Proteus morganii*, *Proteus* spp., *Hafnia alvei*, and *Klebsiella* spp. are able to produce histamine and other biogenic amines. The majority of the studies also concurred that the potential of these microorganisms to produce toxic levels of biogenic amines is enhanced at abusive temperatures.

Tables 6.2, 6.3, and 6.4 summarize research on production of biogenic amines by microorganisms. The tables list studies on production of biogenic amines by bacterial isolates inoculated on different culture media and on fish

Table 6.3
Production of biogenic amines by bacteria isolates incubated on fish.

Bacteria	Fish	Histamine (mg/100 g)	Other biogenic amines (mg/100 g)	Temperature	Reference
Proteus morganii	Tuna	> 5 < 5		24, 30°C 15°C	Eitenmiller et al., 1982
Actinobacter	Spanish mackerel	> 0.1		0°C	Middlebrooks et al., 1988
Aeromonas hydrophilia	Spanish mackerel	> 0.1		0°C	Middlebrooks et al., 1988
Clostridium perfringens	Spanish mackerel	> 0.1		0°C	Middlebrooks et al., 1988
Enterobacter aerogenes	Spanish mackerel	Detectable	> 0.1 Detectable	0°C	Middlebrooks et al., 1988
Enterobacter spp.	Mackerel (Scomber japonicus)	> 0.1			Wendakoon and Sagakuchi, 1992a
Hafnia alvei	Spanish mackerel	> 0.1		0°C	Middlebrooks et al., 1988
Morganella morganii	Spanish mackerel	> 0.1		0°C	Middlebrooks et al., 1988
Proteus spp., Proteus vulgaris, Proteus mirabilis	Spanish mackerel	> 0.1		0°C	Middlebrooks et al., 1988
Pseudomonas spp.	Spanish mackerel	> 0.1		0°C	Middlebrooks et al., 1988
Vibrio alginolyticus	Spanish mackerel	> 0.1		0°C	Middlebrooks et al., 1988
Carnobacterium divergens V41	Smoked salmon		Not detected	3–9°C, 27 days	Connil et al., 2002

that may be cold-smoked, respectively. Studies where isolates from fish have been incubated in media and monitored for histamine production are listed in Table 6.4. Spoilage and toxin formation occur due to a variety of microorganisms, and therefore identical storage times for similar fish species may produce varying levels of scombrotoxin.

Okuzumi et al. (1990) investigated the relationship between microflora on horse mackerel (*Trachurus japonicus*) and the dominant spoilage bacteria. The results of their study showed that *Pseudomonas* I/II, *Pseudomonas* III/IV-NH, *Vibrio*, and *Photobacterium* were dominant when high levels of putrescine, cadaverine, and histamine were detected.

The activity of decarboxylase can be an indirect measurement of the potential for biogenic amine formation. A study by Middlebrooks et al. (1988)

Table 6.4
Production of biogenic amines on culture media by microorganism isolated from fish products.

Microorganism	Fish	Histamine	Temperature and time	Reference
Proteus morganii	Skipjack (*Euthynnus pelamis*)	Detected	35°C for 24 h	Kimata et al., 1960
	Jack mackerel (*Trachurus symmetricus*)	Detected		Kimata et al., 1960
	Sardine	> 100 mg/100 g		Ababouch et al., 1991
Hafnia alvei	Skipjack	Detected		Kimata et al., 1960
	Jack mackerel	Detected		Kimata et al., 1960
Proteus spp.	Skipjack	Detected	35°C for 24 h	Kimata et al., 1960
	Jack mackerel	Detected		Kimata et al., 1960
	Sardine	> 100 mg/100 g		Kimata et al., 1960 Ababouch et al., 1991
Klebsiella spp.	Skipjack	Detected		Kimata et al., 1960
	Jack mackerel	Detected		Kimata et al., 1960
Morganella morganii	Tuna (*Thunnus thunnus*)	> 100 mg/100 g	37°C for 18 h	Lopez-Sabater et al., 1994
	Skipjack tuna (*Katsuwonus pelamis*)	> 100 mg/100 g	7, 19, 30°C for 24 h 15, 25°C	Arnold et al., 1980
	Albacore tuna	> 100 mg/100 g		Kim et al., 2000
Klebsiella spp.	Tuna	> 100 mg/100 g	37°C for 18 h	Lopez-Sabater et al., 1994
Enterobacter aerogenes and *E. cloacae*	Tuna	50 to 100 mg/100 g	37°C for 18 h	Lopez-Sabater et al., 1994
Citrobacter freundii	Tuna	< 25 mg/100 g	37°C for 18 h	Lopez-Sabater et al., 1994
Proteus mirabilis	Tuna	< 25 mg/100 g	37°C for 18 h	Lopez-Sabater et al., 1994

Table 6.4
(Continued)

Microorganism	Fish	Histamine	Temperature and time	Reference
Proteus vulgaris	Tuna	< 25 mg/100 g > 100 mg/100 g	37°C for 18 h	Lopez- Sabater et
	Sardine	10 to 200 mg/ 100 g	7, 19, 30°C 24 h 35°C for 24 h	al., 1994 Arnold et al., 1980 Ababouch et al., 1991
E. agglomerans	Tuna	< 25 mg/100 g	37°C for 18 h	Lopez- Sabater et al., 1994
Serratia liquifaciens	Tuna	< 25 mg/100 g	37°C for 18 h	Lopez- Sabater et al., 1994
Providencia stuarti	Sardine	15 to 100 mg/ 100 g	35°C for 24 h	Ababouch et al., 1991
Vibrio spp.	Sardine	10 mg/100 g	35°C for 24 h	Ababouch et al., 1991
Stenotrophonas maltophilia	Albacore tuna (*Thunnus alalunga*)	2.58 mg/100 g > 100 of other biogenic amines	4°C for 6 d 37°C for 24 h	Ben-Gigirey et al., 1998

showed that 17 bacterial isolates (*Acinetobacter lowffi, Aeromonas hydrophila, Burkordelia cepacia, Clostridium perfringens, Enterobacter aerogenes, Enterobacter* spp., *Hafnia alvei, Morganella morganii, Photobacterium damsela, Proteus mirabilis, Proteus vulgaris, Proteus* spp., *Pseudomonas fluorescens/ putida, Pseudomonas putrefaciens, Pseudomonas* spp., *Shingomonas paucimobilis*, and *Vibrio alginolyticus*) from mackerel tissue were capable of exhibiting decarboxylase activity (production of histamine, cadaverine, and putrescine) when incubated in Spanish mackerel at 0, 15, and 30°C. Other bacteria which also show strong histidine decarboxylase activities include: *Klebsiella pneumonia* (Taylor et al., 1979), *Klebsiella planticola* (Taylor and Lieber, 1979), *Alteromonas putrefaciens* (Frank et al., 1985), *Photobacterium phosphoreum* (Morii et al., 1986), *Staphylococcus xylosus* (Rodriguez-Jerez et al., 1994), *Cedecea lapagei, Cedecea neteri, Plesiomonas shigelloides* (Lopez-Sabater et al., 1994), *Providencia* spp. (Ababouch et al., 1991), *Lactobacillus curvatus* LTH 975, *Lactobacillus buchneri* LTH 1388 (Leuschner and Hammes, 1999), *Serratia* spp. (Lopez-Sabater et al., 1996), and *Escherichia* spp. (Gale, 1946). Wendakoon et al. (1990) reported that most of the bacteria that convert amino acids into nonvolatile amines possess more than one decarboxylase enzyme.

Okuzumi et al. (1984) studied histamine-forming bacteria in addition to other N-group (psychrophilic halophilic, histamine-forming) bacteria in and on fresh fish. The histamine-forming N-group bacteria included *Proteus morganii*, *Proteus vulgaris*, *Hafnia alvei*, *Citrobacter* spp., *Vibrio* spp., and *Aeromonas* spp. For samples taken in the summer, *P. morganii* was found most frequently, followed by the N-group bacteria. For the samples taken during winter, only the N-group bacteria were found (no other histamine bacteria were detected).

Changes in the concentration of tyramine, agmatine, putrescine, cadaverine, spermidine, tryptamine, spermine, histamine, and trimethylamine and the development of the microbial population during the storage of Mediterranean gilt-head sea bream (*Sparus aurata*) were studied in parallel at three temperatures (0°C, 8°C, 15°C) (Koutsoumanis et al., 1999). Pseudomonas and H_2S-producing bacteria were found to be the dominant microorganisms. *Enterobacteriaceae* and lactic acid bacteria were also present in the fish microflora. Among the biogenic amines, putrescine and cadaverine were detected when pseudomonas exceeded 10^6 to 10^7 colony forming units (cfu) per g. Histamine was produced only in samples stored at 15°C and reached levels greater than 5.0 mg per 100 g at 48 h. Putrescine and cadaverine also reached high levels after 120 h at 15°C. Tyramine, tryptamine, agmatine, and trimethylamine were absent regardless of the storage temperature. The authors concluded that only putrescine and cadaverine could be used as an index of freshness. The role and significance of putrescine and cadaverine in food safety and biogenic amine poisoning is yet to be established. Furthermore, in prevalence studies, researchers regularly find it difficult to select or obtain samples that are representative of the total population of fish, muscle, or microorganisms.

6.3.5 EFFECTS OF PROCESSING

6.3.5.1 Effects of Evisceration

The effect of evisceration on biogenic amine production is inconsistently reported in the literature. The rates of cadaverine and putrescine formation can be ranked as follows: whole ungutted fish > fillets from whole ungutted fish; and fillets from gutted fish > whole gutted fish (Haaland et al., 1990). However, this generalized description is heavily dependent upon extrinsic factors, such as harvesting method and procedures for transportation, processing, and retailing. Consequently, literature citations contain contradictory information on the impact of evisceration on biogenic amine formation. Much of the variation reported may result from researchers' failure to obtain fish where the conditions from harvest through processing were known. Unfortunately, much of the data reported included products obtained from retail stores and distributors. Unless samples are obtained from sources where the complete history of the fish is known, conflicting results will continue to be reported in the literature.

6.3.5.2 Effects of Postharvest Handling

The most important factors contributing to the production of biogenic amines during postharvest handling are the duration of storage and the storage temperature. Both the post-mortem formation of amino acids and their rapid decarboxylation are temperature dependent.

The effect of temperature on histamine formation has been the subject of many studies (Table 6.5). Different studies reported 100-fold variations in histamine concentrations in skipjack tuna allowed to spoil under similar conditions. Although the information in Table 6.5 contains substantial variation, it is obvious that longer storage times and higher temperatures seem to induce histamine production. Control of biogenic amine production by low temperatures (for example 0°C) is consistently observed.

Postharvest handling conditions have a significant effect on the presence and concentration of putrescine and cadaverine. Ababouch et al. (1991) reported that bacteria on the skin and gills of freshly harvested sardines (*Sardina pilchardus*) quickly invaded and grew within the muscle tissue, reaching 5×10 cfu per g and 6×10 cfu per g after 24 hours at ambient temperature and eight days of storage in ice, respectively. Histamine, cadaverine and putrescine accumulated to levels of 235 mg per 100 g, 105 mg per 100 g, and 30 mg per 100 g, respectively, after eight days in ice, but reached these levels after only 24 hours at ambient temperature.

Klausen and Huss (1987) found no histamine formation in mackerel stored in ice, whereas a rapid increase was noted at 10°C. Interestingly, after storage at 10°C for two days with no detectable histamine formation, subsequent storage at 0°C for eight days led to formation of 20 mg per 100 g histamine. These studies indicate that although the histamine-forming bacteria will not grow at 0°C, decarboxylase formed during storage at 10°C may remain active at 0°C.

6.3.5.3 Freezing

Freezing has been observed to increase biogenic amines in some fish species and not in others. However, in most of the studies the increases have been minimal. When frozen fish are thawed, the increase in biogenic amines is less than when the fresh fish are incubated for the same time under identical temperature conditions. An explanation that has been offered is that the microflora are reduced as a result of the freezing process. Growth of the microflora may also have been reduced due to DNA injury during the freezing process.

6.3.5.4 Salting

Salt concentrations of up to 2% have been shown to be ineffective in preventing the growth of *Morganella morganii* and *Klebsiella pneumonia*. Higher concentrations of salt (3.5 to 5.5%) could inhibit the histamine production of some histamine-forming bacteria. In one study, the degree of inhibition of bacteria stored for five weeks at 5°C showed a linear relationship with the concentration of salt.

Table 6.5
Biogenic amine formation in fish and fish products.

Fish	Temperature	Time	Histamine (mg/100 g)	Cadaverine	Putrescine
Skipjack tuna	0°C	1 day	< 0.1	< 1	< 1
		24 days	< 0.1	< 1	< 1
	22°C	1 day	> 50	ND	ND
Albacore	0°C	1 day	7.5	ND	ND
		33 days	82.5	ND	ND
	25°C	7 days	100	ND	ND
Atlantic herring	1°C	3 days	ND	< 3	< 3
		7 days	ND	< 3	< 3
Atlantic mackerel	1°C	3 days	ND	< 3	< 3
		7 days	ND	< 3	< 3
Mahi mahi	21°C	2 days	154	ND	ND
	32°C	Market	0.16	ND	ND
		1 day	292	ND	ND
	0°C	Harvest	0.08	0.0	0.7
		6 hours	0.06	0.4	0.7
		12 hours	0.05	0.4	0.7
		17 hours	230.8	70	11
	25°C	Harvest	0.2	0.3	0.7
		6 hours	0.09	0.2	0.7
		12 hours	0.64	2.9	2.0
		15 hours	75.8	66	11
	35°C	Harvest	1.5	4.1	4.9
		6 hours	0.16	2.9	2.9
		12 hours	39.8	12	4.2
		15 hours	262.7	81	29
Yellowfin tuna	0°C	1 day	0.0	0.1	3.9
		3 days	0.0	0.0	5.9
		5 days	0.0	0.0	6.5
		9 days	0.0	0.0	18.0
	4°C	1 day	0.0	0.1	5.0
		3 days	0.0	0.0	21.6
		5 days	0.17	0.0	25.6
		9 days	0.92	12.5	68.8
	10°C	1 day	0.0	0.0	4.0
		3 days	0.0	2.2	125
		5 days	1.71	15.1	281
		9 days	2.39	44.9	564
	22°C	1 day	0.0	0.0	0.6
		3 days	3.58	147	832
		5 days	3.61	165	4533
Hake	0°C	0 day	ND	0.47	ND
		5 days	ND	0.52	ND
		12 days	ND	7.21	ND
		19 days	ND	29.94	ND

Table 6.5
(*Continued*)

Fish	Temperature	Time	Histamine (mg/100 g)	Cadaverine	Putrescine
Hake		25 days	ND	72.1	ND
Kahawai	0°C	2 days	150	ND	NR
		2 days	350	NR	NR
Pink salmon	10°C	14 days	ND	NR	NR
Pacific herring	10°C	14 days	5.5	NR	NR
Sardine marinade,		0 month	4.5	70	575
2% acetic acid		1 month	3.5	40	565
		2 months	2.5	30	400
		3 months	7.0	30	200
		4 months	8.0	37	300
		5 months	8.5	40	280
Sardine marinade,		0 month	7.2	38	360
4% acetic acid		1 month	4.0	24	250
		2 months	3.3	25	200
		3 months	3.5	16	170
		4 months	4.3	20	240
		5 months	4.5	34	325
Bigeye tuna	21°C	0 hour	0.0	0	0
		6 hours	0.0	2	0
		18 hours	0.0	5	2
		28 hours	0.2	8	3
		36 hours	0.7	13	4
		48 hours	3.0	18	32
	22°C	2 days	> 50	NR	NR
Carp fish halves	3°C	0 days	0.001	NR	HR
		2 days	0.028	NR	NR
		4 days	0.015	NR	NR
		6 days	0.162	NR	NR
		8 days	0.001	NR	NR
		10 days	0.001	NR	NR
		13 days	2.01	NR	NR
Carp fish halves	15°C	0 days	0.001	NR	NR
		2 days	0.084	NR	NR
		4 days	4.21	NR	NR
Carp minced meat	3°C	0 days	0.001	NR	NR
		2 days	0.049	NR	NR
		4 days	0.032	NR	NR
		6 days	0.059	NR	NR
		8 days	1.01	NR	NR
		10 days	2.83	NR	NR
		13 days	20.5	NR	NR

Table 6.5
(*Continued*)

Fish	Temperature	Time	Histamine (mg/100 g)	Cadaverine	Putrescine
Carp minced meat	15°C	0 days	0.001	NR	NR
		2 days	18.0	NR	NR
		4 days	17.2	NR	NR

Notes: ND = not detected, NR = not reported.
Sources: Krizek et al. (2002), *J. Sci. Food Acric.*, 82, 1088; Staruszkiewicz et al. (2004), *J. Food. Prot.* 67, 134; Du et al. (2002), *J. Food Sci.*, 67, 292; Flick et al. (2001), *Potential hazards in cold smoked fish: biogenic amines.*

6.3.5.5 Smoking

The production of biogenic amines during chilled storage (5°C) of cold-smoked salmon (*Salmo salar*) from three smoke houses over a two-year period (1997 and 1998) was studied by Jorgensen et al. (2000). Results of that study showed that the production of biogenic amines is unlikely to result in histamine poisoning in humans, as indicated by epidemiological data. Some samples exceeded the defect action level of 5 mg per 100 g established by the FDA for Scombridae and Culpeidae, but no samples reached toxic levels of 50 mg per 100 g, a value at which one would expect illness and that would lead the FDA to undertake legal proceedings (FDA, 1998).

Although the temperatures found in a hot-smoking process may inhibit histamine producers, cold smoking does not expose the fish to temperatures high enough to inhibit histamine-forming bacteria. The effect on histamine formation of hot smoking previously frozen mackerel (*Scomber scombrus*) was reported by Zotos et al. (1995) (Table 6.5). The fish were smoked for a total of seven hours, at sequential temperatures of 30, 40, and 70°C. The study found that a significant ($p > .05$) increase in histamine formation in previously frozen (11 or 33 weeks) mackerel was solely due to the temperature and duction smoking process. The histamine increase appeared to be independent of frozen storage time prior to smoking. Although this example is based on a hot-smoking process, it demonstrates the importance of controlling the temperature and time of the smoking process.

6.4 BIOGENIC AMINES IN CHEESE

6.4.1 Introduction

The number of occurrences of histamine poisoning due to cheese is second only to that for fish (Ordonez et al., 1997; Stratton et al., 1991). The U.S. and the EC have set maximum limits for histamine in fish, but not for cheese. Spanjer and van Roode (1991) therefore suggested a maximum of 900 mg per kg cheese for the sum of tyramine, histamine, putrescine, and cadaverine.

The first reported case of histamine poisoning from cheese was in 1967 and involved Gouda cheese (Doeglas et al., 1964). There have been other reported cases involving Swiss (Sumner et al., 1985), Cheshire (Uragoda and Lodha, 1979), Cheddar (Kahana and Todd, 1981), and Gruyere (Taylor, 1985).

The predominant amines found in cheese are tyramine, cadaverine, putrescine and histamine (Table 6.6) (Stratton et al., 1991; Silla Santos, 1996; Novella-Rodriguez et al., 2002; Novella-Rodriguez et al., 2003). Biogenic amine levels may vary between types of cheese as well as within the varieties themselves. The differences within a variety of cheese may be due to a number of factors, including manufacturing processes, bacterial counts in the milk, heat treatments used, use of starter cultures, and the duration and conditions of the ripening process (Stratton et al., 1991; Pinho et al., 2001; Novella-Rodriguez et al., 2003).

Novella-Rodriguez et al. (2003) studied the content of biogenic amines in different cheese types. The study analyzed 20 unripened cheeses, 20 hard-ripened cheeses made from pasteurized milk, 20 hard-ripened cheeses made from raw milk, 20 goat cheeses, and 20 blue cheeses (Table 6.7).

Ripened cheeses contain higher average concentrations of amines than do unripened cheeses, a difference that could be related to processing (Martelli et al., 1993; Schneller et al., 1997). Casein proteolysis that occurs during cheese manufacture may result in an increased level of free amino acids. These amino acids are then decarboxylated, resulting in the formation of biogenic amines. A

Table 6.6
Principal amines found in cheeses.

Cheese	Amine				
	Cadaverine	Putrescine	Tryptamine	Tyramine	β-phenylethylamine
Brie	•	•			
Brick	•	•			
Camembert	•	•		•	
Cheddar	•	•		•	•
Colby	•	•		•	•
Edam		•	•	•	•
Gouda	•	•	•	•	
Gruyere		•			
Mozzarella	•				
Parmesan				•	
Provolone	•	•			
Romano				•	
Roquefort		•		•	
Swiss	•	•		•	

Source: adapted from Stratton et al. (1991), *J. Food Prot.*, 54, 460.

Table 6.7
Biogenic amine content in different types of cheeses.

	Amine concentration (mg/kg wet extract)				
	Unripened cheese	Hard-ripened cheese, pasteurized milk	Hard-ripened cheese, raw milk	Goat cheese	Blue cheese
Tryptamine	0.6	301	609	830	1585
Histamine	ND	163	391	88	377
β-phenylethylamine	ND	32	28	12	40
Tryamine	ND	45	34	17	129
Putrescine	3.1	612	670	192	257
Cadaverine	1.5	710	369	89	2101

Note: ND = not detected.
Source: adapted from Novella-Rodriguez et al. (2002), *J. Food Sci.*, 67, 2940, Table 1.

longer ripening process may lead to higher concentrations of biogenic amines (Diaz-Cinco et al., 1992; Ordonez et al., 1997; Durlu-Ozkaya et al., 1999).

Very low levels of biogenic amines occur in unripened cheese made from pasteurized milk, due to the pasteurization and the lack of a ripening period. Any high levels that may be found in unripened cheese would most likely be due to the use of poor-quality milk (Novella-Rodriguez et al., 2003).

6.4.2 MICROFLORA

Many different histamine-producing organisms have been isolated from cheeses. A histamine-producing strain of *Lactobacillus buchneri* that was capable of producing 3900 mmol histamine per ml was isolated from Swiss cheese (Sumner et al., 1985). Edwards and Sandine (1981) isolated the following histamine-producing organisms from Swiss cheese: *Streptococcus mitis, Lactobacillus bulgaricus, Lactobacillus plantarum* and propionibacteria. Sumner (1987) identified as histamine producers in commercial Swiss cheese: *Lactobacillus fermentum, Lactobacillus helveticus, Streptococcus faecium,* and two strains of *Streptococcus lactis. Lactobacillus casei, Lactobacillus acidophilus* and *Lactobacillus arabinose* have been identified by Stratton et al. (1991) as histamine producers. *Enterobacteriaceae,* heterofermentative lactobacilli and *Enterococcus faecalis* contribute to production of biogenic amines, including β-phenylethylamine (Nout, 1994).

Novella-Rodriguez et al. (2002) tested *in vitro* the starter bacteria *Lactococcus lactis* subspecies *lactis* combined with *Lactococcus lactis* subspecies *cremoris,* and *Lactococcus lactis* subspecies *lactis,* and found that they did not decarboxylate amino acids or produce amines. The conclusion was that the biogenic amine content found in cheese should be attributed to the presence of non-starter bacteria. Some researchers believe that biogenic amines are produced through the interaction of adventitious microorganisms (Joosten and

Northolt, 1987; Voigt and Eitenmiller, 1978; ten Brink et al., 1990; Straub et al., 1995; Petridis and Steinhart, 1996; Ordonez et al., 1997).

Fernandez-Garcia et al. (1999) studied the effect of quantity of starter used, and found that using 1% starter generated higher levels of biogenic amines than using 0.1%. Starter cultures available for cheese manufacture should be investigated for their capacity to produce biogenic amines before use. Gennaro et al. (2003) examined the use of mesophilic and thermophilic bacteria as starters. The use of raw milk and a mesophilic bacteria increased cadaverine content by 93 mg per kg compared with using thermophilic bacteria, while use of pasteurized milk and a mesophilic bacteria resulted in an amine content decrease of 71 mg per kg.

6.4.3 Effects of Processing

Several factors contribute to the concentration of biogenic amines in cheeses. First, unripened cheese contains lower concentrations of biogenic amines than ripened cheeses. This may be due to the use of pasteurized milk in the manufacture of unripened cheese or the absence of the ripening period. High levels of biogenic amines in unripened cheese may indicate the use of poor quality raw milk; pasteurization of milk can lower the amount of biogenic amines formed. There is a slower rate of proteolysis in pasteurized milk, which can slow down the liberation of free amino acids (Lau et al., 1991). The heat treatment during pasteurization can also inactivate pyridoxal phosphate, a cofactor for decarboxylase activity (Ordonez et al., 1997; Gennaro et al., 2003; Joosten, 1988). Raw milk and partially-pasteurized milk result in higher levels of biogenic amines in cheese products (Chambers and Staruszkiewics, 1978; Gennaro et al., 2003).

Second, the pH value may have a significant effect on the production of biogenic amines. A pH of 5.0 is optimum for tyrosine and histidine decarboxylase activity (Diaz-Cinco et al., 1992). Novella-Rodriguez et al. (2002) reported an increase in biogenic amines after a drop in pH combined with an increase in *Lactobacillus* counts. Joosten (1988) reported that *Lactobacillus buchneri* produced higher levels of histamine in Gouda cheese at pH 5.39 (6.5 mmol histamine per kg) compared with pH of 5.19 (3.4 mmol histamine per kg). The amount of starter culture affects the pH of cheese and therefore the production of amino acids. In another study, Manchego cheese was manufactured using 1.0% and 0.1% mesophilic starter. The cheese made with 1.0% starter had a pH of 5.15 and produced 15% more tryamine and 28% more histamine than the cheese made with 0.1% starter, which had a pH of 5.08 (Fernandez-Garcia et al., 1999). Fernandez-Garcia et al., (2000) reported lower pH values in cheeses made with 1% starter culture compared with 0.1% starter culture (4.90 to 4.96 and 4.95 to 5.04, respectively). A higher pH increases the production of some biogenic amines. The difference in pH may be small, but, along with other factors, can influence the production of biogenic amines.

First, the ripening time, storage time and temperature may also affect the levels of biogenic amines found in cheese. Amine contents range from 10 to 2000 times higher in ripened cheese than in unripened cheese. The variation in amine content is related to the differences in ripening processes (Martelli et al., 1993; Schneller et al., 1997). Prolonged ripening increases the concentration of biogenic amines (Diaz-Cinco et al., 1992; Ordonez et al., 1997; Durlu-Ozkaya et al., 1999). Novella-Rodriguez et al. (2003) reported that ripened hard cheese contained the highest level of tyramine (125.5 mg per kg), with levels of histamine at 18.3 mg per kg and cadaverine at 29.5 mg per kg. Blue cheese was found to contain 14.4 mg per kg of tyramine, 6.6 mg per kg of histamine and 11.3 mg per kg of cadaverine, as well as 3.4 mg per kg of β-phenylethylamine, 3.2 mg per kg of tryptamine and 18.0 mg per kg of putrescine (all values reported as the median). Innocente and D'Agostin (2002) reported that histamine and tyramine concentrations increase during ripening of Montasio cheese (Table 6.8). The concentrations of biogenic amines found in Montasio cheese are well below the values that are considered toxic. Ordonez et al. (1997) found that levels of tyramine, cadaverine, and putrescine in Idiazabal ewe-milk cheese increased over a ripening time of 180 days. Tyramine level started at 2.74 mg per100 g at day 1 and was 23.8 mg per 100 g at day 180. Cadaverine went from 4.1 to 7.71 mg per 100 g and putrescine went from 3.01 to 10.3 mg per 100 g in 180 days. The other amines in montasio cheese all began to decrease in concentration after 15 days. The increase of biogenic amines during the ripening process has also been documented by others (Martelli et al., 1993; Schneller et al., 1997; Ordonez et al., 1997; Pinho et al., 2001).

Temperature of a storage facility can affect the production of biogenic amines. Pinho et al. (2001) conducted a study to investigate the effect of storage

Table 6.8

Average biogenic amine content in Montasio cheeses, after 60, 90, 120 and 150 days of ripening.

Ripening period (days)	Amine content (mg/100 g)					
	Tryptamine	Histamine	Cadaverine	Putrescine	β-phenylethylamine	Tyramine
60	2.07[a]	2.28[a]	0.15[a]	0.27[a]	0.18[a]	0.17[a]
	(3.77)[b]	(3.17)[b]	(3.24)[b]	(19.23)[b]	(0.47)[b]	(5.23)[b]
90	5.19	3.70	0.49	1.151	0.42	0.14
120	6.12	6.78	0.27	0.61	0.57	0.17
150	24.79	21.76	1.37	24.71	1.42	0.37
				(36.36)[b]		

[a]Mean value without outliers of +/− 3 standard deviations (samples 19 and 22 were outliers for the 60 day ripening samples, sample 5 was the outlier for 150 days of ripening, but only for putrescine).
[b]True mean values.
Source: Innocente and D'Agostin (2002), *J. Food Prot.*, 65, 1498.

temperature. Samples of Azeitao cheese were transported at either 4°C or 25°C, held at 4°C for two weeks, then held at 25°C for another two weeks. Biogenic amines were significantly higher in the cheese transported at 25°C than at 4°C. When the 4°C cheese was placed at 25°C for two weeks there was a 37% increase in the concentration of biogenic amines. This demonstrates that it is important that proper storage temperatures be maintained throughout transportation, distribution, purchase, and storage.

Fourth, the salt concentration in cheese also influences the production of biogenic amines (Kebary et al., 1999; Joosten, 1988). Gouda cheese contains 3.5 mmol histamine per kg with a salt:water ratio of 0.048, and 2.1 mmol histamine with a salt:water ratio of 0.026 (Joosten, 1988). Each cheese has its own characteristic free amino acid and biogenic amine profiles, resulting from its specific degradation, interconversion, and synthesis (Polo et al., 1985).

The concentration of biogenic amines in cheese could be used as an indicator for its freshness, and an indicator of the quality of the raw materials and manufacturing processes involved.

6.5 BIOGENIC AMINES IN FERMENTED MEATS

6.5.1 Biogenic Amine Profile

Biogenic amines are commonly found in fermented meats. Histamine poisoning has not been associated with this type of product, however histamine has been found at low levels in some fermented meats (Dierick et al., 1974; Taylor et al., 1978; Vidal et al., 1990; Shalaby, 1993; Maijala et al., 1993). The most common amine found in fermented meats is tyramine (Trevino et al., 1997; Eerola et al., 1998), which is found at higher concentrations than other amines. The toxic level of biogenic amines is 100 mg per 100 g of product (Arnold et al., 1978). Taylor et al. (1978) and Vandekerckhove (1977) found amounts of histamine up to 55 mg per 100 g, putrescine up to 40 mg per 100 g, cadaverine up to 5.6 mg per 100 g, tyramine up to 151 mg per 100 g, and β-phenylethylamine up to 6.1 mg per 100 g in dry sausage. Table 6.9 lists the

Table 6.9
Amines found in dry sausage.

Amine	Quantity (mg/100 g)
Histamine	trace to 55.0
Putrescine	3.1 to 39.6
Cadaverine	trace to 5.6
Tyramine	10.2 to 50.6
β-phenylethylamine	ND to 6.1

Note: ND = not detected.
Source: Stratton et al. (1991), *J. Food Prot.*, 54, 460.

amines found in dry sausage (Stratton et al., 1991). The polyamines spermine and spermidine are naturally occurring in the materials used in fermented meats; therefore the concentrations are not influenced by starter cultures. Fermented meats contain a wide variety of biogenic amines as well as variations in the biogenic amine profile (Bover-Cid et al., 1999; Hernandez-Jover et al., 1997; Vidal-Carou et al., 1990). Hernandez-Jover et al. (1997) proposed that a biogenic amine index (comprising the combined total content of cadaverine, putrescine, tyramine, and histamine) be used to determine the hygienic quality of raw material.

Many factors affect the production of biogenic amines in fermented meats, including the natural microflora present and their ability to decarboxylate, manufacturing processes, type and quality of meat, and the length of maturation (Shalaby, 1995).

6.5.2 MICROFLORA

Many different starter cultures are used in the fermentation process for sausages, and have been found to affect the total amount of biogenic amines in the fermented meats (Buncic et al., 1993; Maijala et al., 1993). *Lactobacillus divergens* and *Lactobacillus carnis* produce tyramine (Edwards et al., 1987), *Enterobacteriaceae* produces cadaverine, and putrescine is produced by *Pseudomonas* (Slemr, 1981). *Lactobacillus plantarum*, however, decreases amine production in dry sausage (Buncic et al., 1993) and is unable to produce either histamine or tyramine. Ansorena et al. (2002) found that spontaneous non-starter lactic acid bacteria and cocci are responsible for tyramine found in Italian sausage, while the tyramine in Belgian South sausage is a product of enterococci and contaminant Gram-positive cocci (Masson et al., 1996; Ansorena et al., 2002). Other authors also believe that natural microflora, lactic-acid bacteria, and contaminant bacteria contribute to the production of biogenic amines (Maijala et al., 1993; Shalaby 1995). Therefore, when choosing a starter culture, a manufacturer should check the individual organism for its amine-producing ability.

6.5.3 EFFECTS OF PROCESSING

There are many different types of fermented meats, each with its own particular process. The microbial and biochemical reactions during fermentation cause the characteristic acidification, proteolysis and drying that make the product safe. The distinctive flavor of sausage is also produced in these processes. The conditions under which fermented meats are produced are very favorable for the production of biogenic amines (Bover-Cid et al., 2000). Many factors contribute to the quality and acceptability of the final product.

The initial and final pH of sausage during ripening plays an important role in the production of biogenic amines. In the early stages of sausage-ripening there is a decrease in pH, if this decrease is not adequate there is an increase in the production of histamine (Eerola et al., 1998). Maijala et al. (1993) and

Ansorena et al. (2002) also found that this change in pH leads to a decrease in the amounts of histamine and putrescine produced. Use of acidulants, such as glucono δ-lactone, may influence amine production by ensuring a drop in pH (Santos et al., 1986; Buncic et al., 1993; Maijala et al., 1993). A gradual increase in pH throughout the ripening process is related to the proteolytic activity of the starter culture as it forms peptides and amino acids (Bover-Cid et al., 1999).

The hygienic quality of the raw material used for the manufacture of sausage is an important factor relating to the production of biogenic amines. High-quality meats with low initial bacterial counts help keep the biogenic amines well below the toxic level (Shalaby 1995; Bover-Cid et al., 2000) and should be used with the addition of a non-amine-producing starter culture.

Bover-Cid et al. (2000) studied the effects of storing a high-quality meat product at 4°C for five days before use. The sausage made from the meat stored at 4°C contained significantly higher levels of tyramine and cadaverine. There were also higher levels of histamine and putrescine present. Significant differences in the concentrations of *Enterobacteriaceae*, lactic acid bacteria, coagulase-negative staphylococci and enterococci were found between the two samples.

The manufacturing process used in meat fermentation can increase or decrease the concentration of biogenic amines in the end product. Semi-dry sausage is fermented for shorter periods and often with the addition of lactic acid starter cultures. Dry sausages are typically allowed to ferment for longer periods, employing natural microflora. During ripening, the histamine level in dry sausage may increase by ten-fold in the first three days (Dierick et al., 1974). Butturini et al. (1995) and Cantoni (2004) agree that dry sausages prepared without a starter culture have different levels and profiles of biogenic amines, which they attribute to the differences in the ripening process and to spontaneous fermentation by natural microflora. Semi-dry sausages typically contain lower concentrations of biogenic amines. Biogenic amine presence in Italian sausage has also been attributed to microflora (Tiecco et al., 1985).

Bover-Cid et al. (1999) examined the effect of sausage diameter versus the concentration of biogenic amines. The larger-diameter sausages contained a significantly higher quantity of tyramine, histamine, β-phenylethylamine, and tryptamine. This may be due to the longer ripening time required for the large-diameter sausages. A difference in the biogenic amines in the center of the sausage compared with the edges of the sausage was also reported. The center was found to contain higher concentrations of biogenic amines than the edges.

Storage time and temperature after manufacturing can also increase the amount of biogenic amines present. Komprda et al. (2001) reported an increase of tyramine content from 15 to 90 mg per kg during ripening, and then another increase from 90 to 200 mg per kg during storage. The samples were then stored for a further 60 days at either 8 or 22°C (representing room temperature and refrigeration). Two types of sausage were used for the study, sausage A (starter culture *Lactobacillus sakei*, *Staphylococcus carnosus*, *S. xylosus*) and sausage B (starter culture *Lactobacillus sakei*, *Staphylococcus carnosus*, *Pediococcus pentosaceus*). Sausage A did not show a significant increase in the level of biogenic amines after either refrigerated or room-temperature storage (236 and 206 mg per kg respectively). Sausage B, however, did show a significant increase in biogenic amine content. From 200 mg per kg after ripening, biogenic amine content increased after refrigerated storage to 304 mg per kg, and after room-temperature storage to 468 mg per kg.

6.6 BIOGENIC AMINES IN FRESH MEATS

High levels of biogenic amines in non-fermented foods indicate undesirable microbial activity (Silla Santos, 1996). Biogenic amines are natural components of many foods, including meat (Kaniou et al., 2001). Biogenic amines have been found in cooked and uncooked beef and pork (Nemeth-Szerdahelyi et al., 1993). Meat and meat products can contain tyramine, cadaverine, putrescine, spermine, and spermidine (Koehler and Eitenmiller, 1978; Nakamura et al., 1979; Edwards et al., 1983; Santos-Buelga et al., 1986; Stratton et al., 1991; Shalaby, 1993; Shalaby, 1995; Shalaby and El-Rahman 1995). Fresh and processed pork is reported to contain high levels of adrenaline and spermine and low levels of noradrenaline, putrescine, histamine, cadaverine, and tyramine (Halasz et al., 1994), while histamine has been found in bovines and sheep (Teodorovic et al., 1994). Storage of meat can increase the level of biogenic amines.

Hernandez-Jover et al. (1997) proposed that the combined total content of putrescine, cadaverine, histamine and tyramine could be used as an index to evaluate meat freshness, where a value of 5.0 µg per g or less is considered high quality.

6.7 BIOGENIC AMINES IN WINE AND BEER

Wine and beer contain low concentrations of biogenic amines (Stratton et al., 1991), a summary is given in Table 6.10. White wines generally contain very low levels of biogenic amines (Littlewood et al., 1988), while red wines have higher levels (Ough, 1971). Wines are reported to generally contain less than 10 mg per liter (Ough, 1971; Pechanek et al., 1983; Baucom et al., 1986), however there have been some reports of much higher biogenic amine content (Baucom et al., 1986; Ough, 1971). Biogenic amine concentrations of 8 mg per liter may cause headaches if large quantities are consumed (Ough, 1971). Soufleros et al. (1998) state that biogenic amine production is dependent on the microflora and the amino-acid composition of the wine after fermentation. The amino-acid composition after fermentation is dependent on the grape variety, vine nutrition, and yeast metabolism. The pH is also an important factor; the higher the pH, the higher the levels of biogenic amines produced (Lonvaud-Funel and Joyeux, 1994). In Burgundy wines, histamine, tyramine, and putrescine are increased during malolactic fermentation (Gerbaux and Monany, 2000).

Histamine has been found in Swedish beer at 2.6 to 4.7 mg per liter, in Danish beer at 3.2 to15 mg per liter, and up to 20 mg per liter in French beers (Zee and Simard, 1981). Canadian, American, and European beers contain

Table 6.10
Amines found in fermented beverages.

Beverage	Amine	Quantity (mg/l)
American red wine	Histamine	0.2 to 15.5
	Cadaverine	4.0 to 47.0
	Putrescine	0.6 to 5.5
	Tyramine	ND to 0.2
American white wine	Histamine	0.2 to 11.4
	Cadaverine	3.2 to 108.3
	Putrescine	0.7 to 11.7
	Tyramine	ND to 0.5
European red wine	Histamine	ND to 30
	Tyramine	0.07 to 25.4
European white wine	Histamine	ND to 20
	Tyramine	0.1 to 6.5
Nigerian palm wine	Tyramine	11.27
Cuban wine	Tyramine	ND to 3.75
Japanese sake	Tyramine	0.21 to 0.51
American beer	Putrescine	3.7 to 7.1
	Tyramine	1.0 to 16.3
Canadian beer	Histamine	4.8 to 5.4
	Putrescine	3.0 to 5.4
	Tyramine	11.7 to 17.6
European beer	Histamine	2.6 to 20
	Cadaverine	ND to 55.2
	Putrescine	2.6 to 6.6
Japanese beer	Tyramine	0.2 to 1.3
Nigerian beer	Tyramine	7.2 to 7.4
Cuban beer	Tyramine	1.2 to 9.3
Nonalcoholic beer	Tyramine	0.5 to 4.0

Note: ND = not detected.
Source: Stratton et al. (1991), *J. Food Prot.*, 54, 460.

histamine at levels of between 4.5 and 7.3 mg per liter. Even though histamine levels in beer are not high, they are still of concern because beer is generally consumed in greater quantities than is wine (Hanna et al., 1988).

6.8 BIOGENIC AMINES IN OTHER FOODS

Biogenic amines have been found in fruits, vegetables, fruit juices and cocoa beans. Juices made from oranges, raspberries, lemons, grapefruit, mandarins, strawberries, currants, and grapes have all been found to contain levels of biogenic amines, with putrescine being the most predominant (Maxa and Brandes, 1993). Tryptamine and noradrenaline have been found in orange juice, while tomato contains tyramine, tryptamine and histamine. Banana

Table 6.11
Amine contents of various vegetables.

Vegetable	Amine	Quantity (mg/100 g)	Reference
Mixed vegetable	Histamine	0.1	(Stratton et al 1991)
	Putrescine	0.3 to 0.7	
	Cadaverine	0.6 to 1.5	
	Tyramine	ND to 0.7	
Ketchup	Tyramine	3.4	(Kalac et al 2002)
	Putrescine	5.3	
Frozen green peas	Spermidine	4.7	(Stratton et al 1991)
Spinach puree	Histamine	1.8	(Kalac et al 2002)

Note: ND = not detected.
Sources: Stratton et al. (1991), *J. Food Prot.*, 54, 460; Kalac et al. (2002). *Food Chem.*, 77, 349.

contains tyramine, noradrenaline, tryptamine, and serotonin, plums contain tyramine and noradrenaline, and spinach was found to contain histamine (Halasz et al., 1994).

Cocoa beans naturally contain phenylethylamine, as do some mushrooms (Pfundstein et al., 1991). Vegetables identified as containing biogenic amines include Chinese cabbage, endive, iceberg lettuce, and radicchio (Simon-Sarkadi and Holzapfel, 1994). Spermidine was the major polyamine found in these vegetables (7 to 17 µg per g). Frozen spinach puree, ketchup, concentrated tomato paste, and frozen green peas were found to contain low amounts of biogenic amines (Table 6.11) (Kalac et al., 2002).

Table 6.12
Amine contents of various fermented vegetables.

Fermented vegetable	Amine	Quantity (mg/100 g)
Sauerkraut	Histamine	0.7 to 20
	Tyramine	2.0 to 9.5
	Cadaverine	0.3 to 3.0
	Putrescine	0.1 to 4.0
Salted black beans	Tyramine	45.0
Shrimp sauce	Tyramine	24.5
Soy sauce[a]	Histamine	ND to 274
	Tyramine	ND to 466
	Tryptamine	ND to 93.0

Note: ND = not detected.
[a]Levels expressed as mg/l.
Source: Stratton et al. (1991), *J. Food Prot.*, 54, 460.

Fermented vegetables often contain histamine (Table 6.12). Taylor et al. (1978) found that sauerkraut contains an average of 5.06 mg per 100 g, but as much as 20 mg per 100 g was reported by Mayer and Pause (1978). Miso and soy sauce, both made from fermented soybeans, contain tyramine and histamine. Inyu, a soy sauce made from black soybeans, generally has higher levels of biogenic amines than does regular soy sauce (Yen, 1986). Yen also reports that other foods made from fermented black soybean products, such as toshi and sufu, contain high levels of biogenic amines, even in excess of 100 mg per 100 g. Tyramine has been found in fermented salted black beans (45 mg per 100 g) and shrimp sauce (24 mg per 100 g) (Mower and Bhagavan, 1988).

Histamine may also be found in egg yolk, although levels are very low. Fresh eggs contain the highest level of histamine, 0.078 mg per 100 g, while stored eggs contain 0.063 mg per 100 g and boiled eggs contain 0.046 mg per 100 g of histamine (Moudgal et al., 1991).

6.9 REFERENCES

Ababouch, L., Afilal, M.E., Rhafiri, and Busta, F.F. (1991). Identification of histamine-producing bacteria isolated from sardine *(Sardina pilchards)* stored at ambient temperature, *Food Microbiol.*, 8, 127, 1991.

Aiso, K., Iida, H., Nakayama, J. and Nakano, K. (1958). Histamine poisoning caused by certain marine fish products and the specific etiological agents. Chiba Daigaku Fuhai, Kenhyusho Hokoku 11, 1–6.

Aksnes, A. (1988). Location of enzymes responsible for autolysis in bulk-stored capelin *(Mallotus villosus)*, *J. Sci. Food Agric.*, 44, 271.

Aksnes, A. and Brekken, B. (1988). Tissue degradation, amino acid liberation and bacterial decomposition of bulk stored capelin, *J. Sci. Food Agric.*, 45, 53.

Ansorena, D., Montel, M.C., Rokka, M., Talon, R., Eerola, S., Rizzo, A., Raemaekers, M. and Demeyer, D. (2002). Analysis of biogenic amines in northern and southern European sausages and role of flora in amine production, *Meat Sci.*, 61, 141.

Arnold, S.H. and Brown, W.D. (1978). Histamine toxicity from fish products, *Adv. Food Res.*, 34, 113–154.

Arnold, S.H., Price, R.J., and Brown, W.D. (1980). Histamine formation by bacteria isolated from skipjack tuna, *Katsuwonas pelamis*. Bull. Jpn. Soc. Sci. Fish. 46, 991–995.

Baranowski, J.D., Frank, H.A., Brust, P.A., Chongsiriwatana, M. and Premaratne, R.J. (1990). Decomposition and histamine content in mahimahi *(Coryphaena hippurus)*, *J. Food Prot.*, 53, 217.

Baucom, T.L., Tabacchi, M.H., Cottrell, T.H.E. and Richmond, B.S. (1986). Biogenic amine content of New York state wines, *J. Food Sci.*, 51, 1376.

Behling, A.R. and Taylor, S.L. (1982). Bacterial histamine production as a function of temperature and time of incubation. *J. Food Sci.* 47, 1311–1317.

Ben-Gigirey, B., Vieties Baptista de Sousa, J.M., Villa, J.M., and Barros-Velaquez, T.G. (1998). Changes in biogenic amines and microbiological analysis in albacore *(Thunnus alalunga)* muscle during frozen storage. *J. Food Prot.*, 61(5), 608–615.

Bermejo, A., Mondaca, M.A., Roeckel, M., and Marti, M.C. (2003). Growth and Characterization of the histamine-forming bacteria of Jack mackerel (*Trachurus symmetricus*). *J. Food Process. Preserv.*, 26, 401–414.

Bjeldanes, L., Shultz, D.E. and Morris, M.M. (1978). On the aetiology of scombroid poisoning: cadaverine potentiation of histamine toxicity in the guinea-pig, *Food Cosmet. Toxicol.*, 16, 157.

Bover-Cid, S., Izquierdo-Pulido, M. and Vidal-Carou, M.C. (2000). Influence of hygienic quality of raw materials on biogenic amine production during ripening and storage of dry fermented sausages, *J. Food Prot.*, 63, 1544.

Bover-Cid, S., Schoppen, S., Izquierdo-Pulido, M. and Vidal-Carou, M.C. (1999). Relationship between biogenic amine contents and the size of dry fermented sausages, *Meat Sci.*, 51, 305.

Buncic, S., Paunovic, L., Teodorovic, V., Radisic, D., Vojinovic, G., Smiljanic, D. and Baltic, M. (1993). Effects of gluconodeltalactone and *Lactobacillus plantarum* on the production of histamine and tyramine in fermented sausages, *Int. J. Food Microbiol.*, 17, 303.

Butturini A., Aloisi, P., Tagliazucchi, P. and Cantoni, P.C. (1995). Ammine biogene prodotte da enterobatteri e batteri lattici issolati de impasti di salame, *Industrie Alimentari*, 24, 105.

Cantoni, C. (2004). Ammine biogene di prodotti carnei nazionali, *Industrie Alimentari*, 34, 9.

Chambers, T. and Staruszkiewics, W.F. (1978). Fluorometric determination of histamine in cheese, *J. Assoc. Off. Anal. Chem.*, 61, 1092.

Chu, C.-H. and Bjeldanes, L.E. (1981). Effect of diamines, polyamines and tuna fish extracts on the binding of histamine to mucin *in vitro*, *J. Food Sci.*, 47, 79.

Clifford, M., Walker, R., Ijomah, P., Wright, J., Muray, C.K. and Hardy, R. (1991). Is there a role for amines other than histamines in the aetiology of scombrotoxicosis?, *Food Addit. Contam.*, 8, 641.

Clifford, M., Wright, R.,Wright, J., Hardy, R. and Murray, C.K. (1989). Studies with volunteers on the role of histamine in suspected scombrotoxicosis, *J. Food Sci.*, 47, 365.

Connil, N., Prevost, H., and Dousset, X. (2002). Production of biogenic amines and in cold smoked salmon inoculated with *Carnobacterium divergens* V41, and specific detection of this strain by multiplex-pcr. *J. Appl. Microbiol.*, 92(4), 611–617.

Diaz-Cinco, M.E., Fraijo, O., Grajeda, P., Lozano-Taylor, X. and Gonzalez de Mejia, E. (1992). Microbial and chemical analysis of Chihuahua cheese and relationship to histamine and tyramine, *J. Food Sci.*, 57, 355.

Dierick, N., Vandekerckhove, P. and Dameyer, D. (1974). Changes in nonprotein nitrogen compounds during dry sausage ripening, *J. Food Sci.*, 39, 301.

Doeglas, H.M.G., Huisman, J. and Nater, J.P. (1964). Histamine intoxication after cheese, *Lancet*, 2, 1361.

Douglas, W. (1970). Histamine and antihistamines; 5-Hydroxytryptamine and antagonists, in Goodman, L. and Gilman, A., eds., *The Pharmacological Basis of Therapeutics*, 5th ed., Macmillan, New York, pp. 621–662.

Du,.W.-X., Lin, C.M., Phu, A.T., Cornell, J.A., Marshall, M.R. and Wei, C.I. (2002). Development of biogenic amines in yellowfin tuna (*Thunnus albacares*): Effect of storage and correlation with decarboxylase-positive bacterial flora, *J. Food Sci.*, 67, 292.

Durlu-Ozkaya, F., Alichanidis, E., Litopoulou-Tzanetaki, E. and Tunail, N. (1999). Determination of biogenic amine content of Beyaz cheese and biogenic amine production ability of some lactic acid bacteria, *Milchwissenschaft-Milk Sci. Int.*, 54, 680.

Edwards, R.A., Dainty, R.H. and Hibbard, C.M. (1983). The relationship of bacterial numbers and types to diamine concentration in aerobically stored beef, pork, and lamb, *J. Food Technol.*, 62, 777.

Edwards, R.A., Dainty, R.H., Hibbard, C.M. and Ramandanis, S.V. (1987). Amines in fresh beef of normal pH and the role of bacteria in changes in concentration observed during storage in vacuum packs at chill temperature, *J. Appl. Bacteriol.*, 63, 427.

Edwards, S. and Sandine, W. (1981). Public health significance of amines in cheese, *J. Dairy Sci.*, 64, 2431.

Eerola, H.S., Sagues, A.X.R. and Hirvi, T.K. (1998). Biogenic amines in Finnish dry sausages, *J. Food Saf.*, 18, 127.

Eitenmiller, R.R., Orr, J.H., and Wallis, W.W. (1982). Histamine formation in fish: microbial and biochemical conditions. In: Martin, R.E., Flick, G.J., Hebard, C.E., Ward, D.R. (Eds.), Chemistry and Biochemistry of Marine Food Products, AVI, Westport, CT, pp. 39–50.

Fernandez-Garcia, E., Tomillo, J. and Nunez, M. (1999). Effect of added proteinases and level of starter culture on the formation of biogenic amines in raw milk Manchego cheese, *Int. J. Food Microbiol.*, 52, 189.

Fernandez-Garcia E., Tomillo, J. and Nunez, M. (2000). Formation of biogenic amines in raw milk Hispanico cheese manufactured with proteinases and different levels of starter culture, *J. Food Prot.*, 63, 1551.

Fernandez-Salguero, J. and Mackie, I.M. (1987). Technical note: Preliminary survey of the content of histamine and other higher amines in some samples of Spanish canned fish, *Int. J. Food Sci. Technol.*, 22, 409.

Flick, G., Oria, M. and Douglas, L. (2001). *Potential hazards in cold smoked fish: Biogenic amines, J. Food Sci.*, 66(7), S-1088-S-1099.

Food and Drug Administration (FDA) (1996). *Fish and Fisheries Products Hazards and Controls Guide*, 1st ed., FDA, Center for Food Safety and Applied Nutrition, Office of Seafood, Washington, D.C.

Food and Drug Administration (FDA) (1998). *Fish and Fisheries Products Hazards and Controls Guide*, 2nd ed., FDA, Office of Seafood, Washington, D.C.

Frank, H., Baranowski, J.D., Chongsiriwatana, M., Brust, P.A. and Premaratne, R.J. (1985). Identification and decarboxylase activities of bacteria isolated from decomposed mahimahi (*Coryphaena hippurus*) after incubation at 0 and 32°C, *Int. J. Food Microbiol.*, 2, 331.

Gale, E. (1946). The bacterial amino acid decarboxylases, *Adv. Enzymol. Relat. Subjects Biochem.*, 6, 1.

Gennaro M.C., Gianotti, V., Marengo, E., Pattono, D. and Turi, R.M. (2003). A chemometric investigation of the effect of the cheese-making process on contents of biogenic amines in a semi-hard Italian cheese (Toma), *Food Chem.*, 82, 545.

Gerbaux, V. and Monany, C. (2000). Les amines biogenes dans les vins de Bourgogne. Teneurs, origine et maitrise dans les vins, *Rev. Fr. Oenol.*, 183, 25.

Gildberg, A. (1978). Proteolytic activity and the frequency of burst bellies in capelin, *J. Food Technol.*, 13, 409.

Gloria, M., Daeschel, M.A., Craven, C. and Hilenbrand Jr., K.S. (1999). Histamine and other biogenic amines in albacore tuna, *J. Aqu. Food Prod. Technol.*, 8, 54.

Granerus, G. (1968). Effects of oral histamine, histidine, and diet on urinary excretion of histamine, methylhistamine, and 1-methyl-4-imidazoleacetic acid in man, *Scand. J. Clin. Lab. Invest.*, 10, suppl., 49.

Haaland, H., Arnesen, E. and Njaa, L.R. (1990). Amino-acid-composition of whole mackerel (*Scomber scombrus*) stored anaerobically at 20-degrees C and at 2-degrees C, *Int. J. Food Sci. Technol.*, 25, 82.

Halasz, A., Barath, A., Simon-Sarkadi, L. and Holzapfel, W.H. (1994). Biogenic amines and their production by microorganisms in food, *Trends Food Sci. Technol.*, 5, 42.

Hanna, P., Glover, V. and Sandler, M. (1988). Tyramine in wine and beer, *Lancet*, 1, 879.

Hernandez-Jover, M., Izquierdo-Pulido, M., Veciana-Nogues, M.T., Marine-Font, A. and Vidal-Carou, M.C. (1997). Effect of starter cultures on biogenic amine formation during fermented sausage production, *J. Food Prot.*, 60, 825.

Hildrum, K., Scanlan, R.A. and Libbey, L.M. (1976). Nitrosamines from the nitrosation of spermidine and spermine, in Walker, E., Bogovski, P. and Griciute. L., Eds., *Environmental N-Nitroso Compounds Analysis and Formation*, Polytechnical Institute Tallinn, Estonia.

Hui, J. and Taylor, S.L. (1983). High pressure liquid chromatographic determination of putrefactive amines in foods, *Journal AOAC*, 66, 853.

Hungerford, J.M. and Arefyev, A.A. (1992). Flow-injection assay of enzyme-inhibition in fish using immobilized diamine oxidase, *Analytica Chimica Acta*, 261, 351.

Ibe, A., Saito, K., Nakazato, M., Kikuchi, Y., Fujinuma, K. and Nishima, T. (1991). Quantitative determination of amines in wine by liquid-chromatography, *J. Assoc. Off. Anal. Chemists*, 74, 695.

Ienistea, C. (1973). Significance and detection of histamine in food, in Hobbs, B. and Christian, J.H.B., eds., *The Microbiological Safety of Foods*, Academic Press, New York, pp. 327–343.

Innocente, N. and D'Agostin, P. (2002). Formation of biogenic amines in a typical semihard Italian cheese, *J. Food Prot.*, 65, 1498.

Joosten, H.M.L.J. (1988). Conditions allowing the formation of biogenic amines in cheese: 3. Factors influencing the amounts formed, *Neth. Milk Dairy J.*, 41, 329.

Joosten, H.M.L.J. and Northolt, M.D. (1987). Conditions allowing the formation of biogenic-amines in cheese: 2. Decarboxylative properties of some nonstarter bacteria, *Neth. Milk Dairy J.*, 41, 259.

Jorgensen, L.V., Dalgaard, P.H. and Huss, H. (2000). Multiple compound quality index for cold-smoked salmon (*Salmo salar*) developed by multivariate regression of biogenic amines and pH, *J. Agric. Food Chem.*, 48, 2448.

Kahana, L.M. and Todd, E. (1981). Histamine intoxication in a tuberculosis patient on isoniazid, *Ca. Dis. Weekly Rep.*, 7, 79.

Kalac, P., Svecova, S. and Pelikanova, T. (2002). Levels of biogenic amines in typical vegetable products, *Food Chem.*, 77, 349.

Kaniou, I., Samouris, G., Mouratidou, T., Eleftheriadou, A. and Zantopoulos, N. (2001). Determination of biogenic amines in fresh unpacked and vacuum-packed beef during storage at 4 degrees C, *Food Chem.*, 74, 515.

Kebary, K.M.K., El-Sonbaty, A.H. and Badawi, R.M. (1999). Effects of heating milk and accelerating ripening of low fat Ras cheese on biogenic amines and free amino acids development, *Food Chem.*, 64, 67.

Kimata, M., Akamatsu, M., and Ishida, Y. (1960). Studies on the classification of the genus *Proteus* I. On the taxonomical situation of *Proteus morganii*. Mem. Res. Inst. Food Sci. Kyoto Univ. 20, 1–7.

Klausen, N. and Huss, H.H. (1987). Growth and histamine production by *Morganella morganii* under various temperature conditions, *Int. J. Food Microbiol.*, 5, 147.

Klausen, N. and Lund, E. (1986). Formation of biogenic amines in herring and mackerel, *Z. Lebensm Unters Forsch.*, 182, 459.

Koehler, P.E. and Eitenmiller, R.R. (1978). High performance liquid chromatographic analysis of tyramine, phenylethylamine and tryptamine in sausages, cheese, and chocolate, *J. Food Sci.*, 43, 344.

Komprda, T., Neznalova, J., Satndara, S. and Bover-Cid, S. (2001). Effect of starter culture and storage temperature on the content of biogenic amines in dry fermented sausage polican, *Meat Sci.*, 59, 267.

Koutsoumanis, K., Lampropoulou, K. and Nychas, G.J.E. (1999). Biogenic amines and sensory changes associated with the microbial flora of Mediterranean gilt-head sea bream (*Sparus aurata*) stored aerobically at 0, 8, and 15 degrees C, *J. Food Prot.*, 62, 398.

Krizek, M., Pavlicek, T. and Vacha, F. (2002), Formation of selected biogenic amines in carp meat, *J. Sci. Food Agric.*, 82, 1088.

Lau, K.L., Barbano, M. and Rasmussen, R.R. (1991). Influence of pasteurization of milk on the protein breakdown in cheddar cheese during aging, *J. Dairy Sci.*, 74, 727.

Leuschner, R.G.K. and Hammes, W.P. (1999). Formation of biogenic amine in mayonnaise, herring and tuna fish salad by lactobacilli, *Int. J. Food Sci. Nutr.*, 50, 159.

Littlewood, J.T., Gibb, C., Clover, V., Sandler, M. and Davies, P.T.G. (1988). Red wine as a cause of migraine, *Lancet*, 1, 558.

Lonvaud-Funel, A. and Joyeux, A. (1994). Histamine production by wine lactic acid bacteria: isolation of a histamine-producing strain of *Leuconostoc oenos*, *J. Appl. Bacteriol.*, 77, 401.

Lopez-Sabater, E., Rodriguez-Jerez, J.J., Hernandez-Herrero, M. and Mora-Ventura, M.T. (1994). Evaluation of histidine decarboxylase activity of bacteria isolated from sardine (*Sardina pilchardus*) by an enzyme method, *Lett. Appl. Microbiol.*, 19.

Lopez-Sabater, E., Rodriguez-Jerez, J.J., Hernandez-Herrero, M. and Mora-Ventura, M.T. (1996). Incidence of histamine-forming bacteria and histamine content in scombroid fish species from retail markets in the Barcelona area, *Int. J. Food Microbiol.*, 28, 411.

Maga, J. (1978). Amines in foods. *Critical Reviews in Food Science and Nutrition*, 10, CRC Press, Boca Raton, pp. 373–403.

Maijala, R.L., Eerola, S.H., Aho, M.A. and Hirn, J.A. (1993). The effect of Gdl-induced pH decrease on the formation of biogenic-amines in meat, *J. Food Prot.*, 56, 125.

Martelli, A., Arlorio, M. and Tourn, M.L. (1993). Determination of amines and precursor amino acids in gorgonzola cheese by ion pair HPLC without derivation, *Li Rivista di Scienza dell'alimentazione*, 3, 261.

Masson, F., Eclache, L., Compte, L., Talon, C. and Montel, C. (1996). Screening of microbial strains producing amines and isolated from meat products. 546–547.

Maxa, E. and Brandes, W. (1993). Biogene Amine in Fruchtsäften, *Mitt. Klosterneuburg*, 43, 101.

Mayer, K. and Pause, G. (1978). Biogene Amine in Sauerkraut, *Leben. Wiss. Technol.*, 5, 108.

Middlebrooks, B., Toom, P.M., Douglas, W.L., Harrison, R.E. and McDowell, S. (1988). Effects of storage time and temperature on the microflora and amine development in Spanish mackerel (*Scomberomorus maculatus*), *J. Food Sci.*, 53, 1024.

Mietz, J. and Karmas, E. (1977). Chemical quality index of canned tuna as determined by high-pressure liquid chromatography, *J. Food Sci.*, 42, 155.

Mietz, J. and Karmas, E. (1978). Polyamine and histamine content of rockfish, salmon, lobster, and shrimp as an indicator of decomposition, *J. AOAC*, 61, 139.

Moudgal, R.P., Panda, J.N. and Mohan, J. (1991). Histamine in egg yolk: Heat resistance and relation to production status, *Br. Poultry Sci.*, 32, 865.

Mower, H.F. and Bhagavan, N.V. (1988). Tyramine content of Asian and Pacific foods determined by high performance liquid chromatography, *Food Chem.*, 31, 251.

Murray, C., Hobbs, G. and Gilbert, R.J. (1982). Scombrotoxin and scombrotoxin-like poisoning from canned fish, *J. Hyg.*, 88, 215.

Nakamura, M., Wada, Y. Saway, H. and Kawabata, T. (1979). Polyamine content of fresh and processed pork, *J. Food Sci.*, 44, 515.

Nemeth-Szerdahelyi, L., Freudenreich, P. and Fisher, K. (1993). Studies on biogenic amines in pork, *Fleischwirtschaft*, 73, 789.

Nout, M.J.R. (1994). Fermented foods and food safety, *Food Res. Int.*, 27, 291.

Novella-Rodriguez, S., Veciana-Nogues, A.J., Trujillo-Mesa, A.J. and Vidal-Carou, M.C. (2002). Profile of biogenic amines in goat cheese made from pasteurized and pressurized milks, *J. Food Sci.*, 67, 2940.

Novella-Rodriguez, S., Veciana-Nogues, M.T., Izquierdo-Pulido, M. and Vidal-Carou, M.C. (2003). Distribution of biogenic amines and polyamines in cheese, *J. Food Sci.*, 68, 750.

Okuzumi, M., Fukumoto I. and Fujii, T. (1990). Changes in bacterial-flora and polyamines contents during storage of horse mackerel meat, *Nippon Suisan Gakkaishi*, 56, 1307.

Okuzumi, M., Yamanaka, H. and Kubozuka, T. (1984). Occurrence of various histamine-forming bacteria on/in fresh fishes, *Bul. Jap. Soc. Sc.i Fish*, 50, 161.

Ordonez, A.I., Ibanez, F.C., Torre, P. and Barcina, Y. (1997). Formation of biogenic amines in Idiazabal ewe's-milk cheese: Effect of ripening, pasteurization, and starter, *J. Food Prot.*, 60, 1371.

Ough, C.S. (1971). Measurement of histamine in California wines, *J. Agric. Food Chem.*, 19, 241.

Pechanek, U., Pfannhauser, W. and Woidich, H. (1983). Determination of the content of biogenic amines in four food groups of Austrian marketplace, *Z. Lebensmittel. Unters. Forsch.*, 176, 335.

Petridis, K.D. and Steinhart, H. (1996). Biogenic amines in Hart cheese production: 2. Control points-study in a standardized Swiss cheese production, *Deutsche Lebensmittel-Rundschau*, 92, 142.

Pfundstein, B., Theobald, A.R., Spiegelharder, B. and Preussmann, R. (1991). Measuring primary and secondary amines from foods and beverages in West Germany in 1989–1991, *Toxic*, 733.

Pinho, O., Ferreira, I.M.P.L., Mendes, E., Oliveira, B.M. and Ferreira, M. (2001). Effect of temperature on evolution of free amino acid and biogenic amine contents during storage of Azeitao cheese, *Food Chem.*, 75, 287.

Polo, M.C., Ramos, M. and Sanchez, R. (1985). Free amino acids by high performance liquid chromatography and peptides by gel electrophoresis in Mahon cheese during ripening, *Food Chem.*, 16, 85.

Rodriquez-Jerez, J., Mora-Ventura, M.T., Lopez-Sabater, E.I. and Hernandez-Herrero, M. (1994). Histidine, lysine, and ornithine decarboxylase bacteria in Spanish salted semipreserved anchovies, *J. Food Prot.*, 57, 784.

Rogers and Staruszkiewicz (1997). Collaborative study-GLC determination of cadaverine and putrescine in seafood; fluorometric method for histamine in tuna and mahimahi, *J. AOAC*, 80, 591.

Santos, C., Pena, M.J. and Rivas, J.C. (1986). Changes in tyramine during chorizo-sausage ripening, *Meat Sci.*, 51, 518.

Santos-Buelga, A., Pena-Egido, M.J. and Rivas-Gonzalo, J.C. (1986). Changes in tyramine during chorizo-sausage opening, *J. Food Sci.*, 51, 518.

Schneller, R., Good, P. and Jenney, M. (1997). Influence of pasteurized milk, raw milk and different ripening cultures on biogenic amine concentrations in semi-soft cheeses during ripening, *Zeitschrift fur Lebensmittel-Untersuchung Und-Forschung A-Food Research and Technology*, 204, 265.

Shalaby, A.R. and El-Rahman, H.A. (1995). Effect of potassium sorbate on the development of biogenic amines during sausage fermentation, *Die Nahrung.*, 39, 310.

Shalaby, A.R. (1993). Survey on biogenic-amines in Egyptian foods - sausage, *J. Sci. Food Agric.*, 62, 291.

Shalaby, A.R. (1995). Multidetection, semiquantitative method for determining biogenic-amines in foods, *Food Chem.*, 52, 367.

Shalaby, A. (1996). Significance of biogenic amines to food safety and human health, *Food Res. Int.*, 29, 675.

Silla Santos, M.H. (1996). Biogenic amines: their importance in foods, *Int. J. Food Microbiol.*, 29, 213.

Simon-Sarkadi, L. and Holzapfel, W.H. (1994). Determination of biogenic amines in leafy vegetables using acid analyser, *Z. Lebensmittel. Unters. Forsch.*, 198, 230.

Sjaastad, O. (1966). Fate of histamine and *N*-acetylhistamine administered into human gut, *Acta Pharmacol. Toxicol.*, 24, 189.

Slemr, T. (1981). Biogene Amine als potentieller chemescher Qualitäts-indicator Für Fleisch, *Fleischwirtschaft*, 61, 921.

Soares, V. and Gloria, M.B.A. (1994). Histamine levels in canned fish available in the retail market of Belo Horizonte, Minas Gerais, Brazil, *J. Food Comp. Anal.*, 7, 102.

Soufleros, E., Barrios, M. and Bertrand, A. (1998). Correlation between the content of biogenic amines and other wine compounds, *Am. J. Enol. Vitic.*, 49, 266.

Spanjer, M.C. and van Roode, B.A.S.W. (1991). Towards a regulatory limit for the biogenic amines in fish, cheese, and sauerkraut, *Chemicus*, 64, 584.

Staruszkiewicz, W., Barnett, J., Rogers, R., Benner Jr, P., Wong, L. and Cook, J. (2004). Effects of on-board and dockside handling on the formation of biogenic amines in mahi mahi (*Coryphaena hippurus*), skipjack tuna (*Katsuwonus pelamis*), and yellowfin tuna (*Thunnus albacares*), *J. Food Prot.*, 67, 134.

Stratton, J.E., Hutkins, R.W. and Taylor, S.L. (1991). Biogenic amines in cheese and other fermented foods: a review, *J. Food Prot.*, 54, 460.

Straub, B.W., Kicherer, M., Schilcher, S.M. and Hammes. W.P. (1995). The formation of biogenic amines by fermentation organisms, *Z. Lebensmittel Unters. Forsch.*, 201, 79–82.

Sumner, S.S. (1987). Histamine production in Swiss cheese, thesis, University of Wisconsin, Madison.

Sumner, S.S., Speckhard, M.W., Somers, E.B. and Taylor, S.L. (1985). Isolation of histamine-producing *Lactobacillus buchneri* from Swiss cheese implicated in a food poisoning outbreak, *Appl. Environ. Microbiol.*, 50, 1094.

Suzuki, S., Matsui, Y. and Takama, K. (1988). Profiles of polyamines composition in putrefactive *Pseudomonas* type III/IV, *Microbios Lett.*, 38, 105.

Suzuki, S., Noda, J. and Takama, K., (1990). Growth and polyamine production of *Alteromonas* spp. in fish meat under modified atmosphere, *Bull. Fac. Fish Hokkaido Univ.*, 41, 213.

Takagi, M., Iiad, A., Murayama, H. and Soma, S. (1969). On the formation of histamine during loss of freshness and putrefaction of various marine products, *Bull. Fac. Fish Hokkaido Univ.*, 20, 227.

Taylor, S.L. (1985). *Histamine Poisoning Associated With Fish, Cheese, and Other Foods*, World Health Organization, pp. 1–47.

Taylor, S. (1986). Histamine food poisoning: toxicology and clinical aspects, *Critical Reviews in Food Science and Nutrition*, 17, CRC Press, Boca Raton, p. 91.

Taylor, S.L., Leatherwood, M. and Lieber, E.R. (1978). Histamine in sauerkraut, *J. Food Sci.*, 43, 1030.

Taylor, S. and Lieber, E.R. (1979). *In vitro* inhibition of rat intestinal histamine-metabolizing enzymes, *Food Cosmet. Toxicol.*, 17, 237.

Taylor, S., Guthertz, L.S., Leatherwood, M. and Lieber, E.R. (1979). Histamine production by *Klebsiella pneumoniae* and an incident of scombroid fish poisoning, *Appl. Env. Microbiol.*, 37, 274.

Taylor, S., Stratton, J.E. and Nordlee, J.A. (1989). Histamine poisoning (scombroid poisoning): an allergy-like intoxication, *Clin. Toxicol.*, 27, 225.

ten Brink, B., Damink, C., Joosten, H.M.L.J. and Huis in't Veld, J.H.J. (1990). Occurrence and formation of biologically active amines in foods, *Int. Food Microbiol.*, 11, 73.

Teodorovic, V., Buncic, S. and Smiljanic, D. (1994). A study of factors influencing histamine production in meat, *Fleischwirtschaft*, 74, 170.

Tiecco, G., Marcotrigiano, G. and De Natale, G. (1985). Detemiazione dell'istamina de altre ammine biogene con la cromatografia liquida ad alta resoluzione negli insaccati, *Industrie Alimentarie*, 24, 122.

Trevino, E., Beil, D. and Steinhart, H. (1997). Formation of biogenic amines during the maturity process of raw meat products, for example of cervelat sausage, *Food Chem.*, 60, 4, 521–526.

Uragoda, C.G. and Lodha, S.C. (1979). Histamine intoxication in a tuberculosis patient after ingestion of cheese, *Tubercle*, 60, 56.

Vandekerckhove, P. (1977). Amines in dry fermented sausage, *J. Food Sci.*, 42, 283.

Veciana-Nogues, M., Marine-Font, A. and Vidal-Carou, M.C. (1997). Biogenic amines as hygienic quality indicators of tuna. Relationships with microbial counts, ATP-related compounds, volatile amines and organoleptic changes, *Jl. Agric. Food Chem.*, 45, 2036.

Vidal, M.C., Izquierdo, M.L., Martin, M.C. and Marine, A. (1990). Histamine and tyramine in meat-products, *Revista de Agroquimica y Tecnologia de Alimentos*, 30, 102.

Vidal-Carou, M.C., Izquierdo-Pulido, M.L., Martin-Morro, M. and Marine-Font, A. (1990). Histamine and tyramine in meat products: relationship with meat spoilage, *Food Chem.*, 37, 239.

Voigt, M.N. and Eitenmiller, R.R. (1978). Role of histidine and tyrosine decarboxylases and mono diamine oxidases in amine build-up in cheese, *J. Food Prot.*, 41, 182.

Wendakoon, C.N. and Sakaguchi, M. (1992). Nonvolatile amine production in mackerel muscle during growth of different bacterial species, *J. Food Hyg. Soc. Jpn.*, 33, 39.

Wendakoon, C., Murata, M. and Sakaguchi, M. (1990). Comparison of nonvolatile amine formation between the dark and white muscles of mackerel during storage, *Nippon Suisan Gakkaishi*, 56, 809.

Wendakoon, C. and Sakaguchi. M. (1992A). Effects of spices on growth of and biogenic amine formation by bacteria in fish muscle, in Huss, H., Jakobsen, M. and Liston, J., *Quality Assurance in the Fish Industry*, Developments in Food Science, Elsevier, Amsterdam, pp. 305–313.

Yen, G. (1986). Determination of biogenic amines in fermented soybean foods by HPLC, *J. Chin. Agric. Chem. Soc.*, 24, 211.

Zee, J.A. and Simard, R.E. (1981). Biogenic amines in Canadian, American, and European beers, *Can. Inst. Food Sci. Tech. J.*, 14, 119.

Zotos, A., Hole, M. and Smith, G. (1995). The effect of frozen storage of mackerel (*Scomber scombrus*) on its quality when hot-smoked, *J. Sci. Food Agric.*, 67, 43.

7

Marine Phycotoxins in Seafood

Lorraine C. Backer, Helen Schurz-Rogers,
Lora E. Fleming, Barbara Kirkpatrick,
and Janet Benson

CONTENTS

7.1   INTRODUCTION

Seafood constitutes a significant proportion of the world food supply, and more than 70 million tons are harvested each year. Per capita global annual seafood consumption averaged about 13 kg in the mid 1990s (Lipp and Rose, 1997) and estimated seafood consumption in the U.S. in 2000 was 9 kg per person per year (Spalding, 1995). Although it is an important and popular food source, seafood ingestion is not free from associated public-health risks. In fact, seafood ranked third on the list of products most frequently associated with foodborne disease (Lipp and Rose, 1997); one type of seafood-related disease, ciguatera fish poisoning, is the most commonly reported food poisoning caused by a chemical toxin (Centers for Disease Control and Prevention, 1996).

The vast majority of food poisoning cases associated with seafood ingestion are caused by postharvest contamination with infectious organisms (e.g., *Salmonella* spp., *Campylobacter* spp., *Clostridium botulinum*, *Shigella* spp., or *Listeria* spp.) or with toxins of bacterial origin (e.g., scombroid poisoning from high levels of histamine produced by *Vibrio* spp.), or are the result of allergies to shellfish (Lipp and Rose, 1997). Other adverse health effects are associated with eating seafood contaminated with chemicals (e.g., mercury). However, there is another group of diseases characterized by both acute and chronic neurologic symptoms of varying intensity and duration that is associated with eating shellfish and large reef fish. These diseases are caused by contamination of seafood with potent neurotoxins that are naturally produced by marine algae.

Algae and microalgae are found in the marine environment throughout the world. Many types of microalgae, such as dinoflagellates and diatoms, produce some of the most powerful known natural toxins. Under certain environmental conditions, algae rapidly multiply to produce blooms. When algal blooms pose environmental or health hazards, they are termed harmful algal blooms (HABs). The reasons why blooms occur are not known, nor are the reasons for why these organisms produce toxins at some times but not at others. However, it is clear that during HABs, or as a normal consequence of bioaccumulation through the marine food chain or web, the toxins produced by these microalgae, called phycotoxins, may accumulate in a variety of marine organisms. Phycotoxins accumulated in seafood can cause a number of human diseases upon ingestion of the contaminated seafood, including neurotoxic shellfish poisoning (NSP), paralytic shellfish poisoning (PSP), amnesic shellfish poisoning (ASP), diarrheic shellfish poisoning (DSP), and azaspiracid shellfish poisoning (AZP), as well as ciguatera fish poisoning (CFP) (Anderson, 1994; Backer et al., 2003; Baden et al., 1995; Clark et al., 1999; Fleming et al., 2001; Fleming et al., 2002; Halstead et al., 1994; Tester, 1994; Van Dolah, 2000).

These potent natural toxins are tasteless and odorless, and contaminated seafood appears to be completely normal. They are not destroyed by cooking or by food preservation (e.g., freezing, drying, or salting). In addition, these toxins are refractory to the action of human digestive enzymes, and there are no antidotes against their biological activity (Schantz, 1973).

Some evidence exists that HABs are now occurring more frequently and over a wider geographic area than in the past (Epstein et al., 1994; Halstead et al., 1994; Tester, 1994; Todd, 1994; Viviani, 1992). Phycotoxin contamination of seafood is therefore a challenge for those people responsible for ensuring seafood quality and has important implications for public health (including nutrition and medical care).

7.2 ORGANISMS, TOXINS, AND SYNDROMES

7.2.1 INTRODUCTION

The syndromes associated with ingestion of seafood contaminated with marine phycotoxins, their symptoms, causative organisms (including geographic distribution), associated toxins, and molecular mechanisms, have been reviewed in the literature (Baden et al., 1995; Baden and Trainer, 1993; Falconer, 1993). The following sections of this chapter provide information about the organisms and toxins associated with PSP, DSP, NSP, ASP, AZP, and CFP, followed by more general information about the clinical and epidemiologic characteristics of these diseases.

Organisms and toxins associated specifically with PSP, NSP, ASP, AZP, and CFP are summarized below. This information and a list of clinical signs and symptoms of these diseases are summarized in Table 7.1.

7.2.2 ORGANISMS AND TOXINS

7.2.2.1 Paralytic Shellfish Poisoning

The paralytic shellfish poisons include at least 20 derivatives of saxitoxin, which is a tetrahydropurine comprising two guanidinium functions (Baden and Trainer, 1993). Saxitoxins are produced by dinoflagellate species from *Alexandrium* (*Gonyaulax*), *Pyrodinium*, and *Gymnodinium* genera. Paralytic shellfish poisons accumulate in bivalves (e.g., clams, mussels), coral reef crabs, and certain gastropods that eat these microalgae (Kotaki et al., 1981; Noguchi

Table 7.1

Characteristics of human diseases and conditions caused by eating seafood contaminated with phycotoxins.

Characteristic	Diseases and conditions						
	Paralytic shellfish poisoning (PSP) and puffer fish poisoning	Neurotoxic shellfish poisoning (NSP)	Diarrheic shellfish poisoning (DSP)	Amnesic shellfish poisoning (ASP)	Azaspiracid shellfish poisoning (AZP)	Ciguatera fish poisoning (CFP)
Main area with endemic disease	Temperate areas worldwide	Gulf of Mexico, southern U.S. coast, New Zealand	Europe, Japan	East and west coasts of North America	Europe	Tropical coral reefs
Associated foods (transvectors)	Bivalve shellfish, primarily scallops, mussels, clams, oysters, and cockles Specific herbivorous fish and crabs	Bivalve shellfish, primarily mussels, oysters, scallops	Bivalve shellfish, primarily scallops, mussels, clams, and oysters	Bivalve shellfish, primarily scallops, mussels, clams, oysters Possibly some fish species	Bivalve shellfish	Large reef fish, e.g., barracuda (most common), grouper, red snapper, and amberjack
Acute symptoms	Gastrointestinal: diarrhea, nausea, vomiting Respiratory: shortness of breath, progressing to paralysis Cardiovascular: arrythmias, hypertension or hypotension Neurologic: paresthesias of mouth and lips, weakness, dysphasia, dysphonia	Gastrointestinal: diarrhea, nausea, vomiting Respiratory: shortness of breath Cardiovascular: arrythmias, hypertension or hypotension Neurologic: paresthesias of mouth lips, tongue, and throat; dizziness; reversal of hot and cold sensations Other: muscular aches	Gastrointestinal: nausea, vomiting, diarrhea, abdominal pain Other: chills, headache, and fever	Gastrointestinal: diarrhea, vomiting, abdominal pain Respiratory: shortness of breath. Cardiovascular: arrythmias, hypertension or hypotension Neurologic: paresthesias (especially reversal of hot and cold sensation), burning in teeth or extremities, confusion, memory loss, disorientation, seizure and coma	Gastrointestinal: diarrhea, vomiting, abdominal pain	*2–6 hr postexposure:* Gastrointestinal: diarrhea, nausea, vomiting *3 hr postexposure:* Neurologic: paresthesias, reversal of hot and cold sensation, pain, weakness *2–5 days postexposure:* Cardiovascular: bradycardia, hypotension, increase in T wave abnormalities

Chronic symptoms	Unknown	Unknown	Unknown Possible carcinogen	Amnesia	Unknown	Paresthesias
Treatment	Supportive care Possibly respiratory support	Supportive care	Supportive care	Supportive care, especially for elderly and people with renal disease	Supportive care	IV Mannitol Supportive care Tricyclic antidepressants Children more vulnerable than adults
Incubation time	5–30 min	30 min–24 hours	<24 hours	<24 hours	<24 hours	<24 hours
Duration	Days	Days	Days	Years	Days	Months
Death rate	1–14%	0%	0%	3%	Unknown	0.1–12%
Toxin (number)	Saxitoxin (≥20)	Brevetoxin (≥10)	Okadaic acid Dinophysistoxins (≥6)	Domoic acid (3)	Azaspiracid (5)	Ciguatoxin (≥10) Maitotoxin Scaritoxin
Toxin-producing organism	Dinoflagellates: *Gymnodinium catenatum*, *Pyrodinium bahamense* var. *compressum*, *Alexandrium* spp.	Dinoflagellate: *Karenia brevis* (formerly *Gymnodinium breve*)	Dinoflagellates: *Dinophysis* spp., *Prorocentrum lima*	Diatoms: *Pseudo-nitzschia* spp.	Dinoflagellates: *Protoperidinium* spp.	Epibenthic dinoflagellates: *Gambierdiscus toxicus* Possibly *Ostreopsis* spp.; *Coolia* spp.; or *Prorocentrum* spp.
Molecular mechanism(s)	Na$^+$ channel blocker	Na$^+$ channel activator	Phosphorylase phosphatase inhibitor	Glutamate receptor agonist	Unknown	Na$^+$, Ca^{++} channel activators

Table 7.1
(Continued)

Characteristic	Diseases and conditions					
	Paralytic shellfish poisoning (PSP) and puffer fish poisoning	Neurotoxic shellfish poisoning (NSP)	Diarrheic shellfish poisoning (DSP)	Amnesic shellfish poisoning (ASP)	Azaspiracid shellfish poisoning (AZP)	Ciguatera fish poisoning (CFP)
Biochemical site of action	Site 1 on voltage-dependent sodium channel	Site 5 on voltage-dependent sodium channel	Catalytic subunit of phosphorylase phosphatases	Kainate receptor in central nervous system	Unknown	Ciguatoxin: site 5 on voltage-dependent sodium channel Maitotoxin: calcium channels
Physiologic effect	Inhibition of ion conductance	Repetitive firing, shift of voltage dependence of activation	Inhibition of phosphorylase phosphatases 1 and 2a	Receptor-induced depolarization and excitation	Unknown	Ciguatoxin: repetitive firing, shift of voltage dependence of activation Maitotoxin: calcium ion influx

Sources: Backer et al. (2003); Baden et al. (1995); Baden and Trainer (1993); Fleming et al. (2001).

et al., 1969; Raj et al., 1983). Evidence from an incident in Indonesia also indicates that these toxins can accumulate in clupeoid fish (Kao, 1993).

Saxitoxin has a relaxant action on vascular smooth muscle (Kao et al., 1971). Specifically, the paralytic shellfish poisons act on membranes to block the inward flow of sodium ions through the voltage-gated sodium channel in a dose-dependent manner. The voltage-gated sodium channel is a protein of approximately 250,000 Da. The sodium (Na) channel is present in many excitable cells, including mammalian nerves, skeletal muscle, and cardiac muscle fibers (Kao, 1993). When a cell is depolarized, the conformation of the sodium channel molecule changes to permit movement of Na^+ into the cell. The toxins bind to resting, active, or inactive Na channels, but they have no effect on resting membrane potential or potassium channels (Baden and Trainer, 1993). Although tetrodotoxin (from puffer fish) possesses a different chemical structure and is not a phycotoxin, it produces nearly identical neurologic effects to those produced by the paralytic shellfish poisons.

Historically, PSP has occurred in North America (the Pacific Northwest and the Northeast) and Europe (Acres and Gray, 1978; Anderson, 1989). More recently, PSP has been reported in Japan, Malaysia, the Philipines, Indonesia, Latin America, and China (Anderson et al., 1996; Kao, 1993). The fatality rate for PSP varies on the basis of local health-care practitioner awareness of the disease and its treatment and on the capacity of the existing medical system to assist one or more poisoning victims needing respiratory support. For example, in recent outbreaks in Europe and North America, no deaths occurred among more than 200 cases. However, in similar outbreaks in southeast Asia and Latin America, where the disease is unfamiliar to local health practitioners and where health-care resources are limited, fatality rates of 2 to 14% have been reported (Kao, 1993).

7.2.2.2 Diarrheic Shellfish Poisoning

The toxins responsible for DSP include a series of polyether molecules (including okadaic acid and six derivatives of dinophysistoxin), four pectenotoxins (polyether lactones), and yessotoxins (including two sulfate esters that resemble brevetoxins) (Murata, 1982; Murata, 1987; Tachibana et al., 1981; Yasumoto, 1989). Diarrhetic shellfish poisons are produced primarily by dinoflagellates from the genera *Dinophysis*, although *Prorocentrum lima* also produces both okadaic acid and dinophysistoxin-1 (Heredia-Tapia et al., 2002).

Okadaic acid is a powerful tumor promoter of a nonphorbol ester type that inhibits protein phosphatase-1 and -2A *in vitro* (Haystead et al., 1989). Okadaic acid directly stimulates smooth muscle contraction (Haystead et al., 1989) and probably causes diarrhea, either by stimulating the phosphorylation of proteins controlling sodium secretion by intestinal cells or by increasing phosphorylation of elements that regulate permeability to solutes, resulting in a passive loss of fluids (Aune and Yndestad, 1993).

The biological activities of the other diarrhetic shellfish poisons are not well understood, and some of the toxins included in the DSP 'complex' may not be associated with adverse health effects in people. Some of the physiologic effects reported after intraperitoneal injection into mice include hepatotoxicity (from pectenotoxin-1), cardiac muscle lesions (from yessotoxin), and intestinal damage (from dinophysistoxin-1) (Terao et al., 1986; Terao et al., 1990).

DSP has been reported in Japan and Europe (Kat, 1983; Yasumoto et al., 1978) as well as in India and North and South America (Aune and Yndestad, 1993). Furthermore, although DSP has not been reported in humans, the toxins have been isolated from *Prorocentrum lima* cultures from the Gulf of California, Mexico (Heredia-Tapia et al., 2002).

7.2.2.3 Neurotoxic Shellfish Poisoning

The ten known brevetoxins associated with NSP are produced by the dinoflagellate **Karenia brevis** (formerly known as *Gymnodinium breve* and *Ptychodiscus brevis*), which is the organism associated with Florida red tides (Steidinger, 1983). Brevetoxins also have been associated with blooms of *Chattonella cf. verruculosa* that were responsible for fish kills in Delaware, U.S., during the summer of 2000 (Naar et al., 2002). Compared with saxitoxins, which block Na^+ ion influx, brevetoxins specifically induce a channel-mediated Na^+ ion influx (Baden and Trainer, 1993). Although evidence suggests that brevetoxins affect mammalian cortical synaptosomes and neuromuscular preparations (Gallagher and Shinnick, 1980; Risk et al., 1982), all of the effects associated with brevetoxins result from the substantial and persistent depolarization of predominantly nerve membranes (Wu and Narahashi, 1988).

NSP has been reported from the southeastern coast of the U.S., the Gulf of Mexico, and New Zealand (Ishida et al., 1996). Few cases of NSP occur in the U.S. because of comprehensive monitoring programs that periodically sample shellfish and the waters where shellfish are harvested. If shellfish or seawater samples are contaminated with brevetoxins, harvesting is stopped until the shellfish have depurated the toxin and are again safe to eat.

NSP has been identified outside the typical geographic area where *K. brevis* is found. In 1987, an unusual movement of ocean currents carried a red tide from the Gulf of Mexico to the coast of North Carolina (Morris et al., 1991). People there were unaware of the risks associated with eating shellfish during a red tide, and an outbreak of NSP associated with eating contaminated shellfish occurred in November.

7.2.2.4 Amnesiac Shellfish Poisoning

ASP is caused by eating shellfish contaminated with one or more of three domoic acid derivatives, which are excitatory neurotoxic amino acids (Baden and Trainer, 1993). Domoic acid is produced by the diatom *Nitzchia pungens* and accumulates in mussels, specifically *Mytilus edulis* (Baden and Trainer, 1993). Domoic acid is similar in structure to the excitatory dicarboxylic amino acid, kainic acid, and has an antagonistic effect at the glutamate receptor. Both of these compounds cause glutamate-induced neuronal depolarization and an excitatory effect in invertebrates (Shinozaki and Ishida, 1976; Takeuchi et al., 1984).

The first cases of ASP were identified after an outbreak associated with eating cultivated mussels harvested from Prince Edward Island, Canada (Perl et al., 1990; Todd, 1990b). Domoic acid also has been implicated in the deaths of marine mammals along the U.S. Pacific coast (Scholin et al., 2000), and human diseases from eating shellfish contaminated with domoic acid have been anecdotally reported in the U.S. Pacific Northwest.

7.2.2.5 Azaspiracid Shellfish Poisoning

AZP, the most-recently characterized marine seafood poisoning, is associated with eating shellfish contaminated with azaspiracids. The first human intoxications attributed to AZP occurred in the Netherlands, and the symptoms included those similar to DSP (i.e., nausea, vomiting, severe diarrhea, and stomach cramps). However, although chemical analyses did not identify significant levels of the diarrhetic shellfish poisons, they identified a new class of toxins (James et al., 2003a).

The azaspiracids are another class of polyether toxins with unique spiro ring assemblies, a cyclic amine and a carboxylic acid. Five analogs have been described (Ofuji et al., 1999, 2001; Satake et al., 1998). Azaspiracids are produced by species of the dinoflagellate *Protoperidinium*, a phytoplankton genus historically thought to be benign (James et al., 2003a).

Little information exists about the mechanism of action of the azaspiracids. The chronic effects observed in mice after oral administration of azaspiracid included interstitial pneumonia, shortened villi in the stomach and small intestine, fatty changes in the liver, and necrosis of lymphocytes in the thymus and spleen (Ito et al., 2002).

The original cases of AZP were reported in the Netherlands in 1995 and were associated with eating mussels harvested in Ireland (McMahon and Silke, 1996, 1998). AZP in humans has been reported throughout Europe since 1995, and azaspiracids have been found in shellfish harvested in Spain, France, and northern Europe (James et al., 2002; Magdalena et al., 2003a).

7.2.2.6 Ciguatera Fish Poisoning

Ten known derivatives of ciguatoxin and maitotoxin are the phycotoxins associated with CFP. They were believed to be produced by the dinoflagellate *Gambierdiscus toxicus* (Bagnis et al., 1980; Yasumoto, 1979). However, scientists now believe that *G. toxicus* actually produces precursors that are metabolized to the toxic ciguatoxins and maitotoxins by predator organisms (Murata et al., 1990). These toxins accumulate in large, primarily predatory, reef fish such as barracuda and grouper. Ciguatoxin and brevetoxin have some immunologic crossreactivity and thus have at least some similar epitopic sites (Hokama, 1984). The effects of ciguatoxin are caused by the opening of Na^+

channels at resting potential and the inability of the open channels to be inactivated during subsequent depolarization (Baden and Trainer, 1993). The physiologic activity of ciguatoxins is thought to involve both α-adrenergic and cholinergic systems (Baden and Trainer, 1993).

Maitotoxin is found with ciguatoxins in ciguateric fish and, along with ciguatoxin, is one of the most potent natural toxins known. It typically is produced by *Gambierdiscus toxicus* in greater quantity than the ciguatoxins (Wu and Narahashi, 1988). In smooth muscle and skeletal muscle *in vitro*, maitotoxin causes calcium ion-dependent contraction (Ohizumi and Yasumoto, 1983; Ohizumi et al., 1983). Maitotoxin may act on membranes to create a pore that allows Ca^+ ions to flow through the membrane (Murata et al., 1991; Wu and Narahashi, 1988).

CFP in humans has been reported in a circumglobal belt extending approximately from latitude 35° north to 34° south (Hessel et al., 1960), which includes Hawaii, the South Pacific, the Caribbean and Indo-Pacific, and the U.S. Virgin Islands (Bagnis et al., 1979; Hokama et al., 1993; Lange, 1987; Morris, Jr. et al., 1982a, 1982b). Although typically not considered important in the Gulf of Mexico, ciguateric fish have been caught off the west coast of Florida (Morton and Burklew, 1970) and the Texas coast (Villareal, 2003).

The risk of CFP and the severity of disease symptoms may be associated with population sensitivity to the disease and a variety of other conditions. These conditions include the location where the fish was caught, the amount and parts of the fish eaten, fish species, fish size, seasonal fish distribution patterns, types of toxins present, and local ecologic reef disturbances (Lange et al., 1992).

7.2.3 CLINICAL ASPECTS OF MARINE SEAFOOD TOXIN SYNDROMES

7.2.3.1 General Issues

In general, the clinical presentation of the human diseases associated with the ingestion of marine seafood toxins is similar to that of any other food poisoning disease. However, a number of clinical issues make these diseases particularly difficult to diagnose and treat. For example, the neurotoxic syndromes associated with CFP, PSP, and NSP represent points along a continuum of disease severity rather than clinically exclusive diseases. Even if fish or other seafood is the suspected source of a disease outbreak, diarrhea associated with the outbreak could be misdiagnosed as originating from bacterial rather than from phycotoxin contamination.

No specific biomarkers of either effect or exposure are available to test for these diseases in people (Backer et al., 2003; Fleming et al., 2001, 2002). Testing the contaminated seafood for toxins is the only definitive way to make a diagnosis; however, this testing is specialized and not readily available in most clinical settings. Seafood poisonings are therefore typically diagnosed on the basis of the clinical report of signs and symptoms and a recent history of eating seafood. Because the transvector (i.e., the specific contaminated food) is the only significant difference between seafood poisoning and other types of food poisoning, food ingestion history is extremely important in diagnosing these diseases. However, except in areas where marine seafood poisonings are endemic, healthcare professionals are not likely to recognize these diseases in their patients. Consequently, rather than being asked a few simple questions about what they ate, people may be subjected to expensive medical evaluations, and even inappropriate treatment, before illness is correctly diagnosed (Lange et al., 1992; Todd, 1990a). Failure to recognize these diseases also may affect the ultimate outcome for a person. For example, rapid, accurate diagnosis and treatment of CFP within the first 72 hours after exposure may be critical in preventing some of the neurologic symptoms that might otherwise become chronic and debilitating.

Other characteristics of the toxins and toxin-contaminated seafood can also complicate diagnoses. For example, although these toxins are typically associated with ingestion of seafood, they can contaminate other species (due to specific environmental conditions or other biologic parameters that are not yet understood). Both gonyautoxin (a paralytic shellfish poison) and tetrodotoxin have been reported in xanthid crabs, with different relative amounts of the two toxins in crabs harvested from different geographic areas, probably depending on the specific exogenous source of the toxins (Tsai et al., 1995, 1997). In an investigation of an outbreak in Taiwan associated with eating mussels, the occurrence of hypertension in the victims led investigators to postulate that tetrodotoxin, and not paralytic shellfish poisons, caused the cases (Yang et al., 1995). Because of the similar biologic activity and because these toxins can be found together in the same animals, some investigators suggested that these diseases be regarded together as a 'pelagic paralysis' (Kanchanapongkul and Tantraphon, 1993).

Differences in geographic distribution of the microalgae, the toxins they produce, and the organisms that feed on them, further complicate correct diagnosis of marine seafood toxin poisonings. Kodama et al. (1989) reported that toxins extracted from groups of fish of two different, but closely related, species caught in Tahiti or Hawaii were pharmacologically similar, but the toxin extracted from the Tahitian fish was more potent than the toxin extracted from the Hawaiian fish. The authors suggested that the toxicity of the fish was therefore related not only to feeding on a particular benthic dinoflagellate species (*Gambierdiscus toxicus*), but also perhaps to feeding on a specific strain of *G. toxicus*. Similar findings have been reported for DSP (Kumagai, 1986; Murata, 1982).

Another complication associated with correct diagnosis of these diseases is international trade and travel. People eating seafood while traveling may not become ill until they return home, and people eating imported seafood may be unaware of the risks associated with certain fish and shellfish. A physician unfamiliar with these diseases and who is faced with diagnosing a patient's illness may therefore misinterpret the severity of symptoms or the history of food consumption and inappropriately eliminate ciguatera or shellfish poisonings from the differential diagnosis, or not even consider them.

7.2.3.2 Signs and Symptoms of Marine Phycotoxin-Associated Diseases

People suffering from signs and symptoms of human illnesses associated with eating seafood contaminated with marine phycotoxins (Table 7.1) typically present at emergency departments or their physicians' offices with the acute onset (within minutes to 24 hours) of gastrointestinal symptoms. Victims also may exhibit a wide range of signs and symptoms involving many organ systems, including respiration (e.g., difficulty breathing), the peripheral nervous system (e.g., diverse paresthesias), the central nervous system (e.g., hallucinations and memory loss), and the cardiovascular system (e.g., labile blood pressure and arrythmias). These signs and symptoms, depending on the particular disease, may last from hours to months.

Originally associated only with acute health effects lasting a few days to a few weeks, several, if not all, of the human diseases associated with eating phycotoxin-contaminated marine seafood now can be associated with chronic disease. For example, CFP may result in prolonged debilitating paresthesias, ranging from extreme fatigue to pain in the joints, and changes in temperature sensation that can last from weeks to months, and possibly to years (Blythe et al., 1994; Glaziou and Legrand, 1994; Lehane and Lewis, 2000; Quod and Turquet, 1996). Also, although no long-term follow-up has been done with ASP victims, the short-term memory loss associated with ASP appears to be permanent (Perl et al., 1990). No systematic studies of the possible chronic health effects associated with the other shellfish poisonings have been conducted.

7.2.3.3 Prevention and Treatment

Primary prevention has been the most frequently recommended and most obvious intervention for the human diseases associated with eating marine seafood contaminated with toxins. The populations most likely to be exposed to, and thus affected by, HAB toxins include: those occupationally involved in seafood harvesting, shipping, and processing; seafood consumers (including those eating seafood they caught or seafood served in a restaurant); environmental workers (especially those collecting samples); persons who work and play on or near the water; and coastal communities, especially indigenous people who rely on seafood for a substantial proportion of their diet. For these groups, primary prevention for CFP, for example, would require that people avoid catching, handling, or eating large reef fish. However, in island communities where fish (including reef fish) is an important source of protein, simply avoiding fish would have significant nutritional implications (Lehane and Lewis, 2000; Lewis, 1986). Banning or severely limiting seafood harvesting would also have a significant impact on commercial and recreational fishing.

Epidemiologic and laboratory methods can help identify food and toxins associated with a particular disease outbreak. However, very little clinical research has been conducted to determine effective treatments for these diseases; and medical care is primarily supportive (Blythe, 2001). The exception is acute CFP where rapidly administering intravenous mannitol has provided symptom relief and possibly prevented development of chronic symptoms. However, a series of clinical trials to examine the efficacy of using intravenous mannitol to treat acute CFP produced controversial and inconsistent results (Blythe, 2001; Palafox et al., 1988; Schnorf et al., 2002; Ting and Brown, 2001). In addition, whether the particular combination or concentrations of ciguatera toxins present have any implications for treatment or recovery is still unclear (Lehane and Lewis, 2000).

7.2.4 EPIDEMIOLOGY

Epidemiologic data are scarce for marine seafood toxin syndromes. Whether HAB-related diseases from eating seafood truly have increased or whether the baseline disease incidence rates are simply unknown is not clear. Part of the difficulty in understanding the baseline incidence and prevalence of these diseases is the geographic variability of the species distributions, toxin characteristics, and the clinical presentation of the diseases themselves. For example, CFP can manifest as primarily gastrointestinal symptoms followed in some victims by neurologic symptoms if the implicated fish was caught in the Caribbean. However, if the fish was a species found in the Pacific, a different toxin profile and clinical presentation (i.e., primarily neurologic symptoms followed by gastrointestinal complaints) might be reported (Lehane and Lewis, 2000).

Diseases associated with marine seafood toxins appear to have high attack rates. An attack rate is the proportion of a well-defined population that develops a disease over a specific period of time (where the numerator is the number of new cases during that period and the denominator is the size of the population at risk, e.g., the number of people who ate a contaminated food at the start of the time period of interest) (Goodman and Peavy, 1996). Physicians therefore need to ask about disease cases among people sharing the same seafood meal.

These diseases have historically been limited to certain geographic areas (such as subtropical and tropical islands for CFP) (Lehane and Lewis, 2000). However, international travel and the global seafood trade have increased the likelihood of these diseases in areas in which they are not endemic (Ting and Brown, 2001). In addition, these diseases may occur more commonly among people in ethnic subpopulations who have risky seafood ingestion patterns (e.g., subsistence fishing), particularly if they are not reached by the public-health authorities (Fleming et al., 2002; Shubat et al., 1996). Healthcare personnel, particularly in areas where these diseases are not endemic, rarely report diagnoses to the public-health authorities, even when reporting is mandatory (Lehane and Lewis, 2000; McKee et al., 2001).

7.2.5 PUBLIC HEALTH IMPACT

Poisonings associated with eating seafood significantly impact public health worldwide. For example during 1971 to 1990, seafood was the most important vehicle in food poisoning outbreaks in Korea (32%) and Japan (22%) and was responsible for 43% and 62%, respectively, of outbreak-related fatalities (Chan, 1995; Lee, 1996).

In the U.S., fish and shellfish caused at least one in six food poisoning outbreaks with known etiologies, and 15% of the deaths associated with these outbreaks during 1988 to 1992. This is a marked increase over the preceding decade, when seafood consumption was associated with 10% of foodborne disease outbreaks that had identified etiologies (Ahmed, 1992; Centers for Disease Control and Prevention, 1996; Lipp and Rose, 1997).

Accurate estimates of the public health costs of human diseases caused by toxins in marine seafood requires a better understanding of their prevalence and incidence, as well as their acute and chronic health effects in humans. For example, CFP, the most commonly reported foodborne disease caused by a chemical toxin, accounts for more than half the food poisonings associated with fish in the U.S. (Lange, 1987). Despite the apparent importance of CFP as a foodborne disease, information about actual disease rates is limited (Gollop and Pon, 1992; Morris, Jr. et al., 1982a; Quod and Turquet, 1996). Even less information is available about PSP (Gessner and Schloss, 1996), and essentially nothing has been published about disease rates for the other shellfish poisonings. Furthermore, any estimates that do exist apply only to specific geographic areas (e.g., island communities) and cannot be extrapolated to estimate disease rates worldwide. Documented cases of disease from marine seafood toxins probably represent only a minute percentage of the cases that occur. Existing data collection mechanisms rely not only on the correct diagnosis but also on reporting of the case to a disease surveillance program. For foodborne diseases in general, and for these associated with contaminated seafood in particular, basic disease reporting is sporadic. For example, during 1988 to 1992, 165 CFP cases and 65 PSP cases were reported to the Center for Disease Control (CDC) (Centers for Disease Control and Prevention, 1996). However, CDC estimates that fewer than 0.3% of disease outbreaks from contaminated food were actually identified and reported to the CDC system. As many as 50,000 unreported cases of ciguatera and PSP may have occurred in the U.S. during those five years.

Even in areas in which shellfish poisonings are endemic, cases of these diseases are substantially under-reported. McKee et al. (2001) studied the diagnosis, treatment, and reporting of CFP in Miami-Dade County, Florida. They found that physicians had little experience of recognizing the disease, were unaware of a possible treatment (i.e., intravenously administered mannitol), and were thus unable to provide information to their patients to prevent further cases of the disease. This suggests that, despite the fact that these diseases have been known for more than 150 years, the diseases associated with phycotoxins in seafood represent a substantial, but as yet undefined, public health risk.

7.2.6 ECONOMIC IMPACT

Historically, marine seafood poisonings were limited to geographic areas where specific algae and host organisms (e.g., clams, mussels, reef fishes) thrived (i.e., temperate to tropical coastlines and coral reefs). However, as seafood consumption, trade, and tourism become global, these diseases are expanding beyond their traditional geographic boundaries and may be increasing in incidence (Hallegraeff, 1992; Ting and Brown, 2001; Van Dolah, 2000). One result of this globalization is the high cost of diagnosis and treatment in areas where these diseases are not endemic. For example, in 1997 Todd reported that approximately 300 cases of CFP in Canada occurred in people who had eaten imported fish or traveled to areas where CFP is endemic or common (Todd, 1997). The cost of diagnosing one of those ciguatera cases was approximately $4000 (Canadian), with a total annual cost as high as $1,236,000 (Canadian).

In addition to the costs associated with acute symptoms, the chronic sequelae from foodborne diseases in general may also have a significant economic impact. Several investigators have estimated that chronic sequelae (including renal disease, cardiac and neurologic disorders, and nutritional and malabsorptive disorders) may occur either directly, because of the acute effects of food poisoning, or indirectly (i.e., triggered by the acute effects), in 2 to 3% of foodborne disease cases (Lindsay, 1997). Based on an annual estimate of 80 million cases of foodborne disease occurring in the U.S., the public-health costs associated with chronic sequelae from foodborne disease in general totals billions of dollars (Bunning et al., 1997).

Anderson et al. (2000) estimated that in the U.S. during 1987 to 1992, $449,291,987 (U.S.) was spent addressing known HAB-related impacts on public health, commercial fisheries, recreation, tourism, monitoring, and bloom management. Public-health impacts were the largest component (45%), followed by commercial fisheries (37%) and tourism (13%). These estimates were believed to be underestimates because they did not include the value of resources that could not be exploited, such as the extensive Alaskan shellfish beds closed to harvesting because of endemic PSP. Nor did the estimates include the public-health impact of people ignoring the official shellfish harvesting closures. Furthermore, effects such as temporary beach closures or delayed shellfish harvests could not be estimated.

Even a single HAB episode can be extremely costly. In Maryland in 1997, reported cases of human disease associated with exposure to water containing *Pfiesteria piscicida* cost the seafood industry alone an estimated $46 million in lost revenue (Anderson et al., 2000). Lewis (1986) found that CFP in the South Pacific depressed both the local and export fishing industries, affected tourism, and indirectly affected human health (because people avoided eating fresh fish).

7.3   TOXIN DETECTION AND MONITORING

7.3.1   INTRODUCTION

One of the most important chemical characteristics associated with the marine phycotoxins is their potency. These compounds are biologically active at concentrations very close to the current analytic limits of detection. One challenge in protecting public health is identifying which toxins are present in food. Another challenge is developing methods to identify the toxins in biological specimens. Even in circumstances where the medical community is aware of marine seafood poisonings, without an assay to evaluate whether a given disease victim actually has been exposed to the toxin, disease diagnosis, treatment, and prognosis still rely on accurate and timely collecting of symptom data and food ingestion history.

7.3.2   DETECTION BY CONSUMERS

People eating fish cannot detect the marine phycotoxins associated with seafood diseases, and preparation procedures do not remove the toxins (Baden et al., 1995; Baden and Mende, 1982; Baden and Trainer, 1993; Sakamoto et al., 1987). Severe heating processes, such as retorting, may reduce the levels of some toxins (U.S. Food and Drug Administration, 2001) but this is not a practical method for protecting public health.

7.3.3   DETECTION IN SEAFOOD

The stability of these toxins allows their detection at very low concentrations in raw and cooked seafood and, in some cases, in biological specimens. Considerable interest exists in developing rapid detection methods than could be performed outside the laboratory setting, such as onboard ship or at the dockside. For example, Hokama (1984) developed an immunoassay stick test to detect ciguatoxins and related polyether toxins in fish tissues. The assay is commercially available for testing for ciguatoxins in fish (under the name Cigua-Check); however, the kit has not been evaluated as a quantitative assay for ciguatoxins. No other methods that can be used on-site to monitor for phycotoxins in seafood are available.

Laboratory methods for detecting marine toxins (Table 7.2) can be characterized into two types of analyses: indirect assays and direct measurement analyses. Indirect assays, or bioassays, measure the biological effect of a toxin on a system and can implicate, but not verify, the presence of a particular toxin. By contrast, direct measurements can both confirm and quantify the amount of a specific toxin in a food or biological specimen.

The mouse bioassay, an indirect assay, historically has been used to evaluate shellfish toxicity (especially for PSP). Other bioassay procedures have been developed but not generally applied for regulatory purposes (Schantz et al., 1958). The mouse bioassay involves intraperitoneal (i.p.)

Table 7.2

Comparison of bioassays and chemical assays for detection of phycotoxins.

Characteristic	Diseases and conditions					
	Paralytic shellfish poisoning (PSP) and puffer fish poisoning	Neurotoxic shellfish poisoning (NSP)	Diarrheic shellfish poisoning (DSP)	Amnesic shellfish poisoning (ASP)	Azaspiracid shellfish poisoning (AZP)	Ciguatera fish poisoning (CFP)
Toxin (primary or class of toxins)	Saxitoxin	Brevetoxin	Okadaic acid, dinophysistoxin	Domoic acid, kainic acid	Azaspiracid	Ciguatoxin
Indirect measurement (bioassay)	Mouse bioassay	Mouse bioassay Neuroblastoma assay (Truman et al., 2002)	Mouse bioassay Protein-phosphatase inhibition assay (Mountfort et al., 2001)	Mouse bioassay	Cytotoxicity assay (Flanagan et al., 2001)	Mouse bioassay Neuroblastoma assay (Matta et al., 2002)
Media measured	Bivalves, puffer fish	Bivalves	Bivalves	Bivalves	Bivalves	Reef fish, coelenterates
Bioassay detection limit	Mouse bioassay: 20 μg STX eq/100 g	Mouse bioassay: 20 μg STX eq/100 g Neuroblastoma assay: 2 μg STX eq/100 g	Mouse bioassay: 20 μg STX eq/100 g Protein-phosphatase inhibition assay: 20 μg STX eq/100 g	Unknown	Unknown	Neuroblastoma assay: 10 ng/mL
Direct measurement (chemical assay)	LC/MS (Dahlmann et al., 2003) ELISA Receptor binding Fluorometric microplate assay (Louzao et al., 2003) MIST Alert (Jellett et al., 2002)	LC/MS (Hua et al., 1995; Nozawa et al., 2003)	LC/MS (Holmes et al., 1999) ELISA (Chin et al., 1995; Imai et al., 2003) Fluorometric microplate assay (Leira et al., 2003) RIA (Levine et al., 1988)	LC/MS (Tor et al., 2003) ELISA (Kawatsu et al., 1999)	LC/MS (James et al., 2003b; Magdalena et al., 2003b)	LC/MS (Lewis et al., 1999) Serum immunoassay (Zlotnick et al., 1995)

Table 7.2
(Continued)

Characteristic	Diseases and conditions					
	Paralytic shellfish poisoning (PSP) and puffer fish poisoning	**Neurotoxic shellfish poisoning (NSP)**	**Diarrheic shellfish poisoning (DSP)**	**Amnesic shellfish poisoning (ASP)**	**Azaspiracid shellfish poisoning (AZP)**	**Ciguatera fish poisoning (CFP)**
Media measured	Shellfish tissue, fish muscle, human urine	Shellfish tissue, algae	Shellfish tissue	Shellfish tissue	Shellfish tissue	Fish muscle, human serum
Chemical assay detection limit	LC/MS: 0.5 ng ELISA: 0.03 ng/mL	LC/MS: 2 ng/g	LC/MS: 0.5 pg ELISA: 7 ng/mL Fluorometric microplate assay: 1 µg/g RIA: 0.2 pmol	LC/MS: 5 ng/ml ELISA: 0.15 ng/mL		LC/MS: 0.1 ng/mL Serum immunoassay: 0.05 ng/mL

Note: LC/MS = liquid chromatography/mass spectrometry.

injection of mice with an extract of the suspected seafood tissue or water sample and carefully monitoring the animals for toxicity symptoms. Toxicity is measured in mouse units (MUs) per 100 g of shellfish meats. An MU is defined as the number of minutes required for a 1 ml injection of the suspected extract to kill a 20 g mouse; the death of 50% of mice in a test in 930 minutes is defined as 1 MU (Steidinger and Penta, 1999). The mouse bioassay can be used to determine whether shellfish are safe to harvest and eat (i.e., if the number of mouse units exceeds a certain threshold, the shellfish beds are closed to harvesting). For example, in Florida, shellfish beds are closed when *K. brevis* cell counts reach approximately 1320 per liter of seawater (typical concentrations are approximately 264 cells or fewer per liter of seawater) (Florida Department of Agriculture and Consumer Services, 2002). The shellfish beds are monitored until the cell counts drop to 1320 or fewer cells per liter of seawater and are reopened when the mouse bioassay detects no toxin in the shellfish. The toxin concentration determined by the mouse bioassay is expressed as equivalents of saxitoxin (i.e., the amount of toxin required to have the same effect in the mouse bioassay as a specified concentration of saxitoxin).

The mouse bioassay is nonspecific and is inherently highly variable, particularly when compared with analytic methods (Sullivan, 1988). In addition, although the i.p. injection is more direct than oral dosing and will give a more sensitive response, this exposure route is not directly relevant for human exposures through seafood ingestion (Yoo et al., 1995). These characteristics, coupled with growing opposition to using mice for testing, have resulted in considerable effort to find an analytic replacement for the mouse bioassay.

Direct measurement analyses applicable for assessing phycotoxins include immunoassays, receptor binding assays, and chromatography methods, alone or in combination with spectrometry. Direct measurement assays are specific for the toxin being measured and are quantitative. On average, detection limits are three orders of magnitude lower than indirect assays; and depending on the method of sample preparation, sample throughput may be higher. However, because of the instrumentation required, these methods are comparatively more expensive than the indirect measurement assays.

Indirect assays and direct measurement analyses used in combination provide powerful tools for determining the identity of toxins in foods implicated during investigations of disease outbreaks. For example, in 2002, consumption of puffer fish from Florida caused neurologic disease in 21 people (Centers for Disease Control and Prevention, 2002). Initially, based on patient symptoms and reported puffer fish ingestion, the outbreak was attributed to tetrodotoxin. A mouse bioassay confirmed the presence of a Na^+-channel blocking toxin, tentatively identified as tetrodotoxin, in unconsumed portions of fish. However, direct measurement analyses (liquid chromatography/mass spectrometry [LC/MS], immunoassay, and receptor binding assay) confirmed the presence of saxitoxin, but not tetrodotoxin, in the fish samples. Analysis of urine samples from the outbreak victims confirmed these findings. This was the first confirmed report of saxitoxin poisoning associated with puffer fish ingestion in North America.

7.3.4 DETECTION IN THE ENVIRONMENT

To assess the risk from eating seafood harvested from a particular area (see below), shellfish monitoring programs rely on finding high numbers of the dinoflagellates or positive results in the mouse bioassay. Therefore, the analytic methods associated with detecting the marine phycotoxins focus primarily on seafood as the medium for analysis. However, as mentioned earlier, the public-health impact of these marine phycotoxin-associated diseases needs further characterization and some of the analytic techniques listed in Table 7.2 have been adapted to analyze environmental samples that may contain low levels of toxin. For example, recent epidemiologic studies have required documentation of human exposure to Florida red tides through seawater and sea-spray aerosols, and so methods have been developed to analyze brevetoxin in seawater and air (Pierce et al., 1992). In addition, the enzyme-linked immunosorbent assay for brevetoxin is being experimentally applied to detect brevetoxin in contaminated seawater and air, as well as in contaminated shellfish (Chu and Fan, 1985; Naar et al., 2002).

7.3.5 MONITORING PHYCOTOXINS IN SEAFOOD

7.3.5.1 Phycotoxin Stability in Seafood

Phycotoxins accumulate in fish and shellfish because of the natural feeding habits of the respective organisms, rather than because of food handling or processing practices. The toxins causing the diseases discussed in this chapter are heat stable (Australia New Zealand Food Authority, 2001; Committee on Evaluation of the Safety of Fishery Products, 1991). Complete inactivation of saxitoxin (associated with PSP) requires at least ten minutes of exposure to 260°C dry heat. Brevetoxins (associated with NSP) were inactivated (i.e., to levels below the limit of assay detection using Japanese medaka [*Oryzias latipes*]) by exposure to 500°C heat for 10 to 15 minutes (Poli, 1988). Complete inactivation required 10 minutes exposure to 2760°C dry heat (Wannamacher, 2000).

7.3.5.2 Phycotoxins in Seafood

Coupled with successful primary prevention are ongoing monitoring programs for the organisms and their toxins, both in the environment and in the seafood. The molluscan shellfish (i.e., oysters, clams, mussels, and scallops) are the species associated with shellfish poisonings. The absence of characteristics such as abnormal taste, smell, or appearance precludes sensory inspection for these toxins. Instead, ensuring seafood safety relies on testing seawater and the seafood itself. The assays used to detect toxins in seafood have evolved as analytic methods and instrumentation have improved. The American Public

Health Association has developed a series of recommendations for conducting and interpreting these assays (Hosty et al., 1970) in an attempt to standardize testing.

In addition to recommendations for seawater and seafood testing, 'shellfish control authorities', which are entities of state or national governments, have the responsibility to determine the risks associated with specific shellfish-harvesting waters based on the presence of natural toxins. As a result of routine monitoring, harvesting of seafood from these areas may be limited to certain times of the year or to specific environmental conditions.

No authorities are officially responsible for monitoring for ciguatera, which is associated with large reef fish, e.g., barracuda, grouper, red snapper, or parrotfish (U.S. Food and Drug Administration, 2001). Some U.S. states release advisories regarding reefs that are known to contain ciguatoxic fish, and commercial fishermen informally share information about the locations of reefs where ciguatoxic fish have been caught (U.S. Food and Drug Administration, 1995). However, because fish are highly mobile, these activities do not ensure that a given fish, even if harvested outside the waters that contain ciguatoxic fish, will be safe to eat.

Local regulations controlling the harvest and sales of seafood may be more specific. For example, based on ciguatera testing in the 1980s, Dade County, Florida, has completely banned the sale of barracuda within the county (Lawrence et al., 1980).

In general, food processing operations, such as those producing meat and dairy products, are monitored for food safety using spot-checks of manufacturing processes and random sampling and analysis of finished products. Shellfish monitoring is much more difficult because of the large number of species involved, the variability of collecting sites, and the diversity of products. Furthermore, shellfish monitoring is not continuous and is typically conducted away from the harvesting area.

This nonsystematic approach to monitoring has proven inadequate for protecting the U.S. food supply. In response, the FDA enacted the Hazard Analysis and Critical Control Points (HACCP) program of 1997 (U.S. Food and Drug Administration, 1995, 2001). In the U.S., the FDA has established action levels in suspect seafood for the toxins causing some of the shellfish poisonings (see Table 7.3). When an action level is reached, the HACCP plan must be followed to prevent unsafe product from reaching consumers.

One important issue associated with these principles is defining an appropriate sampling regime. A sampling regime must account for what is known about the occurrence of these toxins, including the distribution of specific toxins within the flesh of individual fish as well as among individual fish and different fish species. Another difficulty associated with monitoring seafood safety is the large percentage of imported seafood.

Global seafood safety standards have not been established, and the FDA estimates that more than half of the seafood eaten in the U.S. is imported, from a total of 135 countries. The FDA now requires seafood importers to verify that their overseas suppliers comply with the National Shellfish Sanitation

Table 7.3

U.S. Food and Drug Administration (FDA) action levels in seafood for the toxins associated with shellfish poisonings.

Shellfish poisoning	U.S. FDA action level
Paralytic shellfish poisoning	0.8 ppm saxitoxin equivalent[a]
Diarrheic shellfish poisoning	0.2 ppm okadaic acid plus 35-methyl okadaic acid (diphysistoxin-1)
Neurotoxic shellfish poisoning	20 mouse units/100 g shellfish brevetoxin-2 equivalent
Amnesiac shellfish poisoning	20 ppm domoic acid
	30 ppm domoic acid in viscera of Dungeness crab

[a]The amount of total PSP toxins equivalent in toxicity to 0.8 ppm saxitoxin.

Program and that imported seafood is processed under HACCP controls. The World Health Organization also supports the HACCP plan (World Health Organization, 1995). However, because compliance with this program is costly, many countries comply with these standards only for exported shellfish.

One example of a successful monitoring program is that coordinated by the Florida Department of Environmental Protection, mentioned earlier. Because the monitoring program includes analyzing seawater and shellfish for *K. brevis* and brevetoxin concentrations, respectively, and because emergency-response plans require authorities to close shellfish harvesting when the shellfish become toxic, the incidence of NSP in Florida is low.

In summary, monitoring seawater and seafood for phycotoxins is expensive and not entirely successful. For example, environmental monitoring works only if blooms of the HAB organism are recognized as historical or current events. If uncharacterized organisms produce toxins, or if known organisms produce undescribed toxins that contaminate seafood, the impact on people will not be suspected until an actual outbreak is investigated.

7.4 MITIGATING THE IMPACT OF HARMFUL ALGAL BLOOMS

7.4.1 INTRODUCTION

Interest in controlling the growth of HAB-forming marine organisms to protect food supplies has varied over the past 50 years. In 1958, copper sulfate was applied in west Florida waters to control a red tide bloom (U.S. Bureau of Commercial Fisheries, 1958). Although the number of viable organisms decreased immediately, the copper sulfate was not species specific and did not last over time. The Asian aquaculture industry has used clay and clay compounds to coagulate the organisms, causing them to sink (Kim, 1988; Yu et al., 2001). This technique is concurrently being examined in the U.S. under laboratory conditions (Sengco, 2003).

Another control technique under laboratory examination is the addition of a blue-green alga, *Nannochloris*, into a *K. brevis* red-tide culture (Martin and Taft, 1998; Perez et al., 1997). In laboratory studies, *Nannochloris* produces cytolytic agents called 'apparent oceanic naturally occurring cytolin' (APONINs) which react with the *K. brevis* cells and render them into a non-motile or resting form (Derby et al., 2003; Perez et al., 2001). Ongoing studies at Mote Marine Laboratory in Sarasota, Florida, indicate that adding *Nannochlorlis* cells to fish tanks containing *K. brevis* improves the health of the fish.

7.4.2 MANAGING HABs

Although scientists are unlikely to be able to control HAB development and proliferation in the open oceans, they might be able to use management techniques to mitigate the impacts of HABs for coastal aquaculture and harvest sites. These techniques include; improving polluted bottom mud to control the release of nutrients, using ultrasonic waves to destroy the phytoplankton cells, or physically removing the cells by skimming the surface water or using a chemical flocculent that will aggregate and precipitate the cells (Corrales and Maclean, 1995). In addition to limiting bloom development, preventive management strategies could be used to protect aquaculture sites from HABs. These strategies include; adjusting the depths of bivalves in cages so that the contact between toxic algae and shellfish is minimized, using water pumps to circulate water and disperse the algae, towing the aquaculture cages to areas with lower concentrations of algae, and limiting the accumulation of wastes from farmed seafood that would serve as nutrients to support a bloom (Corrales and Maclean, 1995).

7.5 RESEARCH AND PUBLIC-HEALTH ISSUES

7.5.1 MARINE TOXINS IN NEW SEAFOOD SPECIES

This chapter has so far described some of the more well-known human diseases associated with eating seafood contaminated with phycotoxins. There have in addition been reports of human poisonings and fatalities associated with eating other seafoods in which a toxin was identified but the ultimate source of the toxin (e.g., the ingested animal itself, its prey, or an organism closer to the bottom of the food web) was not. For example, fatal poisonings with a clinical presentation similar to that of CFP occurred in Madagascar following ingestion of meat from a shark (Boisier et al., 1995). The poisonings were apparently unique to this individual fish, with patients presenting almost exclusively with neurologic symptoms. Even though the toxins (tentatively named 'carchatoxins') were definitively linked to ingestion of shark meat, they differed in structure from ciguatoxins (which are commonly implicated in outbreaks associated with eating shark). The uniqueness of the outbreak with regard to fish species, symptoms, and fatality rate made it impossible to determine whether the toxins were produced by the shark itself or were bioconcentrated from another source.

Human disease associated with eating fish not previously identified with a particular toxin has also been reported. One example is saxitoxin poisoning associated with eating puffer fish caught in Florida. Another example involves CFP. Ciguatera has not historically been associated with cold-water fish, but Dinubile and Hokama (1995) reported a case of CFP in a woman who had eaten farm-raised salmon.

7.5.2 OTHER TOXICOLOGIC EFFECTS

The increases in the frequencies and durations of HABs, as well as the apparent expansion in the geographic distribution of many of the HAB-causing organisms, are probably increasing the frequencies with which people are exposed to the HAB-related phycotoxins. Reports demonstrating that at least some of these toxins are pharmacologically active, in addition to causing the typical foodborne diseases, indicate that thorough examination of their pharmacology and biologic activity is warranted.

In addition to possible chronic neurologic effects associated with these toxins, evidence suggests other long-term health risks. For example, Aune and Yndestad (1993) reported that okadaic acid and dynophysistoxins are tumor promoters in mice and that okadaic acid is mutagenic and immunotoxic *in vitro*. In addition, Landsberg and others have reported increasing incidence of gonadal tumors in shellfish exposed to these marine seafood toxins (Landsberg, 1996; Van Beneden, 1997). Therefore, although human victims of these diseases typically recover with no reported ill effects after only a few days, these brief exposures, or exposures repeated over time, could increase the long-term risk for cancer, particularly gastrointestinal cancers (Suganuma et al., 1988). Cordier et al. (2000) conducted an ecologic study to assess the association between the duration of shellfish harvesting bans due to okadaic acid in the shellfish (as a proxy for exposure to diarrheic shellfish poisons) and cancer mortality in the coastal populations. They found associations, particularly among men, between the exposure proxy and some gastrointestinal cancers. Despite the study's limitations, including not controlling for other risk factors for gastrointestinal cancers, the possible association between chronic exposure to diarrheic shellfish poisons and the increased risk for some cancers should be evaluated in a comprehensive epidemiologic study.

7.5.3 CLINICAL ISSUES

Specific biomarkers of exposure and effect are needed to improve the diagnosis, prognosis, and prevention of human diseases associated with eating marine seafood toxins. Focused education for healthcare providers concerning the diagnosis and reporting of these diseases also is needed to assess their true public health impact. Given the reported chronic neurologic effects from exposure to these marine seafood toxins and new evidence suggesting that at least some of the toxins are genotoxic and carcinogenic (Cordier et al., 2000; Suganuma et al., 1988) the long-term health of the human populations who eat these potentially carcinogenic organisms is important in terms of defining their public health impact. Specifically, clinical research is needed to develop and evaluate treatment methods, and epidemiologic research is needed to understand the chronic sequellae from these diseases.

Another important emerging issue is the clinical management of diseases in susceptible populations. Compared with younger adults, elderly people are at higher risk from foodborne disease (Institute of Medicine, 1998), and approximately 20% of the U.S. population will be over age 65 years within the next three decades (Federal Agency Forum on Aging-Related Statistics, 1997; Kinsella and Velkoff, 2001). The medical needs of an aging population, coupled with increased risk for exposure as HABs geographically expand, could produce a burden on medical systems, particularly in popular retirement areas with significant HABs, such as Florida. Compared with adults, children may be at higher risk of developing diseases after eating contaminated seafood because their neurologic systems are still developing and because they may eat relatively larger toxin doses (based on body mass) than would adults.

7.5.4 EPIDEMIOLOGY AND ENVIRONMENTAL PUBLIC HEALTH

Improved disease reporting, surveillance, and epidemiologic studies of these diseases are needed. Little information exists about either the chronic effects of acute exposure to these marine toxins or about the long-term effects of chronic exposures, e.g., elderly populations in coastal retirement communities experiencing annual HABs. Little information is available about the environmental health effects, e.g., asthma exacerbations, from exposure to these toxins.

Given the large-scale underreporting and the apparent increase in the incidence of marine seafood toxin syndromes, multifaceted public-health action is urgently needed. Disease reporting and surveillance need to be improved. The current passive systems (e.g., reportable disease status, calls to poison-information centers, general foodborne disease reporting) are inadequate for doing any more than estimating the magnitude of the problem. In some areas, public-health officials have attempted to improve passive disease reporting. For example, in Dade County, Florida, the South Florida Poison Information Center (SFPIC) has established a toll-free seafood toxin hotline which people can use to report cases of disease and to access information about seafood-related diseases and HABs in general (Fleming et al., 1998). After three months of local publicity and education activities, the number of ciguatera cases reported through the SFPIC increased by 2.7 times over the number in the three months before the publicity and education campaigns. However, any passive disease-surveillance system will identify only a fraction of existing cases. Active disease surveillance, e.g., ongoing monitoring and real-time evaluation of the data collected by poison information centers, in the areas most likely to experience outbreaks of marine seafood toxin diseases would allow the public health community to estimate the public health impact of these diseases. Data collected from surveillance activities can be used to determine appropriate public health precaution activities, such as consumer or physician education.

7.5.5 NEW ORGANISMS, NEW TOXINS

Newly identified diatoms and dinoflagellates from estuaries in the U.S. are currently being characterized, and new species are likely to be discovered throughout the world's oceans and estuaries. These microalgae may pose unexpected health risks, and epidemiologic studies will be needed to determine whether exposure to these organisms or their toxins is associated with subsequent adverse human-health effects. For example, *Pfiesteria piscicda* is a dinoflagellate found in estuaries on the eastern seaboard of the U.S. (Burkholder et al., 1992). The presence of this species and the toxins it may produce was reported to be associated with a variety of adverse health effects in both fish and people (Glasgow, Jr. et al., 1995). Although subsequent research has not documented a human-health risk from exposure to *P. piscicida* or related toxins (Centers for Disease Control and Prevention, 2000), the next newly identified microalgae could have an important environmental or human-health impact. However, how this public-health risk would be identified is not clear. Alert physicians who recognize a local increase in an unusual disease, and emergency departments or poison-information centers that undertake routine monitoring, could all be sources of information on human-health impacts of exposure to previously unidentified marine phycotoxins.

7.5.6 EXPANDING GEOGRAPHIC RANGE

HABs appear to be expanding in both intensity and geographic range, and many hypotheses have been proposed to explain these phenomena. Possible causes for the increased frequencies of HABs reported include increases in scientific awareness of toxic species, the use of coastal waters for aquaculture, coastal-water eutrophication, and unusual climate conditions, as well as wetlands loss, altered predation pressures from overfishing and disease, and global climate changes (Corrales and Maclean, 1995). Possible causes of the geographic expansion of HABs include direct movement of the organisms themselves by imported stock for aquaculture or in ballast water in ships involved in international trade and tourism (Iamada N, 2001; Paterson, 2001; Persson, 2003). Although some countries are employing management efforts to minimize the transfer of microorganisms by ballast water, seafood producers must be aware that toxins from nonendemic toxic algae could contaminate fish caught in areas previously assumed to be free of these toxins (Paterson, 2001).

7.6 SUMMARY AND CONCLUSION

There are a number of risks and emerging public health issues associated with eating seafood contaminated with marine phycotoxins. The associations between specific human diseases and eating phycotoxin-contaminated seafood have been recognized for over 200 years, and control programs have existed for decades. However, despite the potential risks, seafood remains a globally important, often vital, food source. Careful monitoring of the types of seafood at risk of contamination with phycotoxins and successful public health efforts to educate consumers about the risks for foodborne diseases will minimize the public health impact of these diseases while helping to maintain a safe food supply.

7.7 ACKNOWLEDGMENTS

The authors thank Ms. Lisa Vallejo for her diligence in assisting in the organization of this manuscript and Karen Foster for her careful editing.

7.8 REFERENCES

Acres, J. and Gray, J., Paralytic shellfish poisoning, *CMAJ*, 119, 1195, 1978.

Ahmed, F., Review: assessing and managing risk due to consumption of seafood contaminated with microorganisms, parasites, and natural toxins in the US, *Int. J. Food Sci. Technol.*, 27, 243, 1992.

Anderson, D., Paralytic shellfish poisoning in northwest Spain: the toxicity of the dinoflagellate *Gymnodinium catenatum*, *Toxicon*, 27, 6, 665, 1989.

Anderson, D., Red tides, *Sci. Am.*, 271, 2, 62, 1994.

Anderson, D., et al., Paralytic shellfish poisoning in southern China, *Toxicon*, 34, 5, 579, 1996.

Anderson, D., Kaoru, Y. and White, A.L., *Estimated annual economic impacts from HABs in the US*, Woods Hole Oceanographic Institution, Woods Hole, Massachusetts, 2000, 97.

Aune, T. and Yndestad, M., Diarrhetic shellfish poisoning, in Falconer, I.R., ed., *Algal Toxins in Seafood and Drinking Water*, Academic Press, San Diego, 1993.

Australia New Zealand Food Authority, *Shellfish Toxins in Food, A Toxicological Review and Risk Assessment*, Australia New Zealand Food Authority, Canberra, 2001.

Backer, L., et al., Epidemiology, public health, and human diseases associated with harmful marine algae, in Hallegraeff, G., Anderson, D. and Cembella, A., eds., *Manual on Harmful Marine Microalgae*, UNESCO Publishing, Paris, 2003.

Baden, D., Fleming, L.E. and Bean, J.A., Marine toxins, in deWoff, F.A., ed., *Handbook of Clinical Neurology: Intoxications of the Nervous System Part II in Natural Toxins and Drugs*, Elsevier Press, Amsterdam, 1995.

Baden, D. and Mende, T.J., Toxicity of two toxins from the Florida red tide marine dinoflagellate, *Ptychodiscus brevis*, *Toxicon*, 20, 2, 457, 1982.

Baden, D. and Trainer, V.L., Mode of action of toxins of seafood poisoning, in Falconer, I.R., ed., *Algal Toxins in Seafood and Drinking Water*, Academic Press, San Diego, 1993.

Bagnis, R., et al., Origins of ciguatera fish poisoning: a new dinoflagellate, *Gambierdiscus toxicus* Adachi and Fukuyo, definitively involved as a causal agent, *Toxicon*, 18, 2, 199, 1980.

Bagnis, R., Kuberski, T. and Laugier, S., Clinical observations on 3,009 cases of ciguatera (fish poisoning) in the South Pacific, *Am. J. Trop. Med. Hyg.*, 28, 6, 1067, 1979.

Blythe, D., Mannitol treatment for acute and chronic ciguatera fish poisoning, *Mem. Queensland Mus.*, 34, 65, 1994.

Blythe, D.G., The medical management of seafood poisoning, in Hui, Kits and Stanfield, eds., *Seafood and Environmental Toxins*, Marcel Dekker, New York, 2001.

Boisier, P., et al., Fatal mass poisoning in Madagascar following ingestion of a shark (*Carcharhinus leucas*): clinical and epidemiological aspects and isolation of toxins, *Toxicon*, 33, 10, 1359, 1995.

Bunning, V., Lindsay, J. and Archer, D., Chronic health effects of food borne microbial disease, *World Health Stat. Quart.*, 50, 51, 1997.

Burkholder, J.M., et al., New 'phantom' dinoflagellate is the causative agent of major estuarine fish kills, *Nature*, 358, 6385, 407, 1992.

Centers for Disease Control and Prevention, Surveillance for foodborne disease outbreaks – United States, 1988–1992, *MMWR Morb. Mortal. Wkly. Rep.*, 45, SS-5, 1, 1996.

Centers for Disease Control and Prevention, Surveillance for possible estuary-associated syndrome – six states, 1998–1999, *MMWR Morb. Mortal. Wkly. Rep.*, 49, 372, 2000.

Centers for Disease Control and Prevention, Neurologic illness associated with eating puffer fish, *MMWR Morb. Mortal. Wkly. Rep.*, 51, 15, 321, 2002.

Chan, T., Shellfish borne illness: A Hong Kong perspective, *Trop. Geogr. Med.*, 47, 305, 1995.

Chin, J.D., et al., Screening for okadaic acid by immunoassay, *JAOAC Int.*, 78, 2, 508, 1995.

Chu, F.S. and Fan, T.S., Indirect enzyme-linked immunosorbent assay for saxitoxin in shellfish, *J. Assoc. Off. Anal. Chem.*, 68, 1, 13, 1985.

Clark, R.F., et al., A review of selected seafood poisonings, *Undersea Hyperb. Med.*, 26, 3, 175, 1999.

Committee on Evaluation of the Safety of Fishery Products, *Seafood Safety*, National Academy Press, Washington, D.C., 1991.

Cordier, S., et al., Ecological analysis of digestive cancer mortality related to contamination by diarrheic shellfish poisoning toxins along the coasts of France, *Env. Res.*, 84, 2, 145, 2000.

Corrales, R. and Maclean, J., Impacts of harmful algae on seafarming in the Asia-Pacific areas, *J. Appl. Phycol.*, 7, 151, 1995.

Dahlmann, J., Budakowski, W.R. and Luckas, B., Liquid chromatography-electrospray ionisation-mass spectrometry based method for the simultaneous determination of algal and cyanobacterial toxins in phytoplankton from marine waters and lakes followed by tentative structural elucidation of microcystins, *J. Chromatogr.*, 994, 1–2, 45, 2003.

Derby, M.L., et al., Studies of the effect of Psi-APONIN from Nannochloris sp. on the Florida red tide organism *Karenia brevis*, *Toxicon*, 41, 2, 245, 2003.

Dinubile, M. and Hokama, Y., The ciguatera poisoning syndrome from farm-raised salmon, *Ann. Intern. Med.*, 122, 2, 113, 1995.

Epstein, P., Ford, T. and Colwell, R., Marine ecosystems, in Epstein, P. and Sharp, D., eds., *Health and Climate Change*, The Lancet Ltd., London, 1994.

Falconer, I.R., ed., *Algal Toxins in Seafood and Drinking Water*, Academic Press, San Diego, 1993.

Federal Agency Forum on Aging-related Statistics, *Data base news in aging*, Washington, D.C., 1997.

Flanagan, A.F., et al., A cytotoxicity assay for the detection and differentiation of two families of shellfish toxins, *Toxicon*, 39, 7, 1021, 2001.

Fleming, L., et al., Seafood toxin diseases: Issues in epidemiology and community outreach, in Reguera, B., et al., eds., *Harmful Algae*, Xunta de Galacia and Intergovernmental Oceanographic Commission of UNESCO, 1998.

Fleming, L.E., et al., The epidemiology of seafood poisoning, in Hui and Stanfield, eds., *Seafood and Environmental Toxins*, Humana Press, Totowa, 2001.

Fleming, L.E., Backer, L.C. and Rowan, A., The epidemiology of human illnesses associated with harmful marine algae, in Baden, D. and Adams, D., eds., *Neurotoxicology Handbook*, Humana Press, Totowa, 2002.

Florida Department of Agriculture and Consumer Services, *Red Tide Regulations*, Florida Department of Agriculture and Consumer Services, Tallahassee, 2002.

Gallagher, J. and Shinnick, G.P., Effect of *Gymnodium breve* toxin in the rat phrenic nerve diaphragm preparation, *Br. J. Pharmac.*, 69, 367, 1980.

Gessner, B.D. and Schloss, M., A population-based study of paralytic shellfish poisoning in Alaska, *Alaska Med.*, 38, 2, 54, 1996.

Glasgow, H.B., Jr., et al., Insidious effects of a toxic estuarine dinoflagellate on fish survival and human health, *J. Toxicol. Env. Health*, 46, 4, 501, 1995.

Glaziou, P. and Legrand, A.M., The epidemiology of ciguatera fish poisoning, *Toxicon*, 32, 8, 863, 1994.

Gollop, J.H. and Pon, E.W., Ciguatera: a review, *Hawaii Med. J.*, 51, 4, 91, 1992.

Goodman, R. and Peavy, J., Describing epidemiologic data, in Gregg, M., ed., *Field Epidemiology*, Oxford University Press, New York, 1996.

Hallegraeff, G., A review of harmful algal blooms and their apparent global increase, *Phycologia*, 32, 2, 79, 1992.

Halstead, B.W., et al., Other poisonous marine animals, in Hui, Y., et al., eds., *Foodborne Disease Handbook*, Marcel Dekker, New York, 1994.

Haystead, T.A., et al., Effects of the tumour promoter okadaic acid on intracellular protein phosphorylation and metabolism, *Nature*, 337, 6202, 78, 1989.

Heredia-Tapia, A., et al., Isolation of *Prorocentrum lima* (Syn. *Exuviaella lima*) and diarrheic shellfish poisoning (DSP) risk assessment in the Gulf of California, Mexico, *Toxicon*, 40, 8, 1121, 2002.

Hessel, D., Halstead, B. and Peckham, N., Marine biotoxins. 1. Ciguatera poisoning – some biological and chemical aspects, *Ann. N.Y. Acad. Sci.*, 90, 788, 1960.

Hokama, Y., An enzyme immunoassay for the detection of ciguatoxin and competive inhibition by related natural polyether toxins, in *Seafood Toxins*, Ragelis, E., ed., American Chemical Society, Washington, D.C., 1984.

Hokama, Y., et al., A survey of ciguatera: assessments of Puako, Hawaii, associated with ciguatera toxin epidemics in humans, *J. Clin. Lab. Anal.*, 7, 147, 1993.

Holmes, M., Teo, S.L. and Khoo, H.W., Detection of diarrheic shellfish poisoning toxins from tropical shellfish using liquid chromatography-selected reaction monitoring mass spectrometry, *Nat. Toxins.*, 7, 6, 361, 1999.

Hosty, T. and et al., *Recommended procedures for the examination of sea water and shellfish*, American Public Health Association, New York, 1970.

Hua, Y., et al., On-line high-performance liquid chromatography-electrospray ionization mass spectrometry for the determination of brevetoxins in "red tide" algae, *Anal. Chem.*, 67, 11, 1815, 1995.

Iamada N, The quantities of *Heterocapsa circularisquama* cells transferred with shellfish consignments and the possibility of its establishment in new areas, in Hallegraeff, G. et al., eds., IOC of UNESCO, Paris, 2001.

Imai, I., et al., Monitoring of DSP toxins in small-sized plankton fraction of seawater collected in Mutsu Bay, Japan, by ELISA method: relation with toxin contamination of scallop, *Mar. Pollut. Bull.*, 47, 1–6, 114, 2003.

Institute of Medicine, *Ensuring safe food from production to consumption*, National Academy Press, Washington, D.C., 1998.

Ishida, H., et al., Study on neurotoxic shellfish poisoning involving oyster, *Crassostrea gigas*, in New Zealand, *Toxicon*, 34, 9, 1050, 1996.

Ito, E., et al., Chronic effects in mice caused by oral administration of sublethal doses of azaspiracid, a new marine toxin isolated from mussels, *Toxicon*, 40, 2, 193, 2002.

James, K.J., et al., First evidence of an extensive northern European distribution of azaspiracid poisoning (AZP) toxins in shellfish, *Toxicon*, 40, 7, 909, 2002.

James, K.J., et al., Ubiquitous 'benign' alga emerges as the cause of shellfish contamination responsible for the human toxic syndrome, azaspiracid poisoning, *Toxicon*, 41, 2, 145, 2003a.

James, K.J., et al., Detection of five new hydroxyl analogues of azaspiracids in shellfish using multiple tandem mass spectrometry, *Toxicon*, 41, 3, 277, 2003b.

Jellett, J.F., et al., Detection of paralytic shellfish poisoning (PSP) toxins in shellfish tissue using MIST Alert, a new rapid test, in parallel with the regulatory AOAC mouse bioassay, *Toxicon*, 40, 10, 1407, 2002.

Kanchanapongkul, J. and Tantraphon, W., Pelagic paralysis from puffer fish poisoning, *J. Med. Assoc. Thai.*, 76, 5, 285, 1993.

Kao, C.Y., Paralytic shellfish poisoning, in Falconer, I.R., ed., *Algal Toxins in Seafood and Drinking Water*, Academic Press, San Diego, 1993.

Kao, C.Y., et al., Vasodilatory effects of tetrodotoxin in the cat, *J. Pharmacol. Exp. Ther.*, 178, 1, 110, 1971.

Kat, M., Diarrheic mussel poisoning in the Netherlands related to the dinoflagellate *Dinophysis acuminate*, 49, 417, 1983.

Kawatsu, K., Hamano, Y. and Noguchi, T., Production and characterization of a monoclonal antibody against domoic acid and its application to enzyme immunoassay, *Toxicon*, 37, 11, 1579, 1999.

Kim, G., *Cochilodinium polykrikoides* blooms in Korean coastal waters and their mitigation, in Requera, B., et al., IOC of UNESCO, Paris, 1988.

Kinsella, K. and Velkoff, A., *An Aging World*, United States Census Bureau Series P95/01-1, U.S. Government Printing Office, Washington, D.C., 2001.

Kodama, A., et al., Comparative immunological, pharmacological and biological characteristics of ciguateric toxin found in *Ctenochaetus* spp. from Tahiti (South Pacific Ocean) and Hawaii (USA), *Food Agric. Immunol.*, 1, 83, 1989.

Kotaki, Y., Oshima, Y. and Yasumoto, T., Analysis of paralytic shellfish toxins in marine snails, *Bull. Jpn. Soc. Sci. Fish.*, 47, 943, 1981.

Kumagai, M., et al., Okadaic acid as the causative toxin of diarrheic shellfish poisoning in Europe, *Agric. Biol. Chem.*, 50, 2853, 1986.

Landsberg, J., Neoplasia and biotoxins in bivalves: is there a connection?, *J. Shellfish Res.*, 15, 2, 203, 1996.

Lange, W.R., Ciguatera toxicity, *Am. Fam. Physician*, 35, 4, 177, 1987.

Lange, W., Snyder, F. and Fudala, P., Travel and ciguatera fish poisoning, *Arch. Intern. Med.*, 152, 2049, 1992.

Lawrence, D., et al., Ciguatera fish poisoning in Miami, *JAMA*, 244, 3, 254, 1980.

Lee, C., Fish poisoning with particular reference to ciguatera, *J. Trop.l Med. Hyg.*, 83, 3, 93, 1996.

Lehane, L. and Lewis, R.J., Ciguatera: recent advances but the risk remains, *Int. J. Food Microbiol.*, 61, 2–3, 91, 2000.

Leira, F., et al., Development of a F actin-based live-cell fluorimetric microplate assay for diarrheic shellfish toxins, *Anal. Biochem.*, 317, 2, 129, 2003.

Levine, L., et al., Production of antibodies and development of a radioimmunoassay for okadaic acid, *Toxicon*, 26, 12, 1123, 1988.

Lewis, N.D., Disease and development: ciguatera fish poisoning, *Soc. Sci. Med.*, 23, 10, 983, 1986.

Lewis, R.J., Jones, A. and Vernoux, J.P., HPLC/tandem electrospray mass spectrometry for the determination of Sub-ppb levels of Pacific and Caribbean ciguatoxins in crude extracts of fish, *Anal. Chem.*, 71, 1, 247, 1999.

Lindsay, J., Chronic sequelae of foodborne disease, *Emerging Infect. Dis.*, 3, 4, 443, 1997.

Lipp, E.K. and Rose, J.B., The role of seafood in foodborne diseases in the United States of America, *Rev. Sci. Tech.*, 16, 2, 620, 1997.

Louzao, M.C., et al., A fluorimetric microplate assay for detection and quantitation of toxins causing paralytic shellfish poisoning, *Chem. Res. Toxicol.*, 16, 4, 433, 2003.

Magdalena, A.B., et al., The first identification of azaspiracids in shellfish from France and Spain, *Toxicon*, 42, 1, 105, 2003a.

Magdalena, A.B., et al., Food safety implications of the distribution of azaspiracids in the tissue compartments of scallops (*Pecten maximus*), *Food Addit. Contam.*, 20, 2, 154, 2003b.

Martin, D. and Taft, W., Management of the Florida red tide-revisited, *Fla. Scientist*, 6, 10, 1998.

Matta, J., et al., A pilot study for the detection of acute ciguatera intoxication in human blood, *J. Toxicol. Clin. Toxicol.*, 40, 1, 49, 2002.

McKee D et al., Ciguatera fish poisoning reporting by physicians in an endemic area, in Hallegraeff, G., ed., *Harmful Algal Blooms 2000*, IOC of UNESCO, Paris, 2001.

McMahon, T. and Silke, J., Winter toxicity of unknown etiology in mussels, *Harmful Algae News*, 14, 2, 1996.

McMahon, T. and Silke, J., Re-occurence of winter toxicity, *Harmful Algae News*, 17, 12, 1998.

Morris, J.G., Jr., et al., Clinical features of ciguatera fish poisoning: a study of the disease in the US Virgin Islands, *Arch. Intern. Med.*, 142, 6, 1090, 1982a.

Morris, J.G., Jr., et al., Ciguatera fish poisoning epidemiology of the disease on St. Thomas, U.S. Virgin Islands, *Am. J. Trop. Med. Hyg.*, 31, 3, part 1, 574, 1982b.

Morris, P.D., et al., Clinical and epidemiological features of neurotoxic shellfish poisoning in North Carolina, *Am. J. Public Health*, 81, 4, 471, 1991.

Morton, R.A. and Burklew, M.A., Incidence of ciguatera in barracuda from the west coast of Florida, *Toxicon*, 8, 4, 317, 1970.

Mountfort, D.O., Suzuki, T. and Truman, P., Protein phosphatase inhibition assay adapted for determination of total DSP in contaminated mussels, *Toxicon*, 39, 2–3, 383, 2001.

Murata, M., Isolation and structural elucidation of the causative toxin of the diarrhetic shellfish poisoning, *Bull. Jpn. Soc.Sci. Fish*, 48, 549, 1982.

Murata, M., Isolation and structure of yessotoxin, a novel polyether compound implicated in diarrhetic shellfish poisoning, *Tet. Lett.*, 28, 5869, 1987.

Murata, M., et al., Structures and configurations of ciguatoxin from the moray eel *Gymnothroax javanicus* and its likely precursor from the dinoflagellate *Gambierdiscus toxicus*, *J. Am. Chem. Soc.*, 112, 4380, 1990.

Murata, M., et al., Effect of maitotoxin analogues on calcium influx and phosphoinositide breakdown in cultured cells, *Toxicon*, 29, 9, 1085, 1991.

Naar, J., et al., A competitive ELISA to detect brevetoxins from *Karenia brevis* (formerly *Gymnodinium breve*) in seawater, shellfish, and mammalian body fluid, *Env. Health Perspect.*, 110, 2, 179, 2002.

Noguchi, T., Konosu, S. and Hashimoto, Y., Short communications identity of the crab toxin with saxitoxin, *Toxicon*, 7, 4, 325, 1969.

Nozawa, A., Tsuji, K. and Ishida, H., Implication of brevetoxin B1 and PbTx-3 in neurotoxic shellfish poisoning in New Zealand by isolation and quantitative determination with liquid chromatography-tandem mass spectrometry, *Toxicon*, 42, 1, 91, 2003.

Ofuji, K., et al., Structures of azaspiracid analogs, azaspiracid-4 and azaspiracid-5, causative toxins of azaspiracid poisoning in Europe, *Biosci. Biotechnol. Biochem.*, 65, 3, 740, 2001.

Ofuji, K., et al., Two analogs of azaspiracid isolated from mussels, *Mytilus edulis*, involved in human intoxication in Ireland, *Nat. Toxins*, 7, 3, 99, 1999.

Ohizumi, Y., Kajiwara, A. and Yasumoto, T., Excitatory effect of the most potent marine toxin, maitotoxin, on the guinea-pig vas deferens, *J. Pharmacol. Exp. Ther.*, 227, 1, 199, 1983.

Ohizumi, Y. and Yasumoto, T., Contractile response of the rabbit aorta to maitotoxin, the most potent marine toxin, *J. Physiol.*, 337, 711, 1983.

Palafox, N.A., et al., Successful treatment of ciguatera fish poisoning with intravenous mannitol, *JAMA*, 259, 18, 2740, 1988.

Paterson, D., An international and Australian agenda for minimzing the spread of harmful algal blooms via ship ballast water, in Hallegraeff, G.M., IOC of UNESCO, Paris, 2001.

Perez, E., Sawyers, W. and Martin, D., Identification of allelopathic substances produced by *Nannochloris aculata* that affects a red tide organism *Gymnodinium breve*, *Biomed. Lett.*, 56, 7, 1997.

Perez, E., Sawyers, W.G. and Martin, D.F., Lysis of *Gymnodinium breve* by cultures of the green alga *Nannochloris eucaryotum*, *Cytobios*, 104, 405, 25, 2001.

Perl, T.M., et al., An outbreak of toxic encephalopathy caused by eating mussels contaminated with domoic acid, *N. Engl. J. Med.*, 322, 25, 1775, 1990.

Persson, A., The use of sediment slurry culture to search for organisms producing resting stages, in Hallegraeff, G.M., IOC of UNESCO, Paris, 2003.

Pierce, R., et al., Evaluation of solid sorbents for the recovery of polyether toxins (brevetoxins) in seawater, *Bull. Env. Contam. Toxicol.*, 49, 479, 1992.

Poli, M., Laboratory procedures for detoxification of equipment and waste contaminated with brevetoxins PbTx-2 and PbTx-3, *J. Assoc. Off. Anal. Chem.*, 71, 5, 1000, 1988.

Quod, J.P. and Turquet, J., Ciguatera in Reunion Island (SW Indian Ocean): epidemiology and clinical patterns, *Toxicon*, 34, 7, 779, 1996.

Raj, U., et al., The occurrence of paralytic shellfish toxins in two species of xanthid crab from Suva barrier reef, Fiji Islands, *Toxicon*, 21, 4, 547, 1983.

Risk, M., et al., Actions of *Ptychodiscus brevis* red tide toxin on metabolic and transmitter-releasing properties of synaptosomes, *J. Neurochem.*, 39, 5, 1485, 1982.

Sakamoto, Y., Lockey, R.F. and Krzanowski, J.J., Jr., Shellfish and fish poisoning related to the toxic dinoflagellates, *South. Med. J.*, 80, 7, 866, 1987.

Satake, M., et al., Azaspiracid, a new marine toxin having unique spiro ring assemblies, isolated from Irish mussels, *Mytilus edulis*, *J. Am. Chem. Soc.*, 120, 9967, 1998.

Schantz, E.J., Seafood toxicants, in National Academy of Sciences, ed., *Toxicants Occurring Naturally In Foods*, National Academy Press, Washington, D.C., 1973.

Schantz, E., et al., Purified shellfish poison for bioassay standardization, *J. Off. Agric. Chem.*, 41, 160, 1958.

Schnorf, H., Taurarii, M. and Cundy, T., Ciguatera fish poisoning: a double-blind randomized trial of mannitol therapy, *Neurology*, 58, 6, 873, 2002.

Scholin, C., et al., Mortality of sea lions along the central California coast linked to a diatom bloom, *Nature*, 403, 80, 2000.

Sengco, M., Removal of red and brown tide cells using clay flocculation: I. Laboratory culture experiments with *Gymnodinium breve* and *Aureococcus anophageﬀerens*, *Mar. Ecol. Prog. Ser.*, 2003.

Shinozaki, Y. and Ishida, M., Inhibition of quisqualate responses by domoic acid or kainic acid in crayfish opener muscle, *Brain Res.*, 109, 435, 1976.

Shubat, P.J., Raatz, K.A. and Olson, R.A., Fish consumption advisories and outreach programs for Southeast Asian immigrants, *Toxicol. Ind. Health*, 12, 3–4, 427, 1996.

Spalding, B., Better tests needed to meet goal of safer food supply, *Am. Soc. Microbiol. News*, 61, 639, 1995.

Steidinger, K., A re-evaluation of toxic dinoflagellates biology and ecology, in Round, F. and Chapman, D., eds., *Progress in Phycological Research*, Elsevier, Amsterdam, 1983.

Steidinger, K. and Penta, H., *Harmful microalgae and assocaited public health risks in the Gulf of Mexico*, U.S. EPA, Gulf of Mexico Program, Stennis Space Center, 1999.

Suganuma, M., et al., Okadaic acid: an additional non-phorbol-12-tetradecanoate-13-acetate-type tumor promoter, *Proc. Natl. Acad. Sci. U.S.A.*, 85, 6, 1768, 1988.

Sullivan, J., Methods of analysis for DSP and PSP toxins in shellfish a review, *J. Shellfish Res.*, 7, 4, 587, 1988.

Tachibana, K., et al., Okadaic acid, a cytotoxic polyether from two marine sponges of the genus *Halichondria*, *JACS*, 103, 2469, 1981.

Takeuchi, H., et al., Effects of alpha-kainic acid, domoic acid and their derivatives on a molluscan giant neuron sensitive to beta-hydroxy-L-glutamic acid, *Eur. J. Pharmacol.*, 102, 2, 325, 1984.

Terao, K., et al., Histopathological studies on experimental marine toxin poisoning. I. Ultrastructural changes in the small intestine and liver of suckling mice induced by dinophysistoxin-1 and pectenotoxin-1, *Toxicon*, 24, 11–12, 1141, 1986.

Terao, K., et al., Histopathological studies on experimental marine toxin poisoning – 5. The effects in mice of yessotoxin isolated from *Patinopecten yessoensis* and of a desulfated derivative, *Toxicon*, 28, 9, 1095, 1990.

Tester, P.A., Harmful marine phytoplankton and shellfish toxicity. Potential consequences of climate change, *Ann. N.Y. Acad. Sci.*, 740, 69, 1994.

Ting, J.Y. and Brown, A.F., Ciguatera poisoning: a global issue with common management problems, *Eur. J. Emerg. Med.*, 8, 4, 295, 2001.

Todd, E., How ciguatera affects Canadians, in Trapido, E.R., ed., *Proceedings of the Third International Conference*, Puerto Rico, 1990a.

Todd, E., Amnesic shellfish poisoning – a new seafood toxin syndrome, in Graneli, E., ed., *Toxic Marine Phytoplankton*, Elsevier Science Publishing, 1990b.

Todd, E., Emerging diseases associated with seafood toxins and other water-borne agents, *Ann. N.Y. Acad. Sci.*, 740, 77, 1994.

Todd, E.C., Seafood-associated diseases and control in Canada, *Rev. Sci. Tech.*, 16, 2, 661, 1997.

Tor, E.R., Puschner, B. and Whitehead, W.E., Rapid determination of domoic acid in serum and urine by liquid chromatography-electrospray tandem mass spectrometry, *J. Agric. Food Chem.*, 51, 7, 1791, 2003.

Truman, P., et al., Determination of brevetoxins in shellfish by the neuroblastoma assay, *JAOAC Int.*, 85, 5, 1057, 2002.

Tsai, Y.H., et al., Occurrence of tetrodotoxin and paralytic shellfish poison in the Taiwanese crab *Lophozozymus pictor*, *Toxicon*, 33, 12, 1669, 1995.

Tsai, Y., Jeng, S. and Hwang, D., Seasonal and regional variations of toxicity in the Xanthid crab, *Zosimus aeneus,* in Taiwan, *Fisheries Sci.*, 63, 2, 313, 1997.

U.S. Bureau of Commercial Fisheries, *Gulf Fisheries Investigations*, 1958.

U.S. Food and Drug Administration (FDA), *Procedures for the safe and sanitary processing and importing of fish and fishery products*, Federal Register, 1995.

U.S. Food and Drug Administration (FDA), *Fish and Fisheries Products Hazards and Control Guide*, 3rd ed., U.S. Food and Drug Administration, Center for Food Safety and Applied Nutrition, Office of Seafood, Rockville, 2001.

Van Beneden, R.J., Environmental effects and aquatic organisms: investigations of molecular mechanisms of carcinogenesis, *Env. Health Perspect.*, 105 (Suppl. 3), 669, 1997.

Van Dolah, F.M., Marine algal toxins: origins, health effects, and their increased occurrence, *Env. Health Perspect.*, 108 (Suppl. 1), 133, 2000.

Villareal T., Personal Communication, 2003.

Viviani, R., Eutrophication, marine biotoxins, human health, *Sci. Total Env.*, Suppl., 631, 1992.

Wannemacher, R., *Procedures for the inactivation and safe containment of toxins*, adapted from a presentation by Wannemacher, R.W., Assistant Chief Toxicology Division, USAMRIID, 2000.

World Health Organization, *Hazard Analysis Critical Control Point System: Concept and Application*, report of a WHO Consultation with the participation of FAO, unpublished WHO document, Geneva, 1995.

Wu, C.H. and Narahashi, T., Mechanism of action of novel marine neurotoxins on ion channels, *Annu. Rev. Pharmacol. Toxicol.*, 28, 141, 1988.

Yang, C., et al., An outbreak of tetrodotoxin poisoning following gastropod mollusc consumption, *Hum. Exp. Toxicol.*, 14, 446, 1995.

Yasumoto, T., Oshima, Y. and Yamaguchi, M., Occurrence of a new type of shellfish poisoning in the Tokohu District, *Bull. Jpn. Soc. Sci. Fish*, 44, 1249, 1978.

Yasumoto, T., Polyether toxins produced by dinoflagellates, in Natori, S., Hashimoto, K. and Ueno, Y., eds., *Mycotoxins and Phycotoxins '88*, Elsevier, Amsterdam, 1989.

Yasumoto, T., et al., A new toxic dinoflagellate found in association with ciguatera, in Taylor, D. and Seliger, H., eds., *Toxic Dinoflagellate Blooms*, Elsevier-North Holland, New York, 1979.

Yoo, R., et al., *Cyanobacterial (Blue-green Algal) Toxins: A Resource Guide*, AWWA Research Foundation, Denver, 1995.

Yu, Z., Sun, X. and Zhou, J., Progress of harmful algal bloom (HAB) mitigation with clays in China, in Hallegraeff, G.M., Bolch, C.J., Blackburn, S.I. and Lewis, R.J., eds., *Harmful Algal Blooms 2000*. Proceedings 9th International Conference on Harmful Algal Blooms, UNESCO, Paris, 2001.

Zlotnick, B.A., et al., Ciguatera poisoning after ingestion of imported jellyfish: diagnostic application of serum immunoassay, *Wilderness. Env. Med.*, 6, 3, 288, 1995.

8

Bacterial Toxins

Waldemar Dąbrowski and Dagmara Mędrala

CONTENTS

8.1 INTRODUCTION

The reported number of cases of bacterial foodborne poisonings (BFBP) and the deaths they cause worldwide is enormous, both in developing and industrialized countries. In the U.S. alone, each year 76 million foodborne illnesses are reported and 325,000 patients are hospitalized, of which 5000 die. The etiological agent is identified only in 18% of cases, the rest remain undiagnosed or misdiagnosed (Mead et al., 1999).

The number of human pathogens found in food is limited. They may be divided into three groups (Table 8.1):

- Group I contains bacteria that do not produce typical toxins, and the diseases they cause are a result of their outgrowth within a host organism. Such microorganisms produce molecules that provide a defense against host immunological mechanisms and transmission within the invaded organism. When the bacteria reach intestinal epithelium, they penetrate tissues by the outgrowth in cell cytosol or vacuoles.
- Group II includes bacteria that produce toxins responsible for the course of disease during gastrointestinal invasion. Disease symptoms are the result of cell destruction caused by extracellular toxins and by elements present in the cell wall, e.g., fimbriae. Such toxins are not

Table 8.1
Bacterial foodborne pathogens.

Group I		Group II		Group III	
Organism	**Effects**	**Organism**	**Toxins and effects**	**Organism**	**Toxins**
Shigella	Colonization and invasion of epithelial cells in large intestine Replication in cytoplasm	*Aeromonas* sp.	Endotoxins, exotoxins, invasins, extracellular enzymes, adhesions, siderophores	*Clostridium botulinum*	Neurotoxins
Salmonella	Colonization of intestinal mucosa, invasion of enterocytes and M cells Replication in vacuoles (diarrhoeogenic enterotoxin, cytotoxin, Vi antigen, LPS, porins)	*Escherichia coli* EHEC	Shiga family toxins (verotoxins): Stx, Stx1, Stx2, Stxc, Stxe; attachment to cells via fimbriae	*Staphylococcus aureus*	Enterotoxins
Listeria monocytogenes	Proliferation in cytoplasm of different tissues (facultative intracellular pathogen)	*Vibrio cholerae* 01, 0139, non-01/ non-0139	Cholera toxin – enterotoxin (main dehydrating diarrhea toxin) Zonula occludens toxin (responsible for increase in permeability of intestinal mucosa) Accessory cholera enterotoxin Hemolysin		
Yersinia enterocolitica	Proliferation in gut associated lymphoid tissue (facultative intracellular pathogen)(heat stable enterotoxin, LPS, invasin, attachment/invasion protein adhesion Ail)	*Bacillus cereus*	Emetic toxin (vomiting) Enterotoxins (diarrheal illness)		
Campylobacter jejuni	May interact and probably invade M cells in the Peyer's patches (cholera like toxin, hepatotoxin, cytolethal distending toxin, heat labile enterotoxin)	*Clostridium perfringens*	Enterotoxin (type A food poisoning) Beta toxin (necrotic enteritis)		

produced outside the host organisms, or their presence in food does not affect consumers.

- Group III comprises bacteria that produce toxins in food outside the host organisms. Disease symptoms are therefore the result of toxin action and, usually, the presence of microorganisms on their own does not lead to poisoning. Two species, *Clostridium botulinum* and *Staphylococcus aureus*, belong to this group. Botulin and staphylococcal toxins are produced only by selected strains and only in specific environmental conditions, other than those which promote the outgrowth of vegetative cells. Such toxins cannot be characterized without their bacterial producers.

This chapter will focus on group III pathogens as this is the most significant group in the context of toxins in food.

8.2 *CLOSTRIDIUM BOTULINUM*

Clostridium botulinum belongs to a Gram-positive *Clostridium* sp. It has two features that make it unique:

- production of spores (*C. botulinum* produces spores, which are in practice resistant to all physical and chemical factors that destroy vegetative cells)
- obligate or facultative anaerobic mode of outgrowth and toxin production

Based on the serological properties of toxins (neurotoxins) produced by various strains of *C. botulinum*, the following serovars were identified: A, B, C1, C2, D, E, F, G.

C. botulinum strains are divided into four types (Hatheway, 1993):

- Type I (so-called 'proteolytic'): produces A, B, and F neurotoxins; harmful for humans; minimum temperature for growth is 12°C.
- Type II (so-called 'non-proteolytic'): produces B, E, and F neurotoxins; harmful for humans; the minimum temperature for growth is 3.3°C.
- Type III: produces C and D toxins; dangerous for birds, minks, and calves; do not affect humans; the minimum temperature for growth is 15°C.
- Type IV: produces G toxin; harmful for humans; the minimum temperature for growth is 12°C.

At present, G-toxin-producing *C. botulinum* is classified as a different species (*C. argentinense*). Neurotoxins may be also produced by *C. butyricum* (E toxin), *C. barati* (F toxin), and *C. novyi* (D and C1 toxins) (Eklund et al., 1974; Hall et al., 1985; McCroskey et al., 1986; Harvey et al., 2002).

The classic foodborne botulism (FBB) poisoning occurs when a botulin toxin of food origin gets into the human body and is spread via gastrointestinal mucous membrane. An ingestion of *C. botulinum* cells or spores is not a risk to healthy individuals, probably due to good immunological status of the hosts or due to the presence of suitable gastrointestinal microflora, but this has not been explained so far. There are, however, three main exceptions: infant botulism, wound botulism, and adult botulism.

The infant botulism syndrome was first described in the U.S. in 1970 and over 1000 cases have been recorded since. Currently, it is the most frequent form of botulism in the U.S., and accounted for about 66% of all diagnosed cases of botulism in 2001. An ingestion of food contaminated with *C. botulinum* spores by infants (up to twelve months of age) results in the outgrowth of pathogen, toxin production, and disease symptoms. Honey, used in honey-containing products and as a flavoring agent, is the most frequent source of infant botulism (Tanzi and Gabay, 2002). *C. botulinum* spores of type A and B have been detected in 7 to 16% of honey samples in Finland (Nevas et al., 2002). It is suggested that a neurotoxin linked to B-type infant botulism demonstrates antigenic and biological properties different to those expressed by the toxin produced by classical strains of foodborne botulism (Tabita et al., 1999). Toxins differ in their amino-acid sequence and binding affinity. Infant botulism is also caused by *C. butyricum*, which produces toxin similar to the type-E neurotoxin of *C. botulinum* (Zhou et al., 1993).

Wound botulism occurs where *C. botulinum* spores germinate in wound infections and develop into vegetative cells. In such cases, neurotoxin is produced which leads to the onset of neurological symptoms. According to the Centers for Disease Control and Prevention, 23 cases of wound botulism (13.6% of all botulism cases) were reported in 2001 in the U.S. Wound botulism has also been diagnosed after intravenous drug injection (Rundervoort et al., 2003).

Adult botulism is a very rare syndrome and its etiology is similar to infant botulism.

Botulin toxin may also act as an inhalation poison. This property has been reveled for both pure and progenitor (a complex with auxiliary proteins) toxins (Park and Simpson, 2003). *C. botulinum* and its toxin were included onto the list of high-priority agents – in the highest 'A' category of agents that may potentially be used in bioterrorism (Khan et al., 2000; Sobel et al., 2002).

Botulism also affects animals, where intoxication is caused by *C. botulinum* types C and D. A bovine disease 'visceral botulism' was reported in Germany (Bohnel et al., 2001). It was caused by a long-lasting exposure to low quantities of botulin toxin that interfered with the neurological control of intestinal physiology. Visceral botulism in cows may pose a health risk for milk consumers, although to date there are no precise data on how serious the problem is (Cobb et al., 2002).

8.2.1 BOTULIN TOXINS

C. botulinum toxins belong to the AB group of toxins, which also includes diphtheria toxin, pseudomonas exotoxin A, anthrax toxin, Shiga(like) toxin, cholera toxin, pertussis toxin, and plant toxins, e.g., ricin. Moiety A has an enzymatic activity and usually modified cellular-target entering cytosol. Moiety B consists of one or more components and binds the toxin to surface receptors, and is responsible for translocation of the A component into cells. AB toxins are produced in a non-active form and are activated by a split between two cysteine residues within a region (Falnes and Sandvig, 2000).

Toxins produced by *Clostridium* sp. may be divided into:

- toxins affecting vesicular membrane and fusion apparatus; which include neurotoxins of a specific metaloprotease character, seven types of *C. botulinum* neurotoxins (BoNTs) and one type of *C. tetani* neurotoxin (TeNT).
- toxins affecting actin cytoskeleton assembly (ADP-ribosyltransferase); which include C2 and C3 toxins produced by *C. botulinum* types C and D, C3 exoenzyme of *C. botulinum* types C and D, iota toxin of *C. perfringens*, and toxins produced by *C. difficile* and *C. spiroformae*.
- toxins affecting membrane permeability; such compounds (thiol-activated toxins) are produced by many genera of aerobes and anaerobes and lead to pore formation in cell membranes, they include hemolysins from *Staphylococcus*, tetanolysin from *C. tetani*, botulysin from *C. botulinum*, and perfringolysin from *C. perfringens*.

BoNTs are produced by bacterial cells in optimal growth conditions, mainly during a log phase and less so during a stationary phase. Botulin toxin is the most toxic of all known poisons. One mg of toxin contains 30 million doses of mouse LD_{50}. A minimum LD_{50} dose for mice in an intraperitoneal or intravenous injection is within the range from 0.4 to 2.5 ng/kg, whereas 1 ng/kg is LD_{50} for humans. Toxin A is more lethal than B and E. BoNTs are destroyed during thermal processing at 80°C for 30 minutes or at 100°C for 10 minutes.

BoNTs (150 kDa) consist of two polypeptide chains: the heavy chain (HC, 100 kDa) and the light chain (LC, 50 kDa), linked with disulfide and non-covalent bonds. The amine end of the LC is responsible for intraneural enzymatic activity. The HC contains a membrane translocation domain (a 50 kDa amino-terminal polypeptide) and a receptor-binding part (a 50 kDa carboxy-terminal polypeptide) (DasGupta, 1990; Krieglstein et al., 1994). BoNT/A forms dimers, trimers, and bigger structures. BoNT/E generally has a monomer structure, but sometimes forms dimers. BoNT/B is a dimer (Ledoux et al., 1994).

BoNTs form complexes with non-toxic proteins called 'progenitor toxin'. Such proteins protect neurotoxins against the negative influences of the stomach environment and proteolytic enzymes. They also play an important role in toxin binding to intestinal epithelium. At pH higher than 7.2, the complexes are split, but they are restored if pH decreases (Maksymowich et al., 1999). Three forms of progenitor neurotoxins have been described; medium (M, 300 kDa), large (L, 500 kDa) and extra large (LL, 900 kDa) (Sakaguchi, 1990).

M toxin (12S) consists of neurotoxin and non-toxic non-hemaglutynin (NTNH) components. It is produced by all types of *C. botulinum*, except *C. botulinum* type G.

L toxin (16S) is composed of neurotoxin, NTNH and hemaglutynins (HA). HA consists of four subcomponents: HA1, HA2, HA3a and HA3b (Sakaguchi et al., 1984; Inoue et al., 1996). HA1 and HA3b play a role in binding toxin to intestinal epithelium by attaching to epithelium microvilli via galactose (HA1) and sialic acid moieties (HA3b). HA2 and HA3 do not display an ability to attach to the intestinal epithelium.

LL toxin (19S) is an L toxin dimer probably crosslinked through HA1 (Fujinaga et al., 2000). The L toxin is produced by types A, B, C, D, and G (Tsuzuki et al., 1992; Eklund et al., 1989).

All botulin neurotoxins act in a similar way. They only differ in the amino-acid sequence of some protein parts (Prabakaran et al., 2001). Botulism symptoms are provoked both by oral ingestion and parenteral injection. Botulin toxin is not inactivated by enzymes present in the gastrointestinal tracts. Foodborne BoNT penetrates the intestinal barrier, presumably due to transcytosis. It is then transported to neuromuscular junctions within the bloodstream and blocks the secretion of the neurotransmitter acetylcholine. This results in muscle limpness and palsy caused by selective hydrolysis of soluble *N*-ethylmalemide-sensitive factor activating (SNARE) proteins which participate in fusion of synaptic vesicles with presynaptic plasma membrane. SNARE proteins include vesicle-associated membrane protein (VAMP), synaptobrevin, syntaxin, and synaptosomal associated protein of 25 kDa (SNAP-25). Their degradation is responsible for neuromuscular palsy due to blocks in acetylcholine transmission from synaptic terminals. In humans, palsy caused by BoNT/A lasts four to six months.

The following steps are subsequently observed in BoNT action (Montecucco and Schiavo, 1994; Montecucco et al., 1994; Boquet et al., 1998):

- Binding: BoNTs adhere via the HC to negatively charged surface of presynaptic membrane (Montecucco *et al.*, 1994; Chaddock et al., 2000). The receptors for neurotoxins are located in motor neuron plasma membranes at the neuromuscular junction (Dolly et al., 1984). There are various receptors for different neurotoxins, which display dissimilar affinities (Agui et al., 1983; Williams et al., 1983; Black and Dolly, 1986; Evans et al., 1986; Yokosawa et al., 1991). All receptors are gangliosides (sialic acid containing glycosphingolipids). Sialic acid specific lectins of plant origin may inactivate BoNT action (Bakry et al., 1991). Additional receptors for toxin A were identified in 80 and 116 kDa synaptosomal glycoproteins (Park et al., 1990, Poulain et al., 1991, Schengrund et al., 1991).

- Internalization: The toxins diffuse laterally in the membrane, bind to protein receptors and are internalized by receptor-mediated endocytosis. After this stage is completed, the toxins are protected against antibody inactivation. The internalized HC forms aggregates and induces pores in endosomal membrane. The pores serve as gates through which the LC enters a cytoplasm (Ledoux et al., 1994).
- Target modification: In the cytoplasm the LC acts as a zinc-dependent endopeptidase with a zinc-binding His–Glu–x–x–His motif (Schiavo et al., 1993, 1994b). Synaptic vesicles (a core of a multicomponent complex that is responsible for a fusion of carrier vesicles to target membranes in eucaryotic cells) are its substrate. BoNTs A and E are specific endopeptidases demonstrating activity towards SNAP-25. BoNTs B, F, D, and G cause degradation of a vesicle membrane protein – synaptobrevin. The activity of those proteases is very specific and hydrolyzes specific sequences, such as Gln–Phe, Gln–Lys or Ala–Ala (Binz et al., 1994; Schiavo et al., 1994a, 1995).

The onset of botulism occurs generally between 18 and 36 hours after consumption of food products containing botulin toxin. However, it may affect patients earlier or later, even on the tenth day after food consumption. The first symptoms include stomach ache, nausea, vomiting, and diarrhea, followed by neurological disorders. Other symptoms include, skin, mouth and throat dryness, diplopia, blurred vision, dysphonia, dysarthria, dysphagia, and peripheral weakness. In lethal cases of botulism, respiratory muscles are involved. This leads to respiratory failure and death. Because all the symptoms are connected with toxemia, the first step of medical treatment is to provide a patient with antiserum.

Toxins of strains type C and D are not harmful for human and their mechanism of action is completely different (Boquet et al., 1998; Busch and Aktories, 2000). Enterotoxin C2 of *C. botulinum* consists of two unlinked proteins (C2II) and C2I enzyme. C2II recognizes a cell surface glycoprotein, translocates C2I-ADP ribosyltransferase to the cytosol of the target cells (Barth et al., 2002; Stiles et al., 2002), and forms haptomers which bind to the carbohydrates on the cell surfaces. The next stage is formation of highly cation-selective and voltage-gated channels in the lipid membrane, which react with the C2I component. The newly formed complex undergoes a receptor-mediated endocytosis. C2IIa haptomer forms pores in the acid environment of endosome and mediates in transmission of C2I to the cytosol. Pore formation mediated by C2II depends on the presence of receptor and acidic pulses. This suggests that acid environment of endosome changes 'pre-pore' conformation of C2IIa into 'pore' conformation before it binds to the membrane (Blöcker et al., 2003).

The gene sequences that encode neurotoxins have been studied thoroughly. Depending on the *C. botulinum* serotype, the sequences are located on chromosomes, bacteriophages, or plasmids. Genes encoding BoNTs A, B, E and F and associated non-toxic proteins are located on a bacterial chromosome. The genes encoding BoNTs C1 and D and their additional proteins were found on bacteriophages, whereas genes responsible for neurotoxin G and non-toxic proteins of *C. argentinense* were traced within a plasmid sequence (Eklund et al., 1972; 1989; Hauser et al., 1992). The *botR* gene encoding regulatory proteins is located in a toxin gene cluster on chromosomes, bacteriophages, or plasmids, again depending on *C. botulinum* serotype (Johnson and Bradshaw, 2001). Genes encoding BoNT A and B are arranged into very similar clusters (East et al., 1994). Genes encoding BoNT C1 and its additional proteins form three transcriptional units creating *botulinum* loci. The 3'-end is conservative whereas changes at the 5'-end are responsible for variations among toxin types. The *ntnh* gene encoding NTNH and accompanied by *bont* gene are located near the 3'-end. Genes encoding hemaglutinins are upstream of the *ntnh-bont* genes. The *botR* gene encoding a 21 to 22 kDa regulatory protein is located either at the 5'-end in serotypes C and D or between *ntnh-bont* and *ha* genes in strains of serotypes A, B and G (Marvaud et al., 2000). It has been determined that gene sequences of *ha*, *botR*, and *bontA* revealed strain variations at flanking regions (Dineen et al., 2003).

8.2.2 CLOSTRIDIUM BOTULINUM IN THE ENVIRONMENT

C. botulinum is widely distributed in the environment. The number of *Clostridium*-positive samples of soil and bottom sediments ranges from 3 to 100%. *C. botulinum* type A dominates in soil from the western states of the U.S., whereas type B is predominant in soil samples from the eastern states. *C. botulinum* type B is most frequently found in European soil, although type A predominates in Italy. In Japanese soil, types C, D or E are prevalent. *C. botulinum* type F dominates in Paraguayan soil (Dodds, 1993 a,b).

Spores may be transferred from soil and plants to the sea via rainwater, causing the prevalence in coastal waters of the same *C. botulinum* types as on the land. Such a correlation was observed in Great Britain, where the type B predominates both in soil and in bottom sediments. Similarly, 71% of fish and bottom-sediment samples collected in southern France were contaminated with type B, while *C. botulinum* type E was found only in 9.6% of samples (Fach et al., 2002). However, it is commonly believed that non-proteolytic type E is characteristic for the marine environment. A distinguishing feature of type E strains is the ability to grow in low temperatures (about 3°C), which are typical for bottom layers of seas and oceans. Moreover, the bottom sediments provide anaerobic conditions for the outgrowth of *Clostridium*. Therefore, the marine environment promotes *C. botulinum* type E distribution. This has been further supported by the rate of fish and seafood contamination; fish and seafood isolated in many countries are most frequently contaminated with *C. botulinum* type E (Dodds, 1993 a,b). Furthermore, epidemiological studies have shown that the majority of botulism cases linked to fish and seafood consumption reported between 1950 and 1996 in the U.S. were caused by *C. botulinum* type E (Centers for Disease Control and Prevention 1998). *C. botulinum* type F, which was involved in the botulism outbreak caused by home-made liver paste, has been also isolated from bottom sediments, crabs, salmons, and venison.

Strains of type G were isolated from Argentinian soil in 1968. It is suggested that type G do not produce sufficiently high levels of toxin, so far no lethal cases caused by type G have been reported (Ciccarelli et al., 1977).

8.2.3 *CLOSTRIDIUM BOTULINUM* IN FOOD

C. botulinum is frequently isolated from human and animal gastrointestinal tracts. Approximately 64% of samples of cow feces contain *C. botulinum*; 73% of which are non-proteolytic type B and only less than 5% are type E or F (Dahlenborg et al., 2003). According to Dahlenborg et al. (2001), *C. botulinum* type B is isolated from 62% of pig feces. Such a frequent occurrence of *C. botulinum* in feces of farm animals leads to meat contamination with its spores. Prior to the introduction of modern methods of meat processing, meat products had been the most frequently implicated source of botulism outbreaks. The Latin word *botulus* means *sausage*, hence *C. botulinum* was named after the meat products that were suspected to be its main source. However, spores may penetrate soil and contaminate plants via animal feces. Since the 1950s, vegetable products, surprisingly, have been the most important vehicles of *C. botulinum* in the U.S. The 'vegetable cases' – caused only by type A (61.1%) and type B (57.4%) – make up the majority of all reported botulism cases. Fruit and spices are also involved, but less frequently. It is significant that majority of cases (65.1%) are usually linked to home-made products.

Fish and seafood are generally responsible for infections caused by *C. botulinum* type E (Centers for Disease Control and Prevention, 1998). Many verified cases of botulism type E have been reported in Japan (166 cases and 58 deaths between 1951 and 1960). In 2003, *C. botulinum* type E was involved in the outbreak in western Alaska linked to consumption of a beached whale (Anonymous, 2003). Many outbreaks were also associated with a Japanese izuschi dish containing fermented raw fish, vegetables, and cooked and malted rice (okji). In Canada, Alaska, or Scandinavia, botulism is caused by consumption of fish and fermented meat dishes, very often prepared as traditional native dishes (Kotev et al., 1987; Knubley et al., 1995).

Uneviscerated salted mullet fish was a source of the outbreak (type E) in Egypt (Weber et al., 1993). The level of carbohydrates in such products is usually too low for lactic acid fermentation. If the pH of the product is not low enough, it will not protect against the outgrowth of *C. botulinum*.

Cucumbers and cabbage fermented by lactobacilli are popular dishes in the central and eastern Europe. Sauerkraut is frequently consumed by low-income communities, especially in winter. Surprisingly, no cases of botulism have been linked to consumption of such products. This observation may be explained based on the results of studies carried out by Braconnier et al. (2003). The authors analyzed germination of spores of *C. botulinum* type A and B, as well as changes in spore counts, in mushroom, broccoli, and potato purees. The addition of mixtures containing L-cysteine, L-alanine, and sodium lactate to vegetable puree induced an increase in germination, which suggests lack of these components in vegetable puree. Most probably, a low pH, lack of particular amino acids, and potential bacteriocin activity of lactobacilli in fermented vegetable products prevent spore germination.

Commercial products usually do not pose health threats to their consumers. However, botulism cases acquired after consumption of commercially prepared canned foods have been reported. In the U.S., 62 outbreaks occurred in the years 1899 to 1973 (Lynt et al., 1975). Only 7% of outbreaks reported between 1950 and 1996 were linked to commercially processed foods (Centers for Disease Control and Prevention, 1998). The implicated foodstuffs included chopped garlic in soy oil stored in glass bottles at room temperature (Louis et al., 1988), sliced roasted eggplant in oil, yogurt with hazelnuts, stuffed lotus rhizome, bottled caviar, and canned peanuts (Chou et al., 1988; D'Argenio et al., 1995).

Canned mushrooms were involved in many cases of botulism. It is suggested that *Agaricus bisporus* may induce *C. botulinum* spore germination due to oxygen consumption (Sugiyama and Yang, 1975).

Some cases are also connected with service establishments and caused mainly by improper temperature of food storage (Dodds, 1990).

Food stored in a proper way and in proper conditions is not a vehicle of *C. botulinum*. Unlike non-proteolytic strains, proteolytic strains will not grow in refrigeration temperatures. The number of spores in meat and poultry is rather low, much higher numbers are observed in fish. If stored at 3 to 5°C, vacuum-packed, not very sour meat products usually remain safe for consumers up to 21 days. Botulin toxin was not detected in raw rockfish fillets or red snapper homogenates after being stored for 21 days at 4°C. None of 1074 samples of commercially packed fresh fish stored for 12 days at 12°C contained botulin toxin (Lilly and Kautter, 1990).

The outgrowth of *C. botulinum* requires a suitable medium, temperature, atmosphere, pH, E_h potential, and water activity. Toxin is usually only produced in optimal or close-to-optimal conditions. Nutrient demands of *C. botulinum* are complex, and include amino acids, B vitamins, and minerals. In broth, non-proteolytic strains of type B and F grow and produce toxin at 4°C, but in crab meat the outgrowth and toxin production occurs solely at 26°C (Alberto et al., 2003).

It is believed that *C. botulinum* does not grow at pH lower than 4.5, yet botulin toxins were detected in sour home-canned foods. In Poland, toxins are sometimes detected in home-canned vinegar-preserved mushrooms. This may be explained by the presence of *Aspergillus* (Odlaug and Pflug, 1979) or other moulds. The outgrowth of moulds increases pH and enables growth of *Clostridium*. The growth of *C. botulinum* and toxin production depend also on the acidifying agent. The addition of even slight amounts of NaCl (3 to 4%) increases the susceptibility of *Clostridium* to pH – growth is inhibited at pH higher than 4.5.

A low water activity (a_w), which for *C. botulinum* ranges from 0.94 (type B) to 0.97 (type E), enables the outgrowth and toxin production in packaged foods and is typical for foodborne pathogens. The actual effect of a_w will depend on the strain properties and the type of agent regulating water activity.

The presence of other microorganisms is also very important for the outgrowth of *C. botulinum*. Botulin toxins in foods are usually inactivated by heat treatments. However, in non-processed food products, the presence of microflora significantly influences the outgrowth of clostridia. The outgrowth and toxin production is promoted by yeasts at pH 4.0. Yeasts produce a factor that enables the outgrowth of *Clostridium* at lower pH. A synergistic effect of clostridia and lactic acid bacilli (LAB) was also observed. However, LABs may also inhibit the outgrowth of *C. botulinum* due to bacteriocin activity. Such properties are revealed by *Lactobacillus*, *Lactococcus*, *Streptococcus* and *Pediococcus* (Rodgers et al., 2003). The outgrowth of *C. botulinum* may be inhibited by the presence of other *Clostridium* spp., e.g., *C. sporogenes*, and *C. perfringens* (Smith,1975). A similar activity was observed in case of *Peanibacillus* and *Bacillus* (Girardin et al., 2002). This is a commonly observed phenomenon of interspecies and intraspecies competition.

8.2.4 DETECTION OF BOTULIN TOXINS

Three types of detection methods are recommended for botulin toxins:

- Biological methods: Despite ethical objections, a biological method employing mice is still applied due to its sensitivity. It enables detection of the presence and type of toxin, and can be used for food as well as in serum, vomit, and stool samples.
- Genetic methods: Polymerase chain reaction (PCR) and its variants, e.g., multiplex PCR, are widely used for *C. botulinum* detection. Reverse-transcriptase PCR is recommended as an alternative to biological tests using mice (McGrath et al., 2000).
- Microbiological methods: classical microbiological tests can be used to detect *C. botulinum*.

8.3 *STAPHYLOCOCCUS AUREUS*

Staphylococcus aureus is known for its ability to produce a variety of toxins and many disease syndromes. One of the most frequently observed diseases is staphylococcal tonsillitis. These bacteria are frequently present on tonsils of healthy carriers. Patients that are affected by tonsillitis swallow staphylococci hidden in tonsil crypts. However, in this case staphylococci do not cause any gastrointestinal symptoms in the host organism, even if they enter the gastrointestinal tract. The barrier of gastric juice and conditions in a small intestine inhibit the outgrowth of staphylococci and toxin production – gastroenteritis is caused solely by a toxin produced outside the host organism.

Staphylococcal food poisonings (SFP) are among the most frequently diagnosed food poisonings, despite the fact that most cases are not reported to the epidemiological services. Over 30 species of *Staphylococcus* sp. are recognized and many of them may produce staphylococcal enterotoxin (SE). A majority of food isolates belongs to *S. aureus* and its toxins are the main cause of food poisonings. Humans are the main reservoir of staphylococci, the bacteria being frequently found in noses, throats and on skin of human carriers (Bustan et al., 1996).

8.3.1 STAPHYLOCOCCAL TOXINS

S. aureus is divided into six biotypes, based on its presence in humans and animals (Devriese, 1984; Hennekinne et al., 2003). The most frequent SEs are produced by a biotype A (human isolates of *S. aureus*) followed by a biotype C (isolated from cases of bovine and ovine mastitis). SEs may be also produced by *S. intermedius* and *S. hicus* (biotype E). Strains of poultry-like avian biotype (frequent among nasal carriers, e.g., food-industry workers) do not produce SEs (Isigidi et al., 1992). SEs are not destroyed by heating at 100°C for 30 minutes – this is the most important aspect of their potential occurrence in food products.

Enterotoxins comprise groups named from A to H: SEA, SEB, SEC (SEC$_1$, SEC$_2$, SEC$_3$), SED, SEE, SEF, SEG. Recently, further toxins have been described: SEH, SEI, SEK, SEL, SEM, SEN, SEO, SEU (Letertre et al., 2003; Orwin et al., 2001, 2003). Over 95% of staphylococcal food poisoning outbreaks have been caused by types from SEA to SEE (Bergdoll, 1983). Regardless of a considerable biological and physico-chemical similarity, toxins demonstrate strain antigenic variances and differ in biological assays. However, they reveal only few differences in amino acid sequences if their sources are considered. SEA had been a dominant toxin before 1971 and later it was surpassed by SED and SEC. After 1977, SEB started to become as frequent as SEA. Currently, SEE is predominant (Jay, 1986).

SEs belong to a large group of pyrogenic toxin superantigens (PTSAgs) produced by *S. aureus* and *Streptococcus pyogenes* (Dinges et al., 2000). All PTSAgs display three unique biological traits: pyrogenity, superantigenity, and the ability to increase the lethality of SEs in rabbits. SEs are also potent emetic agents. Superantigenity means that SEs may stimulate T lymphocytes. This stimulation is induced by the toxin binding to major histocompatibility (MHC) class II proteins present on antigen presenting cells, and to T-cell receptors (TCRs) on T lymphocytes CD4 and CD8. It is a non-specific, non-covalent bond, which occurs in a variable region of TCRs (TCR Vβ region) (Baker et al., 2002). Superantigens activate significantly higher levels of T lymphocytes than conventional antigens, but still lower than commonly used mitogens of T lymphocytes.

SEs are single polypeptides (26 to 28 kDa) displaying a high heterogeneity in isoelectric focusing. Three-dimensional crystal structures of SEA, SEB, and SEC$_3$ have been described (Swaminathan et al., 1992; Hoffmann et al., 1994; Bohach et al., 1995, 1996; Schad et al., 1995). They are thermostable proteins whose enterotoxicity and antigenicity properties are not destroyed during a 30-minute boiling.

SEA, SEE, and SED require zinc binding to MHC class II. Binding of SEC_3 also needs zinc, but is performed by different mechanisms than in SEA and SEE. Toxin has a structure (H–E–x–x–H) similar to metalloenzymes, e.g., thermilysin (Hase and Finkelstein,1993). Similar structures were identified in botulin neurotoxin. The toxin reveals proteolytic activity, which has a fundamental significance for the mode of toxin action (Papageorgiou et al., 1995).

The molecular regions responsible for gastrointestinal symptoms have been also determined. It has been found that a large central and C-terminal fragment of SEA, SEB and SEC_1 causes emesis. The N-terminal part does not trigger any symptoms. The presence of a disulfide loop is also necessary for symptom occurrence. All SEs (except for SEC) contain two cysteine residues, which form –S–S– bonds. Each SE type and subtype is characterized by a high level of structural dissimilarity, which enables production of highly specific antisera. However, crossreactivity is also observed among SEs, and usually affects SEB and SEC. This is troublesome for the development of diagnostic sera for toxin differentiation. Scientists are also on the lookout for polyvalent sequences within SE chains, which could possibly serve as therapeutic agents.

Genes encoding SEA and SEE may be carried by lysogenic phages (Betley and Mekalanos, 1985). However, such a phenomenon is not common as SED is encoded by a 27.5 kb plasmid, which also provides strains with resistance to penicillin and cadmium. Similarly, SEC and SEB are transmitted by plasmid containing penicillin-resistance genes. Other studies highlight that the genes encoding these toxins are located in a bacterial chromosome. Staphylococcal-toxin genes are insertion sites for more virulence factors, such as toxic shock staphylococcal toxin (TSST).

Based on the amino acid sequence, SEs have been divided into three groups. The first group includes SEB and SEC, together with subtypes and molecular variants. The second group consists of SEA, SEE and SED. The third group comprises SEH. There are numerous point mutations within particular groups. For example, SEC isolated from humans reveals a low level of dissimilarity (> 95% of similarity) if compared with bovine and ovine SEC (Marr et al., 1993).

SEs are produced during the late log or stationary phase, and SE production is strain-dependent. SEB and SEC are produced in great quantities. Toxins such as SED occur in small amounts (Su and Wong, 1993), and so cases of poisoning are underreported due to the mild symptoms of intoxication they produce.

Four loci are responsible for SE expression and production. Fifteen genes are regulated by *agr* (accessory gene regulator). Mutations within *agr* reduce SE expression. It also regulates expression of other staphylococcal toxins (Mullarky et al., 2001). However, not all SEs, e.g., SEA, are regulated by *agr*. The production of various SEs is negatively controlled by growth on media containing glucose, which affects *agr*. It is suggested that the glucose metabolism pathway lowers pH, impact on *agr*, and influence SEC production indirectly. There is also an other mechanism of regulation of SE production via glucose, which is neither *agr*- nor pH-dependent. *Staphylococcus* is osmoto-lerant and when bacteria are affected by osmotic stress, the production of SEB and SEC is reduced. Such an effect may be reversed by an introduction of osmoprotectants to the environment. Glycerol monolaurate – an emulsifier – also inhibits SE production (Recsei et al., 1986; Smith et al., 1986; Peng et al., 1988; Cheung et al., 1992; Schlievert et al., 1992).

8.3.2 Mechanism of Toxin Action

Contrary to the other staphylococcal toxins, SEs trigger emetic response after an oral administration (one of the SFP symptoms). Toxins are quickly eliminated from the organism via the renal pathway after being absorbed from the intestines. SEs act on intestinal mucosa after intragastral introduction, however their receptor has not yet been precisely identified. Two hypotheses on the possible mechanism of SE action have been put forward. The first suggests that inflammation is a result of degranulation, which occurs via the receptor on mast cells. The second, neurogenic, hypothesis proposes that mast cells are stimulated by a neuropeptide released by sensory nerves (Scheuber et al., 1987; Dinges et al., 2000). The mucopurulent excretion is produced in the stomach and the inflow of neutrophiles to lamina propria and epithelium (subsequently substituted by macrophages) is observed. A similar phenomenon occurs in the small intestine. Crypts are formed in jejunum, brush border is destroyed and an intensive infiltration of neutrophiles and macrophages to lamina propria occurs. Changes in colon are minimal. An increase in the levels of inflammation mediators (prostaglandin E_2, leukotrien B4 and 5-hydroksyei-cosatetraenoic acid) is observed during the course of inflammation (Kent, 1966; Komisar et al., 1992).

8.3.3 Enterotoxins and Food Products

The primary source of staphylococcal food contamination is human. However, cows are an additional source – staphylococci are causative agents of mastitis in cows and so may contaminate dairy products (Ombui et al., 1992). Although staphylococci are frequently present in pets (e.g., in dogs, which may suffer from mouth acne), these animals are not critical vehicles of food contamina-tion. Besides dairy products, staphylococci are also present in almost 30% of raw pork, salted meat, and uncooked smoked ham (Atanassova et al., 2001). Meat is frequently contaminated with *S. aureus* and may contain high numbers of colony-forming units (cfu) per gram (Surkiewicz et al., 1975). Home-made cakes, creams, and vegetable salads are important vehicles of staphylococci in central Europe.

Compared with other human pathogens, staphylococci are resistant to low a_w and so their outgrowth in cakes and sweets is possible.

Contamination of food products with staphylococci is not synonymous with the presence of enterotoxins. During production and maturation of Burgos cheese prepared from sheep milk, an increase in the number of *S. aureus* cfu by up to $\times 10^3$ to $\times 10^4$ units was observed. However, enterotoxins were not present (Otero et al., 1988). The enterotoxin production in maturing Camembert cheese produced from raw goat milk revealed that it depended on the initial *S. aureus* cfu (Meyrand et al., 1998). The SE synthesis may be inhibited by pH and glucose (Smith et al., 1986). The outgrowth of enterotoxic *S. aureus* is partially inhibited by starters containing *Lactobacillus sake*, *Pediococcus pentosaceus*, and *Staphylococcus xylosus*, used in sausage manufacturing. The production of SEs: A, B, C_1 and D is completely inhibited (Gonzalez-Fandos et al., 1994). SEA production depends on the staphylococcal growth rate.

Temperature also influences the synthesis of enterotoxins – they are usually produced at temperatures close to optimal (Yang et al., 2001). Out of 77 *S. aureus* strains isolated from food, 58% produced SEA, SEB, or SEE. The lowest temperature limit for the growth was 6.5 to 12.5°C, the highest, 39.5 to 48.5°C. The lowest level for enterotoxin production was 14 to 38°C, the highest, 35 to 44°C (Schmitt et al., 1990).

The amino acid composition of the environment also plays an important role. Valine is required for the outgrowth of *S. aureus*, arginine and cysteine, for the production of SEA, SEB, and SEC (Onoue and Mori, 1997). A low concentration of oleuropein (0.1%) – a phenol compound extracted from olives – retards the growth of *S. aureus*. Higher concentrations (>0.2%) inhibit completely the growth and production of enterotoxins (Tranter et al., 1993).

In the U.S., SFPs are not obligatorily reported diseases. SFPs comprise 14% of all foodborne diseases and it is estimated that only a small percentage of cases are noted by official sanitary and medical authorities. In other countries, such as Hungary, the number of cases is estimated to be about 40% of the total (Bergdoll, 1979). The frequency of SFPs in Japan is 20 to 25%, and rice balls are usually responsible for the disease occurrence. Corned beef and, less frequently, milk are reported in many countries as the main sources of infections. As *Staphylococcus* are mesophilic microorganisms, conditions for growth are better in summer. However, the major factors promoting foodborne poisonings are improper hygiene during food processing, distribution, and storage.

The most frequently observed symptoms include vomiting (82%), nausea (74%), abdominal cramps (64%), diarrhea (64%), and also headaches and muscular cramping. The onset of symptoms usually starts after 6 to 10 hours after food ingestion, however they may be reported earlier. The lethal cases are rare and occur among infants and elderly people. Only 10% of affected people need medical treatment – treatments include analgesics, antidiarrheic drugs, and administration of fluids.

The precise infectious dose has not been established. It probably ranges from 10^5 to 10^8 cfu per g and depends on the environmental conditions and strain properties. The SE concentration of 1ng per g of contaminated food is necessary to trigger the disease symptoms. However, some cases have been described where the dose activating disease symptoms was significantly lower. Tests on human volunteers revealed that 20 to 25 μg (0.4 μg per kg of body weight) led to vomiting.

In addition to SFPs, enterotoxins may participate in the development of atopic eczema (Morishita et al., 1999; Wehner and Neuber, 2001) and menstrual toxic-shock syndrome (MTSS) (Morishita et al., 1999).

8.3.4 DETECTION OF STAPHYLOCOCCAL TOXINS

Three groups of methods have been applied to the detection of staphylococcal enterotoxins:

- Biological methods: This is the oldest group of test methods. In the past, cats were administered food filtrates intraperitoneally, and if the samples being tested were contaminated the cats would vomit. Animal tests are no longer used due to ethical and financial considerations. Cell cultures are now recommended. They are sensitive, cheap, and rapid tests – the cytotoxicity effect may be observed after only two hours (Normanno et al., 2001) – however such tests are not widely applied.
- Immunological methods: Methods such as gel-agglutination tests were introduced many years ago (according to Outcherlony) however they are not sufficiently sensitive. Reversed passive latex agglutination kits (SET-RPLA and TST-RPLA) are presently applied for enterotoxin detection and are more sensitive than gel diffusion (Wieneke, 1988). The ELISA technique is also very popular – toxins are detected via VIDAS STAPH ENTEROTOXIN SET and indirect double sandwich ELISA (Meyrand et al., 1998).
- Molecular biology methods: PCR and its variants are employed for direct detection of fragments of SEA, SEB, SEC, SED, SEE, SEG, SEH and SEI genes. PCR is repeatable and is consistent with passive latex agglutination assay for detection of SEs *in vitro* (McLauchlin et al., 2000). PCR detects only the gene encoding toxin, not a toxin itself. To cope with such a limitation, a PCR-ELISA method has been developed, which is a more sensitive test for detecting of SEA and SEB genes than standard ELISA (Gilligan et al., 2000).

8.4 REFERENCES

Agui, T., Syuto, B., Oguma, K., Iida, H. and Kubo, S., Binding of *Clostridium botulinum* type C neurotoxin to rat synaptosomes, *J. Biochem.*, 94, 521–527, 1983.

Alberto, F., Broussolle, V., Mason, D.R., Carlin, F. and Peck, M.W., Variability in spore germination response by strains of proteolytic *Clostridium botulinum* types A, B and F, *Lett. Appl. Microbiol.*, 36, 41–45, 2003.

Anonymous, Outbreak of botulism type E associated with eating a beached whale – Western Alaska, July 2002, *Morbid. Mortal. Weekly Rep.*, 52, 24–26, 2003.

Atanassova, V., Meindl. A. and Ring, C., Prevalence of *Staphylococcus aureus* and staphylococcal enterotoxins in raw pork and uncooked smoked ham – a comparison of classical culturing detection and RFLP-PCR, *Int. J. Food Microbiol.*, 68, 105–13, 2001.

Baker, M.D., Papageorgiu, A.C., Tiball, R.W., Miller, J., White, S., Lingard, B., Lee, J.J., Cavanagh, D., Kehoe, M.A., Robinsonm, J.H. and Acharya, K.R., Structural and functional role of threonine 112 in a superantigen *Staphylococcus aureus* enterotoxin B, *J. Biol. Chem.*, 277, 2756–2762, 2002.

Bakry, N., Kamata, Y. and Simpson, L.L., Lectins from *Triticum vulgaris* and *Umax flavus* are universal antagonists of botulinum neurotoxin and tetanus toxin, *J. Pharmacol. Exp. Ther.*, 258, 830–836, 1991.

Barth, H., Roebling, R., Fritz, M. and Aktories, K., The binary *Clostridium botulinum* C2 toxin as a protein delivery systems. Identification of the minimal protein region necessary for interaction of toxin, *J. Biol. Chem.*, 277, 5074–5081, 2002.

Bergdoll, M.S., Staphylococcal intoxication, in Reimarm, H. and Bryan, F.L., eds., *Food-Borne Infections and Intoxications*, Academic Press, New York, pp. 443–494, 1979.

Bergdoll, M.S., Enterotoxins, in Easton, C.S.F. and Adlam, C., eds., *Staphylococci and Staphylococcal Infections*, Academic Press, London, pp. 559–598, 1983.

Betley, M.J. and Mekalanos, J.J., Staphylococcal enterotoxin A is encoded by phage, *Science*, 229, 185–191, 1985.

Binz, T., Blasi, J., Yamasaki, S., Baumeister, A., Unk, E., Sudhof, T.C., Jahn, R. and Niemann, H., Proteolysis of SNAP-25 by types E and A botulinal neurotoxins, *J. Biol. Chem.*, 269, 1617–1620, 1994.

Black, J.D. and Dolly, J.O., Interaction of 125, I-labelled botulinum neurotoxins with nerve terminals. I. Ultrastructural autoradiographic localization and quantitation of distinct membrane acceptors for types A and B on motor nerves, *J. Cell Biol.*, 103, 521–534, 1986.

Blöcker, D., Bachmeyer, C., Benz, R., Aktories, K. and Barth, H., Channel formation by the binding component of *Clostridium botulinum* C2 toxin: glutamate 307 of C2II affects channel properties *in vitro* and pH–dependent C2I translocation *in vivo*, *Biochem.*, 42, 5368–5377, 2003.

Blöcker, D., Pohlmann, K., Haug, G., Bachmeyer, C., Benz, R., Aktories, K. and Barth, H., Low pH-induced pore formation is required for translocation of the enzyme component C2I into the cytosol of host cells, *J. Biol. Chem.*, 278, 37360–37367, 2003.

Bohach, G.A., Jablonski, L.M., Deobald, C.F., Chi, Y.-I. and Stauffacher, C.V., Functional domains of staphylococcal enterotoxins, in Ecklund, M., Richard and Mise, K., eds., *Molecular Approaches to Food Safety; Issues Involving Toxic Microorganisms*, Alaken Inc. Fort Collins, pp. 339–356, 1995.

Bohach, G.A., Stauffacher, C.V., Ohlendorf, D.H., Chi, Y.-I., Valf, G.M. and Schlivert, P.M., The staphylococcal and streptococcal pyrogenic toxin family, in Singh, B.R. and Tu, A.T., eds., *Natural Toxin II*, Plenum Publishing Corporation, New York, pp. 131–154, 1996.

Bohnel, H., Schwagerick, B. and Gessler, F., Visceral botulism – a new form of bovine *Clostridium botulinum* toxication, *J. Vet. Med. A. Physiol. Pathol. Clin. Med.*, 48, 373–383, 2001.

Boquet, P., Munro, P., Fiorentini, C. and Just, I., Toxins from anaerobic bacteria: specificity and molecular mechanism of action, *Curr. Opin. Microbiol.*, 1, 66–74, 1998.

Braconnier, A., Broussolle, V., Dargaignaratz, C., Nguyen-The, C. and Carlin, F., Growth and germination of proteolytic *Clostridium botulinum* in vegetable-based media, *J. Food Prot.*, 66, 833–839, 2003.

Busch, C. and Aktories, K., Microbial toxins and the glycosylation of Rho family GTPases, *Curr. Opin. Struct. Biol.*, 10, 528–535, 2000.

Bustan al, M.A., Udo, E.E. and Chugh, T.D., Nasal carriage of enterotoxin-producing *Staphylococcus aureus* among restaurant workers in Kuwait City, *Epidemiol. Infect.*, 116, 319–322, 1996.

Centers for Disease Control and Prevention, *Botulinism in the United States, 1899–1996. Handbook for Epidemiologists, Clinicians and Laboratory Workers*, Atlanta, 1998.

Chaddock, J.A., Purkiss, J.R., Friis, L.M., Broadbridge, J.D., Duggan, M.J. Fooks, S.J., Shone, C.C., Quinn, C.P. and Foster, K.A., Inhibition of vesicular secretion in both neuronal and nonneuronal cells by a retargeted endopeptidase derivate of *Clostridium botulinum* neurotoxin type A, *Infect. Immun.*, 68, 2587–2593, 2000.

Cheung, A.L., Koomey, J.M., Butler, C.A, Projan, S.J. and Fishetti, V.A., Regulation of exoprotein expression in *Staphylococcus aureus* by a locus (sar) disting from agr, *Proc. Natl. Acad. Sci. U.S.A.*, 89, 6462–6466, 1992.

Chou, J.H., Hwang, P.H. and Malison, M.D., An outbreak of type A foodborne botulism in Taiwan due to commercially preserved peanuts, *Int. J. Epidemiol.*, 17, 899–902, 1988.

Ciccarelli, A.S., Whaley, D.N., McCroskey, L.M., Gimenez, D.F., Dowell, V.R.Ir and Hatheway, C.L., Cultural and physiological characteristics of *Clostridium botulinum* type G and the susceptibility of certain animals to its toxin, *Appl. Envir. Microbiol.*, 34, 843–848, 1977.

Cobb, S.P., Hogg, R.A., Calloner, D.J., Brett, M.M., Livesey, C.T., Sharpe, R.T. and Jones, T.O., Suspected botulinism in dairy cows and its implications for the safety of human food, *Vet. Rec.*, 150, 5–8, 2002.

D'Argenio, P., Palumbo, F., Ortolani, R., Pizzuti, R., Russo, M., Carducd, R., Soscia, M., Aureli, P., Fenicia, L., Franciosa, G., Parella, A. and Scala, V., Type B botulism associated with roasted eggplant in oil, *Morbid. Mortal. Weekly Rep.*, 44, 33–36, 1995.

Dahlenborg, M., Bach, E. and Radstrom, P., Development of a combined selection and enrichment PCR procedure for *Clostridium botulinum* types B, E and F and its use to determine prevalence in fecal samples from slaughtered pigs, *Appl. Env.. Microbiol.*, 67, 4781–4788, 2001.

Dahlenborg, M., Borch, E. and Radstrom, P., Prevalence of *Clostridium botulinum* types B, E and F in faecal samples from Swedish cattle, *Int. J. Food Microbiol.*, 82, 105–110, 2003.

DasGupta, B.R., Structure and biological activity of botulinum neurotoxin, *J. Physiol.*, 84, 220–228, 1990.

De Boer, M.L., Kum, W.W. and Chow, A.W., *Staphylococcus aureus* isogenic mutant, deficient in toxic shock syndrome toxin-1 but not staphylococcal enterotoxin A production, exhibits attenuated virulence in a tampon-associated vaginal infection model of toxic shock syndrome, *Can. J. Microbiol.*, 45, 250–256, 1999.

Devriese, L.A., A simplified system for biotyping *Staphylococcus aureus* strains isolated from different animal species, *J. Appl. Bacteriol.*, 56, 215–220, 1984.

Dineen, S.S., Bradshaw, M. and Johnson, E.A., Neurotoxin gene clusters in *Clostridium botulinum* type A strains: sequence comparison and evolutionary implications, *Curr. Microbiol.*, 46, 345–352, 2003.

Dinges, M.M., Orwin, P.M. and Schlievert, P.M., Exotoxins of *Staphylococcus aureus*, *Clin. Microbiol. Rev.*, 13, 16–34, 2000.

Dodds, K.L., Restaurant-associated botulism outbreaks in North America, *Food Control*, 1, 139–141, 1990.

Dodds K.L., *Clostridium botulinum* in the environment, in Hauschild, A.H.W. and Dodds K.L., eds., Clostridium botulinum: *Ecology and Control in Foods*, Marcel Dekker, New York, pp. 51–68, 1993a.

Dodds K.L., *Clostridium botulinum* in the environment, in Hauschild, A.H.W. and Dodds K.L., eds., Clostridium botulinum: *Ecology and Control in Foods*, Marcel Dekker, New York, pp. 21–51, 1993b.

Dolly, J.O., Black, J., Williams, R.S. and Melling, J., Acceptors for botulinum neurotoxin reside on motor nerve terminals and mediate its internalization, *Nature*, 307, 457–460, 1984.

East, A.K., Stacey, I.M. and Collins, M.D., Cloning and sequencing of hemagglutinin component of the botulinum neurotoxin complex encoded by *Clostridium botulinum* types A and B, *Syst. Appl. Microbiol.*, 17, 306–312, 1994.

Eklund, M.W., Poysky, F.T. and Reed, S.M., Bacteriophages and toxigenicity of *Clostridium boiulinum* type D, *Nature New Biol.*, 235, 16–17, 1972.

Eklund, M.W., Poysky, F.T., Meyers, J.A. and Pelroy, G.A., Interspecies conversion of *Clostridium botulinum* type C to *Clostridium novyi* type A by bacteriophage, *Science*, 186, 456–458, 1974.

Eklund, M.W., Poysky, F.T. and Habig, W.H., Bacteriophages and plasmids in *Clostridium botulinum* and *Clostridium tetani* and their relationship to production of toxins, in Simpson, L.L., ed., *Botulinum Neurotoxin and Tetanus Toxin*, Academic Press, New York, pp. 25–51, 1989.

Evans, D., Williams, R.S., Shone, C.C., Hambleton, P., Melling, J. and Dolly, J.O., Botulinum neurotoxin type B. Its purification, radioiodination and interaction with rat-brain synaptosomal membranes, *Eur. I. Biochem.*, 154, 409–416, 1986.

Fach, P., Perelle, S., Dilasser, F., Grout, J., Dargaignaratz, C., Botella, L., Gourreau, J.-M., Carlin, F., Popoff, M.R. and Broussolle, V., Detection by PCR-enzyme-linked immunosorbent assay of *Clostridium botulinum* in fish and environmental samples from a coastal area in Northern France, *Appl. Env. Microbiol.*, 68, 5870–5876, 2002.

Falnes, P.O. and Sandvig, K., Penetration of protein toxins into cells, *Curr. Opin. Cell Biol.*, 12, 407–413, 2000.

Fujinaga, Y., Inoue, K., Nomura, T., Sasaki, J., Marvaud, J.C., Popoff, M.R., Kozaki, S. and Oguma, K., Identification and characterization of functional submits of *Clostridium botulinum* type A progenitor toxin involved in binding to intestinal microvilli and erythrocytes, *FEBS Letters*, 467, 179–183, 2000.

Gilligan, K., Shipley, M., Stiles, B., Hadfield, T.L. and Sofi Ibrahim M., Identification of *Staphylococcus aureus* enterotoxins A and B genes by PCR-ELISA, *Mol. Cell Probes*, 14, 71–78, 2000.

Girardin, H., Albagnac, C., Dargaignaratz, C., Nguyen-The, C. and Carlin, F., Antimicrobial activity of foodborne *Paenibacillus* and *Bacillus* spp. against *Clostridium botulinum*, *J. Food Prot.*, 65, 806–813, 2002.

Gonzalez-Fandos, E., Otero, A., Sierra, M., Garcia-Lopez, M.L. and Prieto, M., Effect of three commercial starters on growth of *Staphylococcus aureus* and enterotoxins (A–D) and thermonuclease production in broth, *Int. J. Food Microbiol.*, 24, 321–327, 1994.

Hall, J.D., McCroskey, L.M., Pincomb, B.J. and Hatheway, C.L., Isolation of an organism resembling *Clostridium barati* which produces type F botulinal toxin from an infant with botulism, *J. Clin. Microbiol.*, 21, 654–655, 1985.

Harvey, S.M., Sturgeon, J. and Dassey, D.E., Botulinsm due to *Clostridium baratti* type F toxin, *J. Clin. Microbiol.*, 40, 2260–2262, 2002.

Hase, C.C. and Finkelstein, R.A., Bacterial extracellular zinc-containing metalloproteases, *Microbiol. Rev.*, 57, 823–837, 1993.

Hatheway, C.L., *Clostridium botulinum* and other *Clostridia* that produce botulinum neurotoxin, in Hauschild, A.H.W. and Dodds, K.L,. eds., Clostridium botulinum: *Ecology and Control in Foods*, Marcel Dekker, New York, pp. 3–20, 1993.

Hauser, D., Gibert, M., Boquet, P. and Popoff, M.R., Plasmid localization of a type E botulinal neurotoxin gene homologue in toxigenic *Clostridium butyricum* strains, and absence of this gene in non-toxigenic *C. butyricum* strains, *FEMS Microbiol. Lett.*, 78, 251–255, 1992.

Hennekinne, J.A., Kerouanton, A., Brisabois, A. and De Buyser, M.L., Discrimination of *Staphylococcus aureus* biotypes by pulsed-field gel electrophoresis of DNA macro-restriction fragments, *J. Appl. Microbiol.*, 94, 321–329, 2003.

Hoffmann, M.L., Jablonski, L.M., Crum, K.K., Hackett, S.P., Chi, Y.-I., Stauffacher, D.L., Stevens, D.L. and Bohach, G.A., Predictions of T cell receptor and major histocompatibility complex binding sites on staphylococcal enterotoxin C1, *Infect. Immun.*, 62, 3396–3407, 1994.

Inoue, K., Fujinaga,Y., Watanabe, T., Ohyama, T., Takeshi, K., Morishii, K., Nakajiama, H. and Oguma, K., Molecular composition of *Clostridium botulinum* type A. *Infect. Immun.*, 64, 1589–1594, 1996.

Isigidi, B.K., Mathieu, A.M., Devriese, L.A., Godard, C. and Van Hoof, J., Enterotoxin production in different *Staphylococcus aureus* biotypes isolated from food and meat plants, *J. Appl. Bacteriol.*, 72, 16–20, 1992.

Jay, J.M., *Staphylococcal Gastroenteritis, in Modern Food Microbiology*, 3rd ed., Van Nostrad Reinhold, New York, pp. 437–458, 1986.

Johnson, E.A. and Bradshaw, M., *Clostridium botulinum* and its neurotoxins: a metabolic and cellular perspective, *Toxicon*, 39, 1703–1722, 2001.

Kent, T.H., Staphylococcal enterotoxin gastroenteritis in rhesus monkeys, *Am. J. Pathol.*, 122, 169–176, 1966.

Khan, A.S., Morse, S. and Lillibridge, S., Public health preparedness for biological terrorism in the USA, *Lancet*, 356, 1179–1182, 2000.

Knubley, W., McChesney, T.C. and Mallonee, J., Foodborne botulism – Oklahoma, 1994, *JAMA*, 273, 1167, 1995.

Komisar, J., Revera, J., Vega, A. and Tseng, J., Effects of staphylococal enterotoxin B on rodent mast cells, *Infect. Immun.*, 60, 2969–2975, 1992.

Kotev, S., Leventhal, A., Bashary, A., Zahavi, H. and Cohen, A., International outbreak of type E botulism associated with ungutted, salted whitefish, *Morbid. Mortal. Weekly Rep.*, 36, 812–813, 1987.

Krieglstein, K.G., DasGupta, B.R. and Henschen, A.H., Covalent structure of botulinum neurotoxin type-A-location of sulfhydryl groups, and disulfide bridges and identification of C-termini of light and heavy chains, *J. Protein Chem.*, 13, 49–57, 1994.

Ledoux, D.N., Be, X.H. and Singh, B.R., Quaternary structure of botulinum and tetanus neurotoxins as probed by chemical cross-linking and native gel electrophoresis, *Toxicon*, 32, 1095–1104, 1994.

Letertre, C., Perelle, S., Dilasser, F. and Fach, P., Identification of new putative enterotoxin SEU by the egc cluster, *J. Appl. Microbiol.*, 95, 38–43, 2003.

Lilly, T., Jr. and Kautter, D.A., Outgrowth of naturally occurring *Clostridium botulinum* in vacuum-packaged fresh fish, *J. Assoc. Off. Anal. Chem.*, 73, 211–212, 1990.

Louis St., M.E., Peck, S.H.S., Bowering, D., Morgan, G.B., Blatherwick, J., Banerjee, S., Kettyls, G.D.M., Black, W.A., Milling, M.E., Hauschild, A.H.W., Tauxe, R.V. and Blake, P.A., Botulism from chopped garlic: Delayed recognition of a major outbreak, *Ann. Intern. Med.*, 108, 363–368, 1988.

Lynt, R.K., Solomon, H.M., Lilly, T., Jr. and Kautter, D.A., Botulinism in commercially canned foods, *J. Milk Food Technol.*, 38, 546–550, 1975.

Maksymowich, A.B., Reinhard, M., Malizano, C.J., Goodnough, M.C. and Johnson, E.C., Pure botulinum nerurotoxin is absorbed from the stomach and small intestine and products neuromuscular blockade, *Infect. Immun.*, 67, 4708–4712, 1999.

Marr, J.C., Lyon, J.D., Roberson, J.R., Lupher, M., Davis, W.C. and Bohach, G.A., Characterization of novel type C staphylococcal enetrotoxins: biological and evolutionary implications, *Infect. Immun.*, 61, 4254–4262, 1993.

Marvaud, J.C., Raffestin, S., Gibert, M. and Popoff, M.R., Regulation of the toxinogenesis in *Clostridium botulinum* and *Clostridium tetani*, *Biol. Cell*, 92, 455–457, 2000.

McCroskey, L.M., Hatheway, C.L., Fenida, L., Pasolini, B. and Aureli, P., Characterization of an organism that produces type E botulinal toxin but which resembles *Clostridium butyricum* from feces of an infant with type E botulism, *J. Clin. Microbiol.*, 23, 201–202, 1986.

McGrath, S., Dolley, J.S.G. and Haylock, R.W., Quantification of *Clostridium botulinum* toxin gene expression by competitive reverse transcription PCR, *Appl. Env. Microbiol.*, 66, 1423–1428, 2000.

McLauchlin, J., Narayanan, G.L., Mithani, V. and O'Neill, G., The detection of enterotoxins and toxic shock syndrome toxin genes in *Staphylococcus aureus* by polymerase chain reaction, *J. Food Prot.*, 63, 479–88, 2000.

Mead, P.S., Slutsker, L., Dietz, V., McCaig, L.F., Bresee, J.S., Shapiro, C., Griffin, P.M. and Tauxe, R.V., Food-related illness and death in the United States, *Emerging Infect. Dis.*, 5, 607–625, 1999.

Meyrand, A., Boutrand-Loei, S., Ray-Gueniot, S., Mazuy, C., Gaspard, C.E., Jaubert, G., Perrin, G., Lapeyre, C. and Vernozy-Rozand, C., Growth and enterotoxin production of *Staphylococcus aureus* during the manufacture and ripening of Camembert-type cheeses from raw goats' milk, *J. Appl. Microbiol.*, 85, 537–544, 1998.

Montecucco, C., Papini, E. and Schiavo, G., Bacterial protein toxins penetrate via a four step mechanism, *FEBS Lett.*, 346, 92–98, 1994.

Montecucco, C. and Schiavo, G., Mechanism of action of tetanus and botulinum neurotoxins, *Mol. Microbiol.*, 13, 1–8, 1994.

Morishita, Y., Tada, J., Sato, A., Toi, Y., Kanzaki, H., Akiyama, H. and Arata, J., Possible influences of *Staphylococcus aureus* on atopic dermatitis – the colonizing features and the effects of staphylococcal enterotoxins, *Clin. Exp. Allergy*, 29, 1110–1117, 1999.

Mullarky, I.K., Su, C., Frieze, N., Park, Y.H. and Sordillo, L.M., *Staphylococcus aureus* agr genotypes with enterotoxin production capabilities can resist neutrophil bactericidal activity, *Infect. Immun.*, 68, 45–51, 2001.

Nevas, M., Hielm, S., Lindstrom, M., Horn, H., Koivulehto, K. and Korkeala, H., High prevalence of *Clostridium botulinum* types A and B in honey samples detected by polymerase chain reaction, *Int. J. Food Microbiol.*, 72, 45–52, 2002.

Normanno, G., Celano, G., Dambrosio, A., Lassandro, L. and Buonavoglia, C., Enterotoxins of *Staphylococcus aureus* induce a cytopathic effect in cell lines, *New Microbiol.*, 24, 341–346, 2001.

Odlaug, T.E. and Pflug, I.J., *Clostridium botulinum* growth and toxin production in tomato juice containing *Aspergillus gracilis*, *Appl. Environ. Microbiol.*, 37, 496–504, 1979.

Ombui, J.N., Arimi, S.M. and Kayihura, M., Raw milk as a source of enterotoxigenic *Staphylococcus aureus* and enterotoxins in consumer milk, *East Afr. Med. J.*, 69, 123–125, 1992.

Onoue, Y. and Mori, M., Amino acid requirements for the growth and enterotoxin production by *Staphylococcus aureus* in chemically defined media, *Int. J. Food Microbiol.*, 36, 77–82, 1997.

Orwin, P.M., Leung, D.Y.M., Donahue, H.L., Novick, R.P. and Schlievert, P.M., Biochemical and biological properties of Staphylococcal enterotoxin K, *Infect. Immun.*, 69, 360–366, 2001.

Orwin, P.M., Fitzgerald, J.R., Leung, D.Y.M., Gutierrez, J.A., Bohach, G.A. and Schlievert P.M., Characterization of *Staphylococcus aureus* enterotoxin L, *Infect. Immun.*, 71, 2916–2919, 2003.

Otero, A., Garcia, M.C., Garcia, M.L., Prieto, M. and Moreno, B., Behaviour of *Staphylococcus aureus* strains, producers of enterotoxins C1 or C2, during the manufacture and storage of Burgos cheese, *J. Appl. Bacteriol.*, 64, 117–122, 1988.

Papageorgiou, A.C., Acharya, K.R., Shapiro, R., Passalacqua, E.F., Brehm, R.D. and Tranter, H.S., Crystal structure of the superantigen enterotoxin C2 from *Staphylococcus aureus* reveals a zinc-binding site, *Structure*, 3, 769–779, 1995.

Park, M.K, Jung, H.H. and Yang, K.H., Binding of *Clostridium botulinum* type B toxin to rat brain synaptosome, *FEMS Microbiol. Lett.*, 60, 243–247, 1990.

Park, J.B. and Simpson, L.L., Inhalational poisoning by botulinum toxin and inhalation vaccination with its heavy-chain component, *Infect. Immun.*, 71, 1147–1154, 2003.

Peng, H.L., Novick, R.P., Kreiswirth, B., Kornblum, J. and Schlievert, P., Cloning characterization and sequencing of an accessory gene regulator (*agr*) in *Staphylococcus aureus*, *J. Bacteriol.*, 170, 4365–4372, 1988.

Poulain, B., Mochida, S., Weller, U., Hogy, B., Habermann, E., Wadsworth, J. D., Shone, C.C., Dolly, J.O. and Tauc, L., Heterologous combinations of heavy and light chains from botulinum neurotoxin A and tetanus toxin inhibit neurotransmitter release in Aplysia, *J. Biol. Chem.*, 266, 9580–9585, 1991.

Prabakaran, S., Tepp, W. and DasGupta, B.R., Botulinum neurotoxin types B and E: purification, limited proteolysis by endoproteinase Glu-C and pepsin, and comparison of their identified cleaved sites relative to the three-dimensional structure of type A neurotoxin, *Toxicon*, 39, 1515–1531, 2001.

Recsei, P., Kreiswirth, B., O'Reilly, M., Schkievert, P., Gruss, A. and Novick, R.P., Regulation of exoprotein gene expression in *Staphylococcus aureus* by agr, *Mol. Gen. Genet.*, 202, 58–61, 1986.

Rodgers, S., Peiris, P. and Casadei, G., Inhibition of nonproteolytic *Clostridium botulinum* with lactic acid bacteria and their bacteriocins at refrigeration temperatures, *J. Food Prot.*, 66, 674–678, 2003.

Rundervoort, R.S., van der Ven, A.J., Vermeulen, C. and van Oostenbrugge, R.J., The clinical diagnosis 'wound botulism' in an injecting drug addict, *Ned. Tijdschr. Geneeskd.*, 147, 124–127, 2003.

Sakaguchi, G., Kozaki, S. and Ohshi, I., *Bacterial Protein Toxins*, Academic Press, London, pp. 435–443, 1984.

Sakaguchi, G., Molecular structure of *Clostridium botulinum* progenitor toxins, in Portland, A.L., Dowel, V.R. and Richard, I.L., eds., *Microbial Toxins in Foods and Feeds. Cellular and Molecular Modes of Action*, Plenum Press, New York, pp. 173–180, 1990.

Schad, E.M., Zitseva, I., Zaitsev, V.N., Dohlste Kalland, M., Schlivert, P.M., Ohlendorf, D.H. and Svenson, Crystal structure of the superantigen staphylococcal enterotoxin A, *EMBO J.*, 14, 3292–3333, 1995.

Schengrund, C.L., Ringler, N.J. and DasGupta, B.R., Adherence of botulinum and tetanus neurotoxins to synaptosomal proteins, *Brain Res. Bull.*, 29, 917–924, 1991.

Scheuber, P.H., Denzlinger, C., Wilker, D., Bed Keppler, G. and Hammer, D.K., Staphylococcal enterotoxin B as a nonimmunological mast cell stimulus in primates; the role of endogenous cysteinyl leukotriens, *Int. Arch. Allergy Appl. Immunol.*, 82, 289–291, 1987.

Schiavo, G., Malizio, C., Trimble, W.S., Polverino de Laureto, P., Milan, G., Sugiyama, H., Johnson, E.A. and Montecucco, C., Botulinum G neurotoxin cleaves VAMP/synaptobrevin at a single Ala–Ala peptide bond, *J. Biol. Chem.*, 269, 20213–20226, 1994.

Schiavo, G., Shone, C.C., Rossetto, O., Alexander, F.C. and Montecucco, C., Botulinum neurotoxin serotype 1 is a zinc endopeptidase specific for VAMP/synaptobrevin, *J. Biol. Chern.*, 268, 11516–11519, 1993.

Schiavo, G., Rossetto, O., Benfenati, F., Poulain, B. and Montecucco, C., Tetanus and botulinum neurotoxins are zinc proteases specific for components of the neuroexcytosis apparatus, *Ann. N. Y. Acad. Sci.*, 710, 65–75, 1994.

Schiavo, G., Shone, C.C., Bennett, M.K., Scheller, R.H. and Montecucco, C.M., Botulinum neurotoxin type C cleaves a single Lys–Ala bond within the carboxyl-terminal region of syntaxins, *J. Biol Chem.*, 270, 10566–10570, 1995.

Schlievert, P.M., Deringer, J.R., Kim, M.H., Projan, S.J. and Novick, R.P., Effect of glycerol monolaurate on bacterial growth and toxin production, *Antimicrob. Agents Chemother.*, 36, 626–631, 1992.

Schmitt, M., Schuler-Schmid, U. and Schmidt-Lorenz, W., Temperature limits of growth, TNase and enterotoxin production of *Staphylococcus aureus* strains isolated from foods, *Int. J. Food Microbiol.*, 11, 1–19, 1990.

Smith, L.D.S., Inhibition of *Clostridium botulinum* by strains of *Clostridium perfringens* isolated from soil, *Appl. Microbiol.*, 30, 319–323, 1975.

Smith, J.L., Bencivengo, M.M., Buchanan, R.L. and Kunsch, C.A., Enterotoxin A production in *Staphylococcus aureus*: inhibition by glucose, *Arch. Microbiol.*, 144, 131–136, 1986.

Sobel, J.,A., Khan, S. and Swerdlow, D.L., Threat of a biological terrorist attack on the US food supply: the CDC perspective, *Lancet*, 359, 874–880, 2002.

Stiles, B.G., Blocker, D., Hale, M.L., Guetthoff, M.A. and Barth, H., *Clostridium botulinum* C2 toxin: binding studies with fluorescence-activated cytometry, *Toxicon*, 40, 1135–1140, 2002.

Su, Y.-C. and Wong, A.C.L., Optimal condition for the production of unidentified staphylococcal entrotoxins, *J. Food Prot.*, 56, 313–316, 1993.

Sugiyama, H. and Yang, K.H., Growth potential of *Clostridium botulinum* in fresh mushrooms packaged in semipermeable plastic film, *Appl. Microbiol.*, 30, 964–969, 1975.

Surkiewicz, B.E., Harris, M.E., Elliott, R.P., Macaluso, J.F. and Strand, M.M., Bacteriological survey of raw beef patties produced at establishments under federal inspection, *Appl. Microbiol.*, 29, 331–334, 1975.

Swaminathan, S., Furey, W., Pletcher, J. and Sax, M., Crystal structure of staphylococcal enterotoxin B, a superantigen, *Nature*, 359, 801–806, 1992.

Tabita, K., Sakaguchi, S., Kozaki, S. and Sakaguchi, G., Distinction between *Clostridium botulinum* type A strains associated with food-borne botulism and those with infant botulism in Japan in intraintestinal toxin production in infant mice and some other properties, *FEMS Microbiol. Lett.*, 63, 2–3, 251–256, 1999.

Tanzi, M.G. and Gabay, M.P., Association between honey consumption and infant botulism, *Pharmacotherapy*, 22, 1479–1483, 2002.

Tranter, H.S., Tassou, S.C. and Nychas, G.J., The effect of the olive phenolic compound, oleuropein, on growth and enterotoxin B production by *Staphylococcus aureus*, *J. Appl. Bacteriol.*, 74, 253–9, 1993.

Tsuzuki, K., Kimura, K., Fujii, N., Yokosawa, N. and Oguma, K., The complete nucleotide sequence of *me* gene coding for the nontoxic-nonhemagglutinin component of *Clostridium botulinum* type C progenitor toxin, *Biochem. Biophys. Res. Comm.*, 183, 1273–1279, 1992.

Weber, J.T., Hibbs, R.G., Darwish, A. and Mishu, B., A massive outbreak of type E botulism associated with traditional salted fish in Cairo, *J. Infect. Dis.*, 167, 451–454, 1993.

Wehner, J. and Neuber, K., *Staphylococcus aureus* enterotoxins induce histamine and leukotriene release in patients with atopic egzema, *Br. J. Dermatol.*, 145, 302–305, 2001.

Wieneke, A.A., The detection of enterotoxin and toxic shock syndrome toxin-1 production by strains of *Staphylococcus aureus* with commercial RPLA kits, *Int. J. Food Microbiol.*, 7, 25–30, 1988.

Williams, R.S., Tse, C.-K., Dolly, J.O., Hamblet, P. and Melling, J., Radioiodination of botulinum neurotoxin type A with retention of biological activity and its binding to brain synaptosomes, *Eur. J. Bioch.*, 31, 437–445, 1983.

Yang, S.E., Yu, R.C. and Chou, C.C., Influence of holding temperature on the growth and survival of *Salmonella* spp. and *Staphylococcus aureus* and the production of staphylococcal enterotoxin in egg products, *Int. J. Food Microbiol.*, 63, 99–107, 2001.

Yokosawa, N., Tsuzuki, K., Syuto, B., Fujii, N., Kimi K. and Oguma, K., Binding of botulinum type C1, D and E neurotoxins to neuronal cell lines and synaptosomes, *Toxicon*, 29, 261–264, 1991.

Zhou, Y., Sugiyama, H. and Johnson, E.A., Transfer of neurotoxigenicity from *Clostridium butyricum* to a nontoxigenic *Clostridium botulinum* type E-like strain, *Appl. Env. Microbiol.*, 59, 3825–3831, 1993.

9

Mycotoxins

Ana M. Calvo

CONTENTS

9.1 BIOLOGY AND ECOLOGY OF THE VARIOUS MOLD SPECIES THAT PRODUCE MYCOTOXINS

9.1.1 *ASPERGILLUS*

9.1.1.1 Introduction

Several *Aspergillus spp.* produce mycotoxins that may be toxic, mutagenic, or carcinogenic. *Aspergillus* species are often soil fungi or saprophytes, however some also cause decay of stored foodstuffs and disease in plants, or can be human and animal pathogens. These fungi are difficult to control, spreading efficiently through the production of asexual spores called conidia. Some *Aspergillus* spp. can survive periods of adverse conditions in crop fields or during storage by forming protective structures called sclerotia.

Agricultural commodities that may be colonized by *Aspergillus* include corn, cereal grains, rice, peanuts, tree nuts, and cottonseed. This colonization may occur before or after harvest, depending upon environmental or storage conditions. Other consumer products are affected because mycotoxins are transferred into milk, meat, and eggs when animals ingest contaminated feed. The *Aspergillus* spp. that produce mycotoxins of major health and economic concern are: *Aspergillus flavus, A. parasiticus, A. ochraceus,* and *A. fumigatus.* The mycotoxins produced by these species include: aflatoxins, sterigmatocystin, cyclopiazonic acid, ochratoxin, patulin, citrinin, citreovindin, gliotoxin, penicillic acid, and xanthomegnin.

9.1.1.2 Aflatoxin-Producing Fungi

Aflatoxins were discovered in the early 1960s, following the death of 100,000 turkeys in the United Kingdom. Analysis of the groundnut meal contained in the turkey feed led to the discovery of *A. flavus*, a major aflatoxin-producing fungus. Aflatoxin is a carcinogenic polyketide (Figure 9.1) and is a frequent contaminant of corn, peanuts, cotton, sorghum, and other oil-seeds. Other *Aspergillus* species known to produce aflatoxins are *A. parasiticus* and *A. nomius*. In general, *A. flavus* produces aflatoxin B_1, and B_2, while *A. parasiticus* produces B_1, B_2, G_1, and G_2, however there are exceptions in which some isolates from *A. flavus* may contain both aflatoxin B_1 and G_1. There are also aflatoxigenic isolates that do not produce aflatoxin.

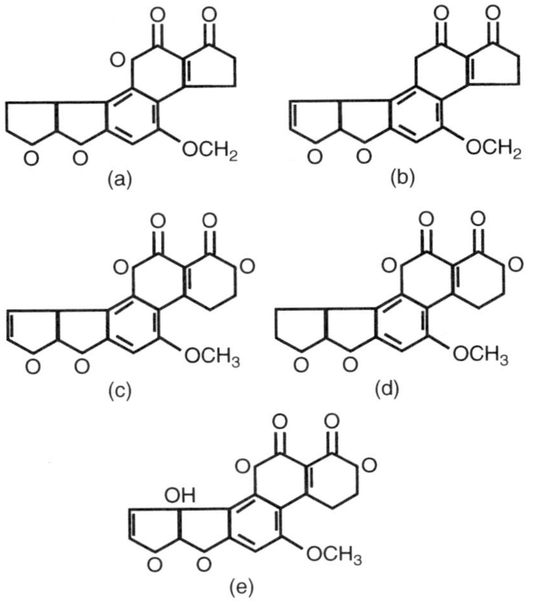

FIGURE **9.1** Different types of aflatoxins: (a) aflatoxin B$_1$, (b) aflatoxin B$_2$, (c) aflatoxin G$_1$, (d) aflatoxin G$_2$, (e) aflatoxin M$_1$.

Soil populations and aflatoxin contamination are influenced by weather patterns, with hot dry soils favoring the *Aspergillus* section Flavi. In terms of geographic location, *A. flavus* incidence is correlated with high minimum temperatures and inversely correlated to latitude. For example, corn ears that develop at temperatures of 28 to 32°C are far more likely to be contaminated by aflatoxin than ears grown later in the season at lower temperatures. However, late planting is not economically feasible due to lower crop yields. Besides hot dry weather, the level of insect and rodent activity in an area may also substantially favor colonization and aflatoxin production. Plant fertility, density, and disease also play roles in the level of aflatoxin contamination.

9.1.1.3 Cyclopiazonic Acid-Producing Fungi

Cyclopiazonic acid is synthesized by a number of *Aspergillus* and *Penicillium* spp. The *Aspergillus* spp. that have been reported as cyclopiazonic-acid producers are *A. flavus* (the most studied cyclopiazonic-acid producer) along with *A. versicolor*, *A. oryzae*, and *A. tamarii*. Among the *Penicillium* spp. producers are *P. verrucosum*, *P. patulum*, *P. camembertii*, and *P. puberulum*. In *A. flavus*, cyclopiazonic-acid production usually occurs in conjunction with aflatoxin production. However, studies of aflatoxin mutants have shown that synthesizing cyclopiazonic acid is independent of the capacity to synthesize aflatoxin (Horn and Dorner, 1999). Little is known about the impact of cyclopiazonic acid on crops or foodstuffs and further investigation into factors governing cyclopiazonic acid incidence is needed.

9.1.1.4 Sterigmatocystin-Producing Fungi

Sterigmatocystin (Figure 9.2a) and aflatoxin are synthesized through a common biosynthetic pathway, where sterigmatocystin is only two enzymatic steps from aflatoxin. Sterigmatocystin is also carcinogenic (Ohtsubo et al., 1978; Xie et al., 1990). *Aspergillus versicolor* can produce sterigmatocystin in postharvest storage affecting corn, rice, wheat, and hay. The other aspergilli that are known to produce sterigmatocystin include *A. flavus*, *A. parasiticus*, *A. rugulosus*, *A. chevalieri*, *A. ruber*, *A. amstelodami*, *A. aurantobrunneus*, *A. quadrilineatus*, *A. sydowii*, *A. ustus*, and the genetically well-studied *A. nidulans*.

Because *A. nidulans* is one of the best characterized eukaryotic systems and because signaling pathways tend to be conserved among *Aspergillus* species, *A. nidulans* is used as a model system. This model system is especially productive in the study of the aflatoxin/sterigmatocystin gene clusters and signal-transduction pathways that lead to mycotoxin production and fungal development (Hicks et al., 1997; Yu and Leonard, 1995). Besides conidiation, *A. nidulans* develops a sexual stage with fruiting bodies called cleistothecia, were sexual spores, or ascospores, are formed. Both asexual and sexual development is linked to sterigmatocystin production (Hicks et al., 1997; Kato et al., in press).

Sterigmatocystin may also be synthesized by the *Penicillium* spp., *P. camembertii*, *P. commune* and *P. griseofulvum*. However, there are few reports of sterigmatocystin contamination of foodstuffs by these fungi.

9.1.1.5 Ochratoxin-Producing Fungi

Aspergillus ochraceus and *A. carbonarius* are ochratoxin producers. Ochratoxin A is derived from isocoumarin linked to phenylalanine (Figure 9.2b). *A. carbonarius* grows at high temperatures and has pigmented spores and hyphae. Due to its ability to withstand heat and ultraviolet (UV) light, *A. carbonarius* colonizes grapes and fruits that mature in direct sunlight. Ochratoxin can be

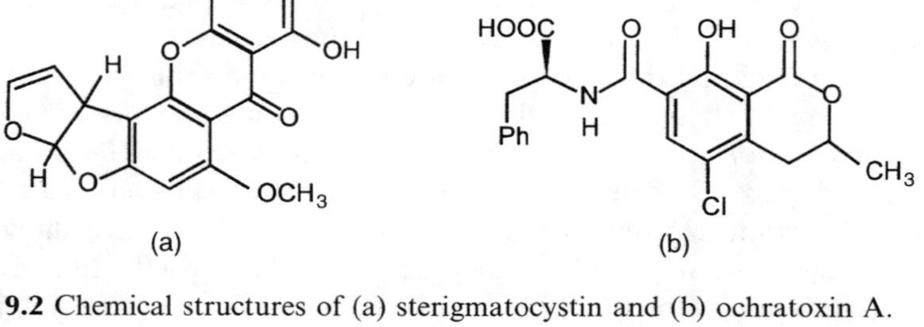

(a)   (b)

FIGURE 9.2 Chemical structures of (a) sterigmatocystin and (b) ochratoxin A.

transmitted to the meat and eggs of animals fed on contaminated grain. *Aspergillus ochraceus* colonizes stored crops and so is an important producer of ochratoxin A. It is likely that colonization by *A. ochracerus* begins in the fields, perhaps during the drying of crops at harvest. *Penicillium verrucosum* also produces ochratoxin A in stored grain, and may be associated with *A. ochraceus* (Frisvad, 1995).

Little is known about field contamination by ochratoxin A. Coffee is one of the crops susceptible to ochratoxin, and contamination is often correlated to insect damage. Ochratoxin-producing *Penicillium* typically infest grain (especially wheat) in temperate zones. Further investigation is required to understand the factors that determine ochratoxin A contamination in coffee and in other susceptible crops.

9.1.2 FUSARIUM

9.1.2.1 Introduction

Fusarium spp. form a diverse group of fungi. One of the most important diseases produced by *Fusarium spp* is fusarium head blight (FHB) in wheat and, less commonly, in barley and triticale. FHB is frequent in temperate regions. Two *Fusarium* spp. have been isolated from FHB, *F. graminearum* and *F. culmorum*. Other species are frequently isolated from affected crops in conjunction with *F. graminearum* and *F. culmorum*, for example, *F. verticillioides*, *Fusarium crookwellense*, and *Fusarium avenaceum*. The following fungi are also found, but at lower frequencies and in grains grown at lower temperature: *Fusarium sporotrichioides*, *Fusarium poae*, and *Fusarium equiseti*.

A number of fusarium mycotoxins are produced, depending upon geographic origin. Among them are deoxynivalenol, zearalenone, fumonisins, and T-2 toxin.

9.1.2.2 *Fusarium graminearum*, Deoxynivalenol and Zearalenone

Besides wheat, *F. graminearum*, along with *Fusarium subglutinans*, also infests corn causing *Gibberella*, or pink ear rot. The main source of inoculum are ascospores of the teleomorph *Giberella zeae* and sometimes conidia of the anamorph *F. graminearum*, which are particularly important during reinfection processes under favorable weather conditions. Infection is brought on by moisture at silking and by heavy precipitation.

The temperature limits for growth have not been reported, although the optimal temperature has been estimated at 24 to 26°C. The relative abundance of the different groups of secondary metabolite depends on O_2 concentration, pH, and osmotic tension. For example, the mycotoxin deoxynivalenol (Figure 9.3a) is synthesized under low oxygen tension (Miller and Blackwell, 1986). However, optimal production for zearalenone (Figure 9.3b) requires oxygen saturation (Hidy et al., 1977).

Deoxynivalenol results in massive electrolyte loss in plant cells upon exposure. *Fusarium graminearum* is a necrotrophic pathogen.

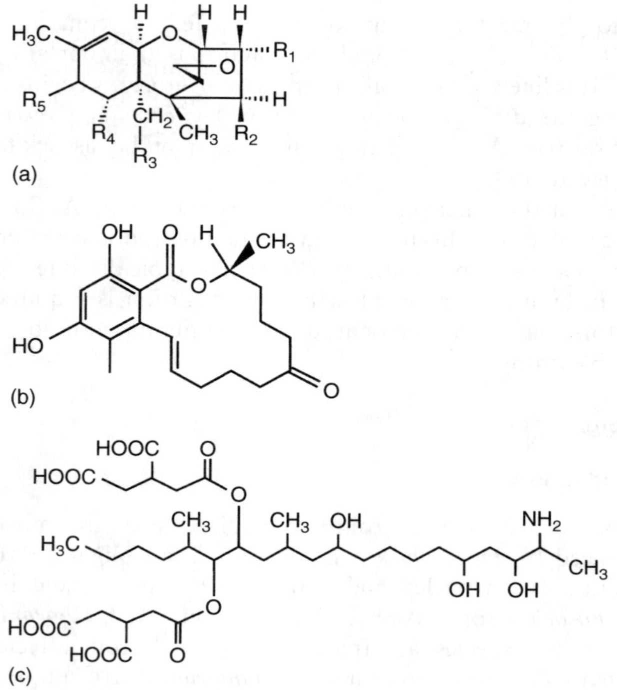

(a)

(b)

(c)

FIGURE 9.3 Chemical structures of (a) thichothecenes (including deoxynivalenol and T-2 toxin), (b) zearalenone, and (c) fumonisin B1.

9.1.2.3 *Fusarium verticillioides* and Fumonisins

Fusarium verticillioides (syn. *F. moniliforme*) causes fusarium ear rot in corn and produces the mycotoxins fumonisins. Fumonisins are amino-polyalcohols (Figure 9.3c) that contaminate corn-based human food and animal feed worldwide. Fumonisins are a health hazard to humans and animals, however their effects have only been recognized in the past 30 years. Recently, genes involved in fumonisin biosynthesis have been identified and described as being organized in a gene cluster (Proctor et al., 2003). *F. verticillioides* disseminates by producing two types of conidia, macroconidia and microconidia. This fungus also has an associated sexual stage that has been described as *Giberella moniliformis*.

Fusarium verticillioides is endemic in corn kernels. The factors that contribute to the occurrence of fusarium ear rot are temperature, drought stress, insect damage, other fungal diseases, and corn genotype. When night temperatures are higher than 25°C, *Fusarium verticillioides* is incapable of growth. However, at temperatures above 25°C, *F. verticillioides* produces fumonisins by invading kernels that are physically damaged by such factors as drought, insect activity, and plant disease.

Solutions containing more than 10^{-4} mol fumonisin are proven to effect negatively the production of amylase and elongation of radicles in seeds (Doehlert et al., 1994). Fumonisin also causes shoot and root length to be decreased (Lamprecht et al., 1994). It is assumed that fumonisins other than fumonisin B_1 and B_2 are much less potent than fumonisin B_1 (which is always prevalent).

9.1.2.4 *Fusarium sporotrichioides* and T-2

When infecting grains such as corn, *Fusarium sporotrichioides* produces the toxin T-2. The minimum, optimum and maximum temperatures for growth are 2.0, 22.5 to 27.5 and 35°C, respectively. T-2 is not normally found in grains because fungal infestation is only possible on grains that are physically damaged. However, T-2 has been frequently isolated from grain dust. Infestation of grain lemmae by *F. sporotrichioides* and *F. poae* may later be colonized by *F. gramineaum* (Sturz and Johnston, 1983), explaining the presence of T-2 in grain dust.

9.1.3 PENICILLIUM

Penicillium spp. produce a wide range of mycotoxins, of which patulin (an unsaturated lactone) is common as a possible food contaminant. The species of this genus disseminate efficiently by the production of airborne conidia.

   Penicillium expansum is the major producer of the mycotoxins patulin and citrinin. Patulin is a mycotoxin mainly found in apple and apple products. *P. expansum* grows from 3 to 35°C, with an optimum of 25°C. Patulin is synthesized from 0 to 25°C with its optimum at 25°C. Citrinin is also produced along with patulin by *P. expansum*.

9.2 THE EFFECTS OF PROCESSING, HANDLING, AND STORAGE ON TOXIN STABILITY

9.2.1 AFLATOXIN

The stages in commodity handling at which aflatoxin and other mycotoxins can be detected and their amounts modified are shown in Figure 9.4. *Aspergillus* spp. thrive in hot, humid, subtropical and tropical climates. When environmental conditions favor aflatoxin production, accumulation is rapid, both in the field and in storage.

   Most manufacturing processes do not detoxify aflatoxin and therefore if the aflatoxins are not detected, products will be marketed. One of the processes used for reducing aflatoxin levels is nixtamalization (alkaline cooking), which is used during the making of corn tortillas, tortilla chips, and corn chips, and gives a 51 to 78% reduction in aflatoxin levels (Torres et al., 2001).

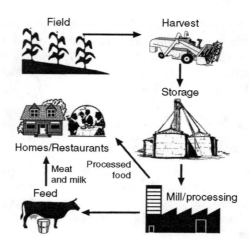

FIGURE 9.4 Different control points at which mycotoxin contamination can be prevented

Humans are also exposed to the aflatoxins when consuming animal products that were contaminated because the animal ate feed containing aflatoxin. Aflatoxin contamination can be passed to milk and dairy products as aflatoxin M (Figure 9.1).

9.2.2 OCHRATOXIN

It has long been established that ochratoxin can be transferred to body fluids and eggs. Important ochratoxin-contaminated foods, in which the effects of processing have been studied, are cereals and coffee. Delay in drying grain after harvesting results in an increase of ochratoxin.

In cereal processing, parts of the wheat kernel are removed to reduce ochratoxin A levels in flour. A 65% reduction was reported in wheat that was milled to produce white flour, and an additional 10% reduction was achieved when the flour was used in baked products (Osborne et al., 1996). Wholegrain breads benefit from milling and baking to a much lesser degree (approximately 10% and 4% respectively) because less kernel is removed. When using contaminated grain for brewing, from 2 to 7% of ochratoxin is passed to beer after fermentation. It is also notable that the production process for breakfast cereals and biscuits leads to considerable reduction of ochratoxin A; however the production processes for pasta have little or no effect on toxin content.

Coffee has been the focus of many studies regarding formation of ochratoxin A, its destruction during roasting, and its presence in brews. Mechanical color sorting leads to minor reductions in ochratoxin A levels, however steaming produces approximately 25% reduction. The effect of heat on stability is considerable, 80% of ochratoxin is destroyed during bean roasting, however decaffeination is the most effective process for removing ochratoxin, achieving 92% elimination.

9.2.3 TRICHOTHECENES: DEOXYNIVALENOL AND T-2

Kernels damaged by trichothecene contamination can be removed by the use of gravity separators reducing inoculum and humidity in storage. Separation of shriveled kernels and washing of grain have been reported as eliminating up to 74% of deoxynivalenol.

Milling results in a higher concentration of deoxynivalenol in bran and shorts, and in lower concentrations in straight-grade flour. The distribution of trichothecenes (deoxynivalenol and T-2) in the different milling fractions of wheat depends on the degree of fungal penetration in the endosperm (Nowicki et al., 1988). Endosperm penetration is dependent on wheat variety. Milling grain that has only surface contamination results in low trichothecene concentration.

Deoxynivalenol and T-2 toxin levels may be reduced in pasta during boiling as toxins are passed into the cooking water (Scott, 1991). In tortilla production, only 18 to 28% of trichothecene content remained after boiling in a calcium hydroxide solution as part of the tortilla-making process (Abbas et al., 1988). Trichothecenes are unstable in the presence of alkali.

Trichothecenes are stable at 120°C and relatively stable at 180°C, however they are destroyed at 210°C after 40 min (Kamimura, 1989). A reduction in deoxynivalenol levels of 44% in dough and baked products has been reported by Neira et al. (1997), with dough fermentation accounting for roughly 50% of this reduction. The combination of high-temperature and pressure, commonly utilized in extrusion or autoclaved food preparation, has proven far less effective, with the best results being a 12% reduction of deoxynivalenol in autoclaved cream corn (Wolf-Hall et al., 1999).

9.2.4 ZEARALENONE

Zearalenone is a compound that is stable during storage and milling, and also during processing and cooking of food (Gajecki, 2002). Studies of heat stability of zearalenone have shown that less than 23% is lost at temperatures lower than 125°C, 34 to 68% at 150°C, and greater than 92% at temperatures higher than 175°C (Ryu et al., 2003).

9.2.5 FUMONISINS

After commercial dry milling, fumonisins were found in grits, flour, germ, and bran. The distribution pattern after milling varied slightly depending on the type of corn, however fumonisin content was usually lower in grits and higher in germ or bran. Although germ and bran are not a major part of the human diet, they still pose a considerable threat as components in animal fodders. In laboratory-scale wet milling, starch fractions were shown not to contain detectable levels of fumonisin B_1, and 22% of the toxin was found in processing waters. The other fractions also showed a reduction in fumonisins, containing approximately 10 to 40% of the original concentration in the corn.

Fumonisins are relatively heat stable and significant removal only occurs during processes in excess of 150°C. It has been shown that the type of cooking process greatly affects the temperature required to achieve a reduction of more than 50% in fumonisin content: 190°C for frying of corn chips (Jackson et al., 1997), 160°C for extrusion of corn grits (Katta et al., 1999), 218°C for roasting corn meal (Castelo et al., 1998)(the reported temperatures refer to the heating medium). The cooking time also affects the stability of the fumonisins (Jackson et al., 1997).

The temperature and pH level of alcohol fermentation are reported as having a limited effect on fumonisin content (Bothast et al., 1992; Hlywka and Bullerman, 1999).

9.2.6 PATULIN

During processing, affected fruit is generally removed or pressurized-water jets are utilized to remove damaged portions of fruit and contaminations (or both). These processes effectively eliminate patulin. However, if these procedures are not done properly, patulin may remain in the processed apple juice and apple products, where it is very stable. Pasteurization at 90°C only causes a reduction of 10%, however patulin is not stable in the presence of sulfur dioxide or sulfydryl compounds. The fermentation process for cider eliminates 99% of patulin.

9.3 MEDICAL AND FINANCIAL ASPECTS OF MYCOTOXIN POISONINGS

9.3.1 MEDICAL ASPECTS

9.3.1.1 Aflatoxin

Aflatoxin has long been recognized as a human mutagen and carcinogen. Ingestion of aflatoxin is directly correlated to human liver cancer. It has also been demonstrated that aflatoxin induces a high incidence of mutation in the *p53* tumor repressor gene and K-ras and H-ras proto-oncogenes (Denissenko et al., 1999; Lasky and Magder, 1997; Riley et al., 1997; Shen et al., 1996; Wang and Groopman, 1999). Altered sequences of these specific genes have been detected at high frequency in a wide variety of human cancers (Kiaris and Spandidos, 1995; Semenza and Weasel, 1997; Sidransky and Hollstein, 1996) and are considered to be among the basic molecular events in the multistep mechanism of carcinogenesis.

9.3.1.2 Ochratoxin

The International Agency for Research on Cancer has classified ochratoxin as a possible human carcinogen. In all mammal species assayed, the toxin produced kidney lesions, either through high dosage or through prolonged consumption (Harwig et al., 1983). The presence of ochratoxin A has been detected in grain products, the meat of animals fed on grain, in human blood samples (Breitholtz et al., 1991; Hald, 1991), and in breast milk (Skaug et al., 2001).

9.3.1.3 Deoxynivalenol

Deoxynivalenol can cause reduction of body weight and reduction of pregnancies in rats, and in humans it can cause depression of immune responses, nausea, vomiting, abdominal pain, dizziness, headache, and fever. Experiments on pigs given fodder containing pure deoxynivalenol indicate that feed with less than 2 mg per kg deoxynivalenol has little impact on growth. However, naturally-contaminated grains with a low deoxynivalenol content are often more toxic than the low deoxynivalenol content might seem to indicate. This may be due to an additive effect of minor toxins, such as culmorin and sambucincol from *F. graminearum*. These toxins may boost the potency of deoxynivalenol (Rotter et al., 1992).

9.3.1.4 Zearalenone

Zearalenone is an estrogenic compound that competitively binds to the estrogen receptors and causes hyperestrocism; the dietary no-effect level in female pigs is less than 1 mg per kg. Cattle are also impacted by the estrogenic effects of this toxin, displayed as depressed ovulation and increased embryolethal resorptions. Non-human primates and humans are also sensitive to the estrogenic effects of zearalenone (Kuiper-Goodman et al., 1987). There are also reports that high levels of this toxin can cause infertility in both male and female pigs.

9.3.1.5 Fumonisin and Related Toxins

Fumonisin B_1 (FB_1) is the major and most toxic fumonisin produced by *F. verticillioides*, and has been described as causing leukoencephalomalacia in horses, pulmonary edema in pigs, and liver and kidney cancer in rats (Gelderblom et al., 1988; Yoshizawa et al., 1994). It has also been established that FB_1 causes esophageal cancer in humans (Gelderblom et al., 1988; Yoshizawa et al., 1994). Mechanistic studies indicate that ceramide synthase, an enzyme involved in sphingolipid synthesis, is one cellular target for fumonisin toxicity and carcinogenicity, resulting in inhibition of sphingolipid biosynthesis (Wang et al., 1991). The disruption to sphingolipid metabolism increases the ratio of two sphingoid precursors, sphinganine and sphingosine. Current reports probably underestimate the role of mycotoxins in disease and as a cause of human mortality. Fumonisins are commonly detected worldwide.

9.3.1.6 T-2 toxin

The T-2 toxin is the probable cause of alimentary toxic aleukia (ATA). The symptoms of ATA include vomiting, fever, acute inflammation of the digestive tract, atrophy of bone marrow, agranulocytosis, necrotic angina, sepsis, and hemorrhagic diathesis. T-2 is responsible for outbreaks of hemorrhagic disease in animals and is associated with neurotoxic effects and oral lesions in birds. The most significant effect of T-2 (and other trichothecenes) is immunosuppressive activity, which has been clearly demonstrated in animal experiments, and is probably linked to the inhibitory effect of this toxin on the biosynthesis of macromolecules. There is limited evidence from animal experiments that T-2 may be carcinogenic.

9.3.1.7 Patulin

Patulin causes oxidative damage to DNA (Liu et al., 2003). In addition to being mutagenic, carcinogenic, and teratogenic for animals, patulin induces intestinal injuries, including epithelial cell degeneration, inflammation, ulceration, and hemorrhages (Mahfoud et al., 2002).

9.3.2 FINANCIAL ASPECTS

Contamination of the world's crops by aflatoxin is estimated to cost $10 billion annually, due not only to the direct loss of crops and animals, but also to the maintenance of toxin monitoring services and the indirect cost of human and animal health care (Trail et al., 1995). Strict legislation will protect the public health in developed countries; however, many countries do not have such legislation or testing capacity. Even if such legislation and testing could be implemented, they would reduce the health risk but could not eliminate large-scale economic losses similar to those currently faced by the U.S., the European Union, and other developed countries.

In general, mycotoxin contamination of foods and feeds and the associated problems are primarily influenced by the location of production, storage, and marketing. The *Aspergillus* species that produce mycotoxins are more common in the warmer, subtropical and tropical areas than in the temperate areas of the world. However, stringent government regulations for mycotoxins and risk analyses are more common in temperate areas than in the warmer areas of the world, where it becomes both a health and a financial problem.

9.4 SELECTED CASES OF FOODBORNE MYCOTOXIN POISONING

9.4.1 T-2 CONTAMINATION DURING WORLD WAR II

The toxin T-2 was isolated from the 'strain T-2' of *F. sporotrichioides*, which has been associated with cattle mortalities. The compound has been the subject of considerable toxicological interest because it is easy to isolate and purify. Although T-2 poising is uncommon because colonization by *F. sporotrichioides* is only possible when grain is physically damaged, it has affected both animals and humans. During World War II, large-scale poisonings occurred in the Soviet Union, caused by the consumption of grains damaged by wintering in the fields. This poisoning affected thousands of people, leading to the disappearance of entire villages.

9.4.2 'RED MOLD POISONING'

A disease known as 'red mold poisoning' affected Japan throughout the 1950s. The mycotoxin deoxynivalenol was later isolated from grains causing the illness and identified as the cause.

Deoxynivalenol has not been known to produce deaths in humans, but has a significant impact on agriculture due to feed refusal. Pig and horse refusal of moldy grain was reported as early as 1928, and cases of complete refusal have been associated with wheat containing 34 mg per kg of deoxynivalenol (Moore et al., 1985).

9.5 DETECTION, IDENTIFICATION, AND DETERMINATION OF MYCOTOXINS IN FOODS AND SEEDS

Aflatoxin is one of the most mutagenic and carcinogenic natural compounds described to date. Traditional methods for the measurement of aflatoxins fall into two groups:

- chromatographic methods
- enzyme-linked immunosorbent assays (ELISAs)

ELISAs exist in many different formats, such as microwell assays (microtiter plates, strips), dipstick assays, and immunofiltration assays.

The continued impact of aflatoxin on food safety and on economies has motivated the development of new technologies in aflatoxin monitoring. In particular, several research groups have developed biosensors for detection of the toxins, as well as presumptive tests for fungal infection. The biosensor platforms that have been tested range from hand-held to bench-top devices and employ many technologies, such as fiber optics, liposomes, small particles (beads), surface plasmon resonance, and microcapillaries. These devices show considerable promise as rapid and sensitive methods for mycotoxin measurement.

Presumptive tests are also being utilized to detect the presence of fungi. By detecting fungal presence rather than toxin content, such tests can eliminate the major drawback of the mycotoxin assay – the laborious and time-consuming extraction process. The most widely used presumptive test for the aflatoxins has been the bright greenish-yellow fluorescence test, which is used to grade cereal grains. Under UV light (365 nm), corn infected with *A. flavus or A. parasiticus* fluoresces. Fluorescence should be used for detecting possible aflatoxin content and for sorting commodities. It should not be viewed as an analytical method because the correlation between fluorescence and actual aflatoxin content is not accurate. Precise measurements are important due to the toxicity of aflatoxin, even at very low levels. A second method of presumptive testing detects fungal infection through changes in seed color.

Various testing methods have also been applied for other mycotoxins. Deoxynivalenol and T-2 can be detected by thin-layer chromatography (TLC), high-performance liquid chromatography (HPLC), and gas chromatography (GC), and an ELISA is also available (Krska et al., 2001). Zearalenone can be measured by TLC and HPLC and immunoaffinity columns coupled with liquid chromatography (LC) (Fang et al., 2002; Fazekas and Tar, 2001). Ochratoxin is detected by TLC, immunoaffinity chromatography, LC, by tandem mass spectrometry (MS), and by ELISA (Scott, 2002). In the case of fumonisin, HPLC is the most widely used method, however, the flow-injection liposome immunoanalysis (FILIA) recently seems to have shown a lower detection limit and is a faster and easier method (Ho and Durst, 2003).

9.6 OFFICIAL REGULATION REGARDING MYCOTOXIN CONTENT IN FOOD AND METHODS FOR ITS CONTROL

9.6.1 WORLDWIDE LEGISLATION

The Hazard Analysis Critical Control Point system (HACCP) has been incorporated in legislation as the method of control for food contamination by the European Commission's General Hygiene Regulations and by the U.S. Department of Agriculture. This system attempts to follow foodstuffs from growth through all stages of handling and processing right up to their consumption (Figure 9.4). Due to the multiple factors affecting contamination and the numerous occasions when it may occur, HACCP incorporates the following well-known business practices: good manufacturing practice (GMP), good hygienic practice (GHP), good agricultural practice (GAP), and good storage practice (GSP). One potential problem with using the HACCP system in the control of commodities is that it requires the commitment of many different owners of processing and handling companies.

For descriptions of the exact procedures for the application of HACCP to mycotoxin prevention, and case studies involving application, see Pineiro et al. (2001), sponsored by the Food and Agriculture Organization of the United Nations (FAO) and the International Agency for Atomic Energy (IAEA) through their joint FAO/IAEA Training and Reference Centre for Food and Pesticide Control.

Regulatory limits for aflatoxin content in food have been established in the U.S. at 20 ppb for food consumed by humans, 0.5 ppb for milk, and 20 to 300 ppb for animal feed. Current European Commission regulatory limits for aflatoxin content in foodstuffs for direct human consumption has been set at 2 ppb, and at 0.05 ppb for milk. EC limits for animal feed are 5 ppb. Contaminated harvests that are not under these maximum limits are to be disposed of. There are also elaborate sampling plans in many regulations (Park et al., 1998).

Mycotoxins occur in many crops and stored seeds as well as in processed and formulated products. According to the FAO, seventy-seven countries have legislation governing mycotoxin content in food and feedstuffs (Table 9.1). An additional thirteen countries are known to have no legislation relating to toxins, while forty other nations have made no response to FAO inquiries. However, according to the most recent FAO survey (1995) the total number of countries with mycotoxin legislation has increased 36% since the previous survey (1987).

The following four mycotoxins have for some time been recognized as being of major agricultural significance: aflatoxin, deoxynivalenol, zearalenone, and ochratoxin. Nevertheless, only aflatoxin is widely regulated, with all

Table 9.1
Mycotoxins currently controlled by legislation.

Mycotoxins controlled for	Number of countries with legislation
Aflatoxin	77
Deoxynivalenol	4
Zearalenone	5
Ochratoxin A	5
Patulin	11
T-2	3
Phomopsin	1
Diacetoxyscirpenol	2
Stachyobotriotoxin	1
Chetomin	1
Fumonisin	1

Source: Worldwide regulations for mycotoxins 1995. A compendium, by the Food and Agriculture Organizations of the United Nations (1997), Rome, Italy.

seventy-seven countries having legislation to control it. The effects of aflatoxins at low doses and the large number of products that may contain aflatoxins illustrate the severity of the problem and the need for legislation. However even aflatoxin regulation is far from uniform, in many cases only a few of its forms are controlled and each country has different allowable limits.

Although other toxins, such as fumonisin B_1, are now considered carcinogenic, government regulation of these metabolites has not kept pace, however some governmental organizations do have advisory levels.

9.6.2 Control Methods for Mycotoxins

Currently, technologies to reduce levels of fungal infection and toxin accumulation are categorized as either preharvest or postharvest. During preharvest, the most important factors controlling contamination include soil moisture, soil temperature, and insect activity. Late season irrigation increases soil moisture and decreases soil temperature, and so is an effective way to lower aflatoxin content in mature kernels. Management factors other than irrigation, such as plant nutrition, fungicide applications, insecticide applications, and harvesting techniques, can all have an effect on aflatoxin content.

Other preharvest techniques include the development of more resistant crops (e.g., Becker, 1999; Guo et al., 1998), and biological control with atoxigenic *A. flavus* strains (Cotty, 1990; Dorner et al., 1998). Atoxigenic *A. flavus* competed successfully with a toxic isolate when they were grown in mixed culture, obtaining a reduction of the aflatoxin content by 82 to 100%. This is a worthwhile approach for control, however possible side effects caused by a preemptive application of *A. flavus* in the environment must be studied to determine potential risks to human and animal health.

Postharvest approaches include control of moisture and temperature and proper ventilation. Treatment of contaminated corn with 2% ammonia reduces aflatoxin levels (Park et al., 1988), however this treatment changes the nutritional value of the seed and causes an ammonia odor and a change in color. Ammoniation is not an FDA-approved detoxifying procedure for crops intended for interstate commerce – it can be used only for crops to be used within the confines of a farm. Furthermore, ammoniation is a hazardous procedure for those conducting treatment.

None of the preharvest or postharvest techniques is completely effective and aflatoxin contamination continues to be a health and economic threat.

In the case of deoxynivalenol contamination, the reduction of toxin levels during cleaning of grain, such as by removal of infected kernels and washing, has been reported to be in the range of 42–100% (Charmley and Prelusky, 1994).

Some cultivars that have shown resistance to FHB are ten times more resistant to mycotoxin contamination (Wang and Miller, 1988). This was due to the presence of a modified peptidyl transferase (at protein synthesis). Early studies had suggested that wheat appeared able to metabolize deoxynivalenol in the field (Miller and Young, 1985; Scott et al., 1984). This was shown later to be the case *in vitro* in an FHB-resistant cultivar (Miller and Arnison, 1986). This implied that one component of resistance to FHB is related to the reduction of the phytotoxic impact of deoxynivalenol.

Some microorganisms are also able to transform trichothecenes into less toxic compounds. For example, rumenal bacteria, bacteria from the large intestine of chickens, and bacterial populations from soil samples, were capable of transforming deoxynivalenol into 3-acetyldeoxynivalenol or 3-keto-4-deoxynivalenol (Binder et al., 2000; Swanson et al., 1987; He et al., 1993; Shima et al., 1997). Therefore, it seems likely that the development of wheat crops with the capability of eliminating this mycotoxin or bio-treatments could possibly be developed as a feasible strategy.

Contamination of crops and products with ochratoxin A and related metabolites is not as directly associated with a particular fungus as is the case with the aflatoxins. Ochratoxin A is also likely to occur with other mycotoxins, such as citrinin and penicillic acid or patulin. In addition, it is not certain whether ochratoxin A contamination is only a storage problem or perhaps a dual field and storage problem. In cases such as coffee crops, the use of insecticides might help to control insect activity and consequently fungal infection. Coffee-berry borers are a major insect pest which can act as vectors to carry fungal spores, resulting in crop infection and ochratoxin accumulation.

In the case of fumonisin control, there is also a strong relationship between insect damage and fusarium ear rot. Corn genotypes containing the anti-insectant protein Bt had lower fumonisin content (Munkvold et al., 1997, 1999).

Controlling for patulin contamination by *P. expansum* can be accomplished through the removal of damaged fruit, or the elimination of the fungi and toxins with water jets and subsequent drying.

9.7 REFERENCES

Abbas, H.K. et al., Decomposition of zearalenone and deoxynivalenol in the process of making tortilla from corn, *Cereal Chem.*, 65, 15, 1988.

Becker, H., USDA researchers create highly aflatoxin-resistant corn. *USDA ARS News.* March 18, 1999.

Binder, E.M. et al., *Microbial detoxification of mycotoxins in animal feed.* Presentation at the X International IUPAC symposium on mycotoxin and phycotoxins, Guaraja, May 21–25, 2000.

Bothast, R.U. et al., Fate of fumonisin B1 in naturally contaminated corn during ethanol fermentation, *Appl. Env. Microbiol.*, 58, 233, 1992.

Breitholtz, A. et al., Plasma ochratoxin A levels in three Swedish populations surveyed using an ion-pair HPLC technique, *Food Addit. Contam.*, 8, 183, 1991.

Castello, M.M., Sumner, S.S. and Bullerman, L.B., Stability of fumonisins in thermally processed corn products, *J. Food Prot.*, 61, 1030, 1998.

Charmley, L.L. and Prelusky, D.B., Decontamination of *Fusarium* mycotoxins, in Miller, J.D. and Tremholm, H.L., eds., *Grain – compounds Other Than Aflatoxin Mycotoxins*, Eagan Press, St. Paul, 1994.

Cotty, P.J., Effect of atoxigenic strains of *Aspergillus flavus* on aflatoxin contamination of developing cottonseed, *Pl. Dis.*, 74, 808, 1990.

Cotty, P.J., Aflatoxin-producing potential of communities of *Aspergillus* section Flavi from cotton producing areas in the Unite States, *Mycol. Res.*, 6, 698, 1997.

Denissenko, M.F. et al., Quantitation and mapping of aflatoxin DNA damage in genomic DNA using aflatoxin B_1-8,9-epoxide and microsomal activation systems, *Mutat. Res.*, 425, 205, 1999.

Doehlert, D.C., Knutson, C.A. and Vesonder, R.E., Phytotoxic effects of fumonisin B, on maize seedling growth, *Mycopathologia*, 127, 117, 1994.

Dorner, J.W., Cole, R.J. and Blankenship B.D., Effect of inoculum rate of biological control agents on preharvest adflatoxin contamination of peanuts, *Biol. Contr.*, 12, 171, 1998.

Fang, X. et al., Detection and identification of zeranol in chicken or rabbit liver by liquid chromatography-electrospray tandem mass spectrometry, *J. AOAC Int.*, 85, 841, 2002.

Fazekas, B. and Tar, A., Determination of zearalenone content in cereals and feedstuffs by immunoaffinity column coupled with liquid chromatography, *J. AOAC Int.*, 84, 1453, 2001.

Foster, B.C. et al., Evaluation of different sources of deoxynivalenol (vomitoxin) fed to swine, *Can. J. Anim. Sci.*, 66, 1149, 1986.

Frisvad, J.C., Mycotoxins and mycotoxigenic fungi in storage, in Jayas, D.S., White, N.D.G, and Muir, W.E., eds., *Stored-Grain Ecosystems*, Marcel Dekker, New York, 1995.

Gajecki, M., Zearalenone-undesirable substances in feed, *Pol. J. Vet. Sci.*, 5, 117, 2002.

Gelderblom, W.C. et al., Cancer promoting potential of different strains of *Fusarium moniliforme* in a short-term cancer initiation/promotion assay, *Carcinogenesis*, 9, 1405, 1988.

Guo, B. Z. et al., Protein profiles and antifungal activities of kernel extracts from corn genotypes resistant and susceptible to *Aspergillus flavus*, *J. Food Prot.*, 61, 98, 1998.

Hald, B., Ochratoxin A in human blood in European countries, in M., Plestina, R., Dirheimer, G., Chernozemsky, I.N. and Bartsch, H., eds., *Mycotoxins, Endemic Nephropathy and Urinary Tract Tumours*, IARC Scientific Publications No. 115, IARC Press, Castegnaro, Lyon, 1991.

Harwig, J., Kuiper-Goodman, T. and Scott, P.M., Microbial food toxicants: Ochratoxins, in Rechcigl, M., ed., *Handbook of Foodborne Diseases of Biological Origin*, CRC Press, Boca Raton, 1983.

He, P., Young, L.G. and Forsberg, C., Microbially detoxified vomitoxin-contaminated corn for young pigs, *J. Anim. Sci.*, 71, 963, 1993.

Hicks, J.K. et al., *Aspergillus* sporulation and mycotoxin production both require inactivation of the *FadA* G protein-dependent signaling pathway, *EMBO J.*, 16, 4916, 1997.

Hidy, P.H. et al., Zearalenone and derivatives: production and biological activities, *Adv. Appl. Microbiol.*, 22, 54, 1977.

Hlywka, J.J. and Bullerman, L.B., Occurrence of fumonisin B_1 and B_2 in beer, *Food Addit. Contain.*, 16, 319, 1999.

Ho, J.A. and Durst, R.A., Detection of fumonisin B1: comparison of flow-injection liposom immunoanalysis with high-performance liquid chromatography, *Anal. Biochem.*, 312, 7, 2003.

Horn, B.W. and Dorner, J.W., Soil populations of *Aspergillus* species from section Flavi along a transect through peanut-growing regions of the United States, *Mycologia*, 90, 767, 1998.

Jackson, L.S. et al., Effect of baking and frying on the fumonisin B_1 content of corn-based foods, *J. Agric. Food Chem.*, 45, 4800, 1997.

Kamimura, H., Removal of mycotoxins during food processing, in Natori, S., Hashimoto, K. and Ueno, Y., eds., *Mycotoxins and Phycotoxins '88*, Elsevier Science, Amsterdam, 1989.

Kato, N., Brooks, W. and Calvo, A.M., Sterigmatocystin and penicillin pene expression is controlled by *veA*, a gene required for sexual development in *Aspergillus nidulans*, *Eukaryotic Cell*, in press.

Katta, S.K. et al., Effect of temperature and screw speed on stability of fumonisin B1 in extrusion-cooked corn grits. *Cereal Chem.*, 76, 16, 1999.

Kiaris, H. and Spandidos, D.A., Mutations of *ras* genes in human tumors, *J. Oncology*, 7, 413, 1995.

Krska, R., Baumgartner, S., Josephs, R., The state-of-the-art in the analysis of type-A and -B trichothecene mycotoxins in cereals. Fresenius, *J. Anal. Chem.*, 371, 285, 2001.

Kuiper-Goodman, T., Scott, P.M. and Watanabe, H., Risk assessment of the mycotoxin zearalenone, *Regul. Toxicol. Pharmacol.*, 7, 253, 1987.

Lamprecht, S.C. et al., Phytotoxicity of fumonisins and TA-toxin to corn and tomato, *Phytopathology*, 84, 383, 1994.

Lasky, T. and Magder, L., Hepatocellular carcinoma *p53* G > T transversions at codon 249: the fingerprint of aflatoxin exposure? *Env. Health Perspect.*, 105, 392, 1997.

Lepom, P. and Kloss, H., Production of sterigmatocystin by *Aspergillus versicolor* isolated from roughage, *Mycopathologia*, 101, 25, 1988.

Liu, B.H. et al., Evaluation of genotoxic risk and oxidative DNA damage in mammalian cells exposed to mycotoxins, patulin and citrinin, *Toxicol. Appl. Pharmacol.*, 191, 255, 2003.

Mahfoud, R. et al., The mycotoxin patulin alters the barrier function of the intestinal epithelium: mechanism of action of the toxin and protective effects of glutathione, *Toxicol. Appl. Pharmacol.*, 181, 209, 2002.

Miller, J.D. and Arnison, P.G., Degradation of deoxynivalenol by suspension cultures of the *Fusarium* head blight resistant cultivar Frontana, *Can. J. Plant. Pathol.*, 8, 147, 1986.

Miller, J.O. and Blackwell, B.A., Biosynthesis of 3-acetyl-deoxynivalenol and other metabolites by *Fusarium culmorum* HLX 1503 in a stirred jar fermentor, *Can. J. Bot.*, 64, 1, 1986.

Miller, J.O., Young, I.C. and Trenholm, H.L., *Fusarium* toxins in field corn. I. Parameters associated with fungal growth and production of deoxynivaneol and other mycotoxins, *Can. J. Bot.*, 61, 3080, 1983.

Moore, C.J. et al., Rejection by pigs of mouldy grain containing deoxynivalenol, *Aust. Vet. J.*, 62, 60, 1985.

Munkvold, G.P., Hellmich, R.L. and Showers, W.B., Reduced *Fusarium* ear rot and symptomless infection in kernels of maize genetically engineered for European corn borer resistance, *Phytopathology*, 87, 1071, 1997.

Neira, M.S. et al., The effects of bakery processing on natural deoxynivalenol contamination, *Int. J. Food Microbiol.*, 37, 21, 1997.

Nowicki, T.M. et al., Retention of the *Fusarium* mycotoxin deoxynivalenol in wheat during processing and cooking of spaghetti and noodles, *J. Cereal Chem.*, 8, 189, 1988.

Ohtsubo, K., Saito, M. and Kimura, H., High incidence of hepatic tumors in rats fed mouldy rice contaminated with *Aspergillus versicolor*, *Food Cosmet. Toxicol.*, 16, 143, 1978.

Osborne, B.G. et al., The effects of milling and processing on wheat contaminated with ochratoxin A, *Food Addit. Contain.*, 13, 141, 1996.

Park, D.L., Perspectives on mycotoxin decontamination procedures, *Food. Addit. Contain.*, 10, 49, 1993.

Park, D.L. et al., Review of the decontamination of aflatoxins by ammoniation: current status and regulation, *J. Assoc. Anal. Chem.* 71, 685, 1988.

Park, D.L., Njapau, H. and Coker, R.D., Sampling programs for mycotoxins: perspectives and recommendations, in Miraglia, M., van Egmond, H.P., Brera C. and Gilbert, J., eds., *Mycotoxins and Phycotoxins: Developments in Chemistry, Toxicology and Food Safety*, Alaken Inc, Colorado, 1998.

Pineiro, M.S. et al., *Manual on the application of the HACCP system in mycotoxin prevention and control.* Food and Agriculture Organization of the United Nations and the International Atomic Energy Agency, 2001.

Proctor, R.H. et al., Co-expression of 15 continuous genes delineates a fumonisin biosynthetic gene cluster in *Gibberella monilifromis*, *Fungal Genet. Biol.*, 38, 237, 2003.

Rabie, C.J., Lubben, A. and Steyn, M., Production of sterigmatocystin by *Aspergillus versicolor* and *Bipolaris sorokiniana* on semisynthetic liquid and solid media, *Appl. Env. Microbiol.*, 32, 206, 1976.

Riley, J. et al., *In vitro* activation of the human Harvey-ras proto-oncogene by aflatoxin B_1, *Carcinogenesis*, 18, 905, 1997.

Rotter, B.A. et al., Investigations in the use of mice exposed to mycotoxins as a model for growing pigs, *J. Toxicol. Env. Health*, 37, 329, 1992.

Ryu, D. et al., Heat stability of zearalenone in an aqueous buffered model system, *J. Agric. Food Chem.*, 51, 746, 2003.

Scott, P.M., Decline in deoxynivalenol (vomitoxin) concentrations in 1983 Ontario winter wheat before harvest, *Appl. Env. Microbiol.*, 48, 884, 1985.

Scott, P., Possibilities of reduction or elimination of mycotoxins present in cereal grain, in Chenkowski, J., ed., *Cereal Grain: Mycotoxins, Fungi and Quality in Drying and Storage*, Elsevier, Amsterdam, 1991.

Scott, P.M., Methods of analysis for ochratoxin A, *Adv. Exp. Med. Biol.*, 504, 117, 2002.

Semenza, J.C. and Weasel, L.H., Molecular epidemiology in environmental health: the potential of tumor suppressor gene *p53* as a biomarker, *Env. Health Perspect.*, 105, 155, 1997.

Shen, H.-M. and Ong, C.-N., Mutations of the *p53* tumor suppressor gene and *ras* oncogenes in aflatoxin hepatocarcinogenesis, *Mutat. Res.*, 366, 23, 1996.

Shima, J. et al., Novel detoxification of the trichothecene mycotoxin deoxynivalenol by a soil bacterium isolated by enrichment culture, *Appl. Env. Microbiol.*, 63, 3825, 1997.

Sidransky, D. and Hollstein, M., Clinical implications of the *p53* gene, *Annu. Rev. Med.*, 47, 285, 1996.

Skaug, M.A. et al., Presence of ochratoxin A in human milk in relation to dietary intake, *Food Addit. Contam.*, 18, 321, 2001.

Sturz, A.V. and Johnston, H.W., Early colonization of the ears of wheat and barley by *Fusariurn poae*, *Can. J. Plant Pathology*, 5, 107, 1983.

Swanson, S.P. et al., Metabolism of three trichothecene mycotoxins, T-2 toxin, diacetoxyscirpenol and deoxynivalenol, by bovine rumen microorganisms, *J. Chromatogr.*, 414, 335, 1987.

Torres, P., Guzman-Ortiz, M. and Ramirez-Wong, B., Revising the role of pH and thermal treatments in aflatoxin content reduction during the tortilla and deep frying processes, *J. Agric. Food Chem.*, 49, 2825, 2001.

Vesonder, R.F., Ciegler, A. and Jensen, A.H., Isolation of the emetic principle from *Fusarium*-infected corn, *Appl. Microbiol.*, 26, 1008, 1973.

Vesonder, F. and Horn, B.W., Sterigmatocystin in dairy cattle feed contaminated with *Aspergillus versicolor*, *Appl. Env. Microbiol.*, 49, 243, 1985.

Wang, E. et al., Inhibition of sphingolipids biosynthesis by fumonisin, implication for diseases associated with *Fusarium moniliforme*, *J. Biol. Chem.*, 266, 14486, 1991.

Wang, J.S., and Groopman, J.D., DNA damage by mycotoxins, *Mutat. Res.*, 424, 167, 1999.

Wang,Y-Z. and Miller, J.D., Effects of *Fusarium graminearum* metabolites on wheat tissue in relation to *Fusarium* head blight resistance, *J. Phytopathology*, 122, 118, 1988.

Wolf-Hall, C.E., Hanna, M.A. and Bullerman, L.B., Stability of deoxynivalenol in heat-treated foods, *J. Food Prot.*, 62, 962, 1999.

Xie, T.X., Sterigmatocystin induced adenocarcinoma of the lung and atypical hyperplasia of glandular stomach in mice, *Zhonghua Zhong Liu Za Zhi*, 12, 21, 1990.

Yoshizawa, T., Yamashita, A. and Luo, Y., Fumonisin occurrence on corn from high-risk and low-risk areas for human esophageal cancer in China, *Appl. Env. Microbiol.*, 60, 1626, 1994.

Yu, J.H. and Leonard, T.J., Sterigmatocystin biosynthesis in *Aspergillus nidulans* requires a novel type I polyketide synthase, *J. Bacteriol.*, 177, 4792, 1995.

10

Heavy Metals

Mikołaj Protasowicki

CONTENTS

10.1 INTRODUCTION

Foods of animal and plant origin contain many chemical elements, which combine to form the building materials of proteins, lipids, carbohydrates, vitamins and other complex compounds. Among these elements, carbon, hydrogen, nitrogen, and oxygen form the largest group. In addition to these, tissues contain many elements which, depending on their amount, are termed either macroelements or microelements (the latter are also known as trace elements).

Macroelements, as well as basic elements are essential for plant and animal organisms. They are the building materials that support tissue, teeth, skin, and hair, play an important role in water-electrolyte management and pH regulation, and are parts of many active compounds vital for metabolic processes.

Microelements are important because of two aspects:

- Some microelements are essential for the normal functions of organisms. They participate in numerous important processes, e.g., enzymatic reactions (Zn, Co, Ni, Mn, Fe, Cr, Al), glycolysis (Mn, Zn), nucleotide synthesis (Mg, Fe), erythropoesis (Fe, Cu), organic acid transformation (Fe, Zn, Ni, Mn), nitrogen exchange (Fe, Mo, Cu, Mn, V, Co), photosynthesis (Fe, Ti, Mg, Mn), and their lack or excess may be a cause of many serious diseases.

- Trace elements, which are not considered essential, may cause severe poisonings if administered in amounts equal to or higher than the minimal dose.

Determination of the roles of microelements and the human daily requirements can be very difficult due to their low concentrations in the human body and problems connected with the elimination of their constant inflow. Throughout the evolution process, the human body developed mechanisms to regulate the absorption of microelements and balance their levels within required ranges. Therefore, human bodies are adjusted to the natural levels at which those elements are present in the non-polluted environment and in non-contaminated foodstuffs. However, human industrial and economic activities are frequently and widely disturbing the environmental balance and leading to contamination of the environment, including foods, with trace elements.

The content of trace elements in foods depends on their concentration in the raw materials and additives used in food production. In addition, trace elements may be transmitted to food from the equipment used during food processing and from the packaging material during storage.

Trace elements include heavy metals, some of which have recently received particular attention. Many definitions of 'heavy metals' have been put forward. The simplest and most precise describes heavy metals as all metal compounds of atomic weight over 20. Other definitions are based on the specific weight, and give the lower limits for heavy metals as 4.5, 5, or even 6 g per cm^3. Due to toxicity of some heavy metals and the possibility of environmental contamination, the potential for high risk is linked to Hg, Cd, As, Pb, as well as Cu, Zn, Sn, Cr, Ni.

All elements are present in the environment (and also in plant and animal organisms, and in water and food) as salts or as metalo-organic compounds, and only in such forms are they biologically active.

To limit the possibilities of food poisoning in humans caused by ingestion of excessive amounts of trace elements via food and water, highest allowable concentrations of trace elements are fixed. The Joint Food and Agriculture Organization/World Health Organization (FAO/WHO) Expert Committee on Food Additives makes global recommendations for general norms, and publishes values of provisional tolerable weekly intake (PTWI) for particular toxic metals based on the results of actualized study results.

10.2 MERCURY

Mercury has been known since ancient times. As early as in the 7th Century B.C., Assyrian medics applied it to cure skin diseases. Mercury compounds were also used by Arabs in the 6th Century B.C. for therapeutic reasons. Mercury was mentioned by Aristotle and Hippocrates (the 4th Century B.C.) who described cinnabar (HgS) as a dye. Mercury and its compounds have also been used in appropriate ways much more recently. The application of cinnabar to color rinds of cheese in England in the 19th Century serves as an example, while the first agricultural application of mercury compounds (seeds treated with phenylmercury) took place in Germany in 1914 (Krenkel, 1973).

Toxic properties of some mercury compounds have been known for a long time. There are theories that mercury compounds were used to poison Ivan the Terrible, Napoleon Bonaparte, and Charles II of England. Improper handling and treatment of samples during the synthesis of organic mercury compounds was the cause of lethal poisonings of chemists in both the 19th and 20th centuries.

The first outbreak of food poisoning caused by mercury compounds was reported in 1953 in Japan. The outbreak was caused by the ingestion of fish containing significant amounts of methylmercury. As the outbreak affected the population living at the Minamata Bay, the disease was named Minamata disease; the name now frequently used as a general name for any foodborne form of mercury poisoning. Other outbreaks of Minamata disease, also of fish origin, have been reported in Japan (Kurland et al., 1960; Harada, 1995). However, the most tragic outbreaks happened in Iraq, from 1955 to 1960, and later from 1971 to 1972. A total of approximately 8000 people became sick after ingestion of bread prepared from grain treated with methylmercury. Similar cases were reported in Guatemala, Pakistan, and Ghana (Al-Tikriti and Al-Mufti, 1976). A surprising case of mercury poisoning occurred in the Åland Islands, Finland. The patient affected was a female who had consumed merganser eggs that contained significant amounts of methylmercury.

Most cases of mercury poisoning led to handicap, chronic disease, or death. The most frequent symptoms include: numbness of limbs, lips and tongue, speech abnormalities, limb function disorders, visual acuity disorders, deafness, and muscular atrophy. Insomnia, hyperactivity, and coma have also been reported. Methylmercury penetrates the blood–brain barrier and causes central nervous system injuries. Mercury also has a teratogenic effect, leading to congenital abnormalities or congenital Minamata disease.

Mercury has been always present in the environment and as a result, mercury is naturally found in living organisms, where it can occur in methylmercury form. In the case of aquatic organisms, methylmercury may comprise up to 100% of total mercury content. The range of natural mercury content that is observed in food of animal and plant origin from non-polluted environments has been measured as from < 0.001 to about 0.05 µg per g. Fish are the exception, where the amount of mercury in muscles, even in non-contaminated environments, may reach up to 0.2 µg per g.

Despite the significant decrease during past decades of the anthropogenic emission of mercury into the environment (due to the restriction or prohibition of its application), there is still a need for control of mercury levels in food. This is because of the significant toxicity of its compounds and their high mobility in the environment. Therefore, in many countries the highest admissible level of mercury in food is regulated by law and, depending on the type of food, such limits are within the range from 0.003 to 0.05 µg per g.

Dried fungi, fish and fish products are the exception, and may contain from 0.5 to 1.0 μg per g (Dz. U., 2003).

The Joint FAO/WHO Expert Committee determined that PTWI for mercury via all possible physiological routes should not exceed 5 μg per g of body weight, and only two thirds may be in the form of a methyl derivative (WHO, 1993).

10.3 CADMIUM

Cadmium was isolated for the first time in 1817 by Strohmeyer. In nature, cadmium is usually present in the form of sulfides accompanying zinc and copper ores. The application of cadmium in various branches of industry started at the beginning of the 20th Century. It is widely used in metallurgy (as a component of alloys and to coat surfaces of other metals) and electro-technics, and in the production of pigments, plastics (as a stabilizer), gum, and pesticides. This industrial use leads to food contamination via the ecosystem. Other sources of cadmium contamination include the burning of coal, oil, and waste. Significant amounts of cadmium are also found in some mineral fertilizers, as well as in industrial and municipal waste used as manure (McLaughlin et al., 1999; WHO, 1992a,b).

The toxicity of cadmium compounds has been known since the first publication by Marmé in 1867. Although acute cadmium poisonings are usually rare, chronic diseases caused by a long-term exposure occur quite frequently. Symptoms include: nausea, vomiting, stomachache, headache, and lowered body temperature. Poisoning leads to acute gastroenteritis and renal, liver, testicle, and prostate disorders. Anemia, hypertension, cardiovascular changes, pregnancy complications, and bone decalcification are also reported. Cadmium is also suspected to be a factor that increases the frequency of prostate cancer, although its carcinogenic effect has not been confirmed. In tests on animals poisoned with cadmium during pregnancy, congenital defects in fetuses were observed.

Toxicity of cadmium increases in cases of zinc deficiency, due to the zinc substitution in biological systems, which leads to functional disorders. Cadmium reduces assimilation of vitamins C and D. However, a large amount of these vitamins in the diet will decrease the toxicity of cadmium through the reduction of its absorption from the intestinal tract (Friberg et al., 1986; Hill, 1996; McLaughlin et al., 1999).

Many cases of foodborne cadmium poisonings were reported in 1940s in England, France, New Zealand, the U.S., the U.S.S.R., and other countries. They were caused by consumption of lemonade, coffee, wine, and other products that had been prepared or stored in cadmium-coated containers, or in refrigerators with cadmium-coated freezers.

The Japanese disease 'itai-itai' (ouch-ouch) is a particular syndrome caused by chronic cadmium poisoning. It leads to fractures of long bones due to decalcification, and to muscular dystrophy. The first time the disease was reported was after World War II, within a population in the lower basin of the Jintzu river, Japan. It was caused by consumption of rice that contained cadmium at a level of 0.6 to 1.1 µg per g. Undoubtedly, other plants that are cultivated in environments highly contaminated with cadmium may also be the cause of poisonings, as would foods of animal origin.

Cadmium poisonings are particularly dangerous as the daily excretion of assimilated cadmium is minimal (0.5% of the total intake). The biological half-life of cadmium is very long, about 33 years. Cadmium is therefore accumulated in humans throughout their whole lifetimes. Although only 5 to 10% of cadmium is absorbed from the gastrointestinal tracts of adults, a daily dose of 66 to 132 µg is sufficient to result in a critical value of 6 µg per g in the kidneys at the age of 50. These factors cause the high level of concern regarding the risks for human health posed by cadmium – cadmium is considered more dangerous than mercury and lead.

The amounts of cadmium found in food from non-contaminated areas do not exceed 0.05 µg per g of products. Exceptions are the livers and, especially, the kidneys of slaughtered animals, which may contain even up to a few µg per g.

Polish legislation sets limits for the maximum amount of cadmium in food, depending on the kind of food products, but within a range from 0.005 to 1.0 µg per g. Extremely high contents of cadmium are allowed only in dried fungi, kidneys, molluscs and cephalopods (up to 1 µg per g), liver and shellfish (up to 0.5 µg per g), dried vegetables, herbs and spices (up to 0.3 µg per g), and dried potatoes (up to 0.2 µg per g) (Dz. U., 2003). The Joint FAO/WHO Expert Committee suggests that PTWI for cadmium should not exceed 7 µg per kg of body weight (WHO, 1993).

10.4 LEAD

Lead was known and mined in the ancient times, and its ease of use promoted its wide application. Lead was used for water-supply systems, first in ancient Greece, later in the Roman Empire. Wealthy Romans used lead wine cups, kitchen utensils, decorations, and other paraphernalia, and it is suggested that this might have led to chronic poisoning (Gilfillan, 1965). Although the toxic properties of lead had already been known in ancient Greece, Egypt, and Rome, where lead poisoning was known as 'saturnism', the metal was not identified as a toxic component of food until the 11th Century (Landrigan, 1990; Mahaffey, 1990). Despite this knowledge, in England in the 19th Century, candies were colored with lead chromate and white lead, and the use of lead for water pipes has survived up to the present time. Tea was also regenerated using lead chromate, and minium (Pb_3O_4) was applied to cheese to make the rind red.

At present, lead is used for production of accumulators, petrol, crystal glass, matches, paints, pesticides, and printing types, hunting ammunition (with arsenic), and anti-corrosive coatings. It is also used in the chemical, rubber, textile, and ceramic industries, and in many other branches of human economic activity.

To date there is no proof for the inevitability of lead for plant and animal organisms (including humans), whereas its toxic activity is widely known. More reported poisonings involved lead than any other elements (Philip and Gearson, 1994a,b). As early as in 1774, Lind noted that lemon juice stored in lead-enameled containers may cause poisoning. A special royal commission was appointed to study the problem four years later.

Food contamination may result from transmission of lead from glaze, enamel, or tinning on kitchen dishes, or from the lead on surfaces of containers or pipes used for storage, processing and transportation of food products. The occurrence of lead in food can also result from environmental contamination, as plants and animals may assimilate lead during growth and incorporate it into their tissues. The level of lead found in plant tissues is proportional to its concentration in the environment, and in cases of animals, the feed and water supplies also play important roles (Vreman et al., 1988; McLaughlin et al., 1999; Sedki et al., 2003).

Symptoms of lead poisoning occur after a daily dose of 2 to 4 mg is ingested for a period of a few months, while daily doses of 8 to 10 mg will cause poisoning after only three to four weeks.

At the onset of poisoning, symptoms include chronic headaches, hyper-activity, muscle tremor, lead colic, and lead line (1 to 2 mm) on gums. Hyperactivity and intelligence-quotient decrease are observed in cases of chronic poisoning in children. Lead poisonings result in anemia due to hemoglobin synthesis disorders. Neurological, encephalopathic, enzymatic, and mutagenic changes, as well as liver, kidney, spinal medulla, and brain damage, are also observed. Lead may be transmitted from the blood of pregnant women to their fetuses, which may result in congenital defects (teratogenic effect). Lead compounds may also exert carcinogenic effects (Philip and Gerson, 1994b; Johnson, 1998; Silbergeld, 2003).

All food products contain some lead. They usually do not exceed the level of 0.1 to 0.2 µg per g, although venison may contain up to several µg per g due to its contamination via ammunition. In order to lower lead intake in Poland, the highest allowed concentrations have been established for various food products, within a range from 0.2 µg per g (for milk) to 2 µg per g (dried fungi). For most products, the values are set between 0.1 and 0.3 µg per g (Dz. U., 2003). The Joint FAO/WHO Expert Committee calculated that lead PTWI should not exceed 25 µg per g of body weight (WHO, 1993). It is particularly important that infants and children should be protected against the possibility of lead uptake.

10.5 ARSENIC

Arsenic is a metalloid, yet it is still classified as a heavy metal. Arsenic compounds have also been known since ancient times, but was described for the first time by Albert the Great in the 13th Century (Sullivan, 1969). Auripigment and realgar were used as yellow paints, and arsenic was one of the most widely known and widely used poisons.

Pure arsenic is presently used as a component of alloys (e.g., with lead to produce hunting ammunition). Arsenic compounds are also used in the chemical, pharmaceutical, and tanning industries, in the manufacture of glass and ceramics, and as pesticides in agriculture and fruit-farming (Nriagu and Azcue, 1990).

The toxicity of arsenic action depends on types of bonds present: non-organic compounds are significantly more toxic than organic ones, whereas As^{+3} salts are more toxic than As^{+5} salts. Small amounts of arsenic exert a stimulating effect on human and animal organisms. Antagonistic properties of this element against selenium and iodine have also been revealed. Hypersensitivity to arsenic, or arsenicphagia, which is typical of miners and consumers of sea fish (who get used to the presence of arsenic), has been described.

Excessive amounts of arsenic can cause skin, lung, and heart diseases, and gastrointestinal disorders, and it is known to have a carcinogenic influence. As^{+3} compounds, which are bound by erythrocytes, affect the activity of numerous enzymes – especially those involved in respiratory processes (Cebrian et al., 1983; Done and Peart, 1971; National Academy of Sciences, 1977; WHO, 2001).

Over 80% of the total arsenic content of aquatic organisms is present as organic compounds. During digestion of such organic arsenic compounds, arsenic is not released or is only released gradually. This explains why no cases of arsenic poisoning have been reported among seafood consumers despite the high levels observed in seafoods (Lawrence et al., 1986).

The levels of arsenic in food do not generally exceed 0.1 µg per g, although higher amounts (even up to several µg per g) have been found in kidneys and livers of slaughter animals and in fish. In Poland, the highest permissible levels of arsenic in foods are within the range of 0.02 to 4.0 µg per g. The lowest levels are applied to fresh herbs, and slightly higher levels (0.05 µg g) to milk. In most products, the maximum amount of arsenic must not exceed 0.2 µg per g. The highest levels relate to fish and fish products (Dz. U., 2003). The Joint FAO/WHO Expert Committee suggests that the PTWI for arsenic should not exceed 15 µg per kg of body weight (WHO, 1989).

10.6 COPPER

Copper is inseparably linked to the history of human civilization. According to suggested standards, the daily physiological demand of copper is from 1.5 to 2.7 mg per person (Ziemlański, 2001). The basic physiological importance of copper is connected with erythropoetic processes and tissue respiration. Copper is essential for catalysis of processes of food-originated iron binding into organic bonds. It stimulates maturation of reticulocytes and their transformation into erythrocytes, and is a constituent of oxidation enzymes, such as polyphenoloxidase, lactase, tyrosinase, ascorbinase, and cytochrome C oxidase. Copper acts similarly on insulin – diabetics administered copper salts, from 0.5 to 1 µg daily, demonstrate clear evidence of improvement.

Copper exerts an effect on the activity of excretory glands, increases the phagocytic properties of leukocytes, therefore promoting human immunity, and also boosts antibiotic activity.

Animal tests have proven that copper is essential for the growth of organisms. If insufficient doses of copper are administered with food, the inhibition of growth is observed.

Large amounts of copper are found in the liver, larger amounts in young individuals than in old. In cases of copper deficiency, anemia, hair discoloration, and other pathological symptoms have been observed. Increased levels of copper, which result from defense mechanism actions of the immune system, have been reported in infectious and cancer diseases (Sarkar, 1995).

Despite the positive effects of optimal levels of copper, deleterious effects may occur if a threshold level is exceeded. Wilson's disease (hepatolenticularic degeneration) is one of the diseases linked to the excess of copper in the body. It results from a dysfunction of the copper transmission process, which occurs due to a lack of suitable enzyme to catalyze the process of copper deletion from detached bonds with albumins and binding to ceruloplasma. The condition leads to neuron degradation, liver cirrhosis, and occurrence of colorful rings on the cornea (DiDonato and Sarkar, 1997).

Foodborne poisonings due to copper and copper compounds can be caused by the improper use of copper dishes (Tanner et al., 1983; Müller et al., 1996; Müller et al., 1998). They may also be caused by breaches of carency period after the application of copper-based pesticides.

Copper is usually present in food at levels of 1 to 2 µg per g, the higher levels are found in animal livers. The highest levels of copper are present in shellfish, this is because copper is a component of their blood pigment, haemocyanin.

A copper complex of chlorophyll in amounts not higher than 1 µg per g of product is used for coloring preserved vegetables, however the complex cannot contain more copper than 200 µg per g (Dz. U., 2003). Non-organic copper compounds were used in the past for food coloration; in the 19th Century in England, copper salts were used to color food products and condiments.

Symptoms of copper poisoning include: metallic taste, salivation, stomach-aches, blue vomiting, diarrhea, reduced blood tension, and tachycardia. Acute cases may also include symptoms of paralysis of the central nervous system, cardiovascular failure, hepatitis, anemia, and uremia.

Polish standards only set maximum accessible levels of copper for plant and animal fats, plant oils, margarine, butter, and mayonnaise. The established values are in the range 0.1 to 1.0 µg per g (Dz. U., 2003). The Joint FAO/WHO Expert Committee recommends that the PTWI should not exceed 3500 µg per g (3.5 mg per g) of body weight (WHO, 1989).

10.7 ZINC

Alloys of zinc were used for brass production as early as in the ancient times. Trials of zinc production were conducted in Europe in the 6th century, however it had been produced earlier in China and India. Zinc is widely applied, i.e., in metallurgy, electrotechnics, printing, rubber production, production of articles of daily use, paints, drugs, disinfectants, and impregnates, as well as in microfertilizers and pesticides.

Zinc is a microelement essential for proper functioning of the human body. The level of daily demand for zinc was established as 13 to 16 mg (Ziemlański, 2001). Zinc plays a role in protein and carbohydrate metabolism and is a component of over 60 metaloenzymes, including: alkaline phosphatase, pancreatic carboxypeptidases A and B, alcoholic and lactic dehydrogenases, carbonate anhydrase, and proteases. It also forms bonds with nucleic acids – which is very important for their functioning (Prasad, 1983; Valee and Falchuk, 1993).

Human food, both plant and animal, usually contains satisfactory amounts of zinc to cover the requirement for this metal, which is present within the range of few to several µg per g of product. Zinc deficiencies are usually caused by a reduction of its absorption in the gastrointestinal tract rather than by its lack. Reduction in absorption may be caused by antagonistic activity of cadmium, calcium or phytates. A decrease in assimilation of zinc is also observed among alcoholics.

Zinc deficiency causes growth inhibition, depigmentation of dark hair, balding, corneous and thick epithelium and skin desquamation. Acute deficiencies of zinc lead to testicular atrophy and to sterility (Shils et al., 1994).

An excess of zinc will cause problems in humans. Excessive doses can lead to biochemical control system damage, while doses slightly higher than optimal can cause disorders in iron and copper metabolism, resulting in incurable anemia, decrease in activity of zinc protein enzymes, and pancreas and kidney damage (Boularbah et al., 1999; Seiler et al., 1994). Increased levels of zinc have been observed in nuclei of neoplastic cells and in cases of acute dental caries, however its role in these diseases has not been explained.

Zinc poisoning may occur after consumption of products stored in zinc-coated containers. For instance, a dish of curried poultry, which was a source of zinc poisoning, was found to contain 1.0 µg per g. Poisoning may be also caused if the carency period after application of zinc pesticides is not observed.

Symptoms of acute zinc poisoning include acute gastroenteritis, vomiting, diarrhea, dizziness, and heaviness in chest.

At present, Polish standards only limit zinc content in juices and nectars. The maximum limit for zinc in these products is 5 µg per g (Dz. U., 2003). The Joint FAO/WHO Expert Committee recommends the PTWI should not exceed 7000 µg per g (7 mg per g) of body weight (WHO, 1989).

10.8 TIN

Tin, similarly to copper, has been known since the Bronze Age and is still widely used today. Tin compounds are used in the production of plastics, antilichenic paints, pesticides, wood preservatives, and antiparasitic drugs for animals (Ebdon et al., 1998). In some countries, inorganic tin compounds ($SnCl_2$) are added to vegetable preserves packed in glass jars to preserve the natural colors of vegetables. Tin-coated metal cans, commonly used for packing foods, may lead to food contamination. Tin compounds may be leached from the tin coating if the food has a low pH. It should be noted that tin-organic pesticides, which are currently in use, may enter food products if improperly handled.

If ingested, inorganic salts are poorly assimilated and are almost completely excreted from the human body via stools and so their toxicity is low. Organic compounds display higher toxicity, and alkyl derivatives, e.g., tributylocin (TBT), are particularly dangerous. The toxicity therefore depends on the type of tin compound. After the consumption of large quantities of tin, enzymatic and ingestion processes are distorted. Long-term exposure to organic tin derivatives leads to sexual gland atrophy and to changes in the nervous system (Saxena, 1987; WHO, 1980; WHO, 1990).

It is estimated that the average daily tin uptake per adult is approximately 4 mg, however tin is not accumulated in the body. So far, the role of tin in the human body has not been completely understood, although some data lead to the conclusion that it is involved in oxidation-reduction processes. Some authors suggest that the lack of tin in the fodder of test animals causes reduced growth and tooth depigmentation (Schwartz et al., 1970).

At present, Polish standards limit the content of tin only in food products packed in tin-coated containers, and in fruit and vegetable preserves, and products including such preserves, packed in other materials (Dz. U., 2003). The content of tin in products intended for children up to the age of three must not exceed 10 µg per g, and for other products it must not exceed 100 µg per g (for food in tin-coated packing) or 20 µg per g (for food in other types of packing). The Joint FAO/WHO Expert Committee established the PTWI value for tin as 14,000 µg per g (14 mg per g) of body weight (WHO, 1989).

10.9 CONCLUSIONS

Studies on the content of heavy metals in food are conducted in the majority of countries worldwide. Toxic heavy metals attract particular attention. Studies carried out on a range of foods and on daily food intakes have revealed that the amounts of heavy metals found in foods are within acceptable limits and do not exceed values observed in other European countries. The present daily uptake of heavy metals has decreased when compared with the values reported in the 1980s.

Alarmingly, higher uptake of lead and cadmium (when compared to PTWI) has been observed in children, especially in industrial areas, and in people who require high food intakes (e.g., manual workers). The PTWI for cadmium and lead may also be exceeded due to consumption of foods containing the highest concentration of these toxic metals.

10.10 REFERENCES

Al-Tikriti, K. and Al-Mufti, A.W. (1976). An outbreak of organomercury poisoning among Iraqi farmers, *Bull. WHO*, 53, 15–21.

Boularbah, A., Bitton, G. and Morel, J.L. (1999). Assessment of metal and toxicity of leachates from teapots. *Sci. Total Environ.*, 227, 69–72.

Cebrian, M.E., Albores, A., Aguilar, M. and Blakeley, E. (1983). Chronic arsenic poisoning in the North Mexico, *Human Toxicol.*, 23, 121–133.

DiDonato, M. and Sakar, B. (1997). Review. Copper transport and its alterations in Menkes and Wilson diseases, *Biochim. Biophys. Acta*, 1360, 3–16.

Done, A.K. and Peart, A.J. (1971). Acute toxicities of arsenical herbicides, *Clin. Toxicol.*, 4, 343–355.

Dz. U. (2003). *Newsletter of Current Legislation* 37, 326. [The Instruction of the Polish Minister of Health on 13th January 2003 regarding maximum levels of chemical and biological contamination that may be present in food, food components, allowed additional substances, auxiliary substances applied in processing or on food surfaces.]

Ebdon, L., Hill, S.J. and Rivas, C. (1998). Organotin compounds in solid waste: a review of their properties and determination using high-performance liquid chromatography, *Trends Anal. Chem.*, 17, 5, 278–288.

Forsyth, D.S., Sun, W.F. and Dalglish, K. (1994). Survey organotin compounds in blended wines, *Food Add. Contam.*, 11, 343–350.

Friberg, L. Elinder, C.G., Kjellstrom, T. and Nordberg, G. (1986). *Cadmium and Health: A Toxicological Appraisal. Vol. II. Effects and Response*, CRC Press, Boca Raton.

Gilfillan, S.C. (1965). Lead poisoning and the fall of the Roman Empire, *J. Occup. Med.*, 7, 53–60.

Harada, M. (1995). Minamata disease: methylmercury poisoning in Japan caused by environmental pollution, *Crit. Rev. Toxicol.*, 25, 1–24.

Hill, R.J. (1996). Risks to humans – an overview, in *Sources of Cadmium in the Environment*. Organization for Economic Co-Operation and Development, Paris, pp. 84–94.

Krenkel, P.A. (1973). Mercury: environmental considerations. Part I. Statement of the problem, *CRC Critical Rev. Environ. Contr.*, 5, 303–373.

Kurland, L.T., Faro, S.N. and Seidler, H. (1960). Minamata disease, *World Neurol.*, 1, 5, 370–395.

Landrigan, P.J. (1990). Current issues in the epidemiology and toxicology of occupational exposure to lead, *Environ. Health Perspect.*, 89, 61–66.

Lawrence, J.F., Michalik, P., Tam, G. and Conacher, H.B.S. (1986). Identification of arsenobetain and arsenocholine in Canadian fish and shellfish by high-performance liquid chromatography with atomic absorption detection and confirmation by fast atom bombardment mass spectrometry, *J. Agric. Food Chem.*, 34, 315–319.

Mahaffey, K.R. (1990). Environmental lead toxicity: Nutrition as a component of intervention, *Environ. Health Perspect.*, 89, 75–78.

McLaughlin, M.J, Parker, D.R. and Clarke, J.M. (1999). Metals and micronutrients – food safety issues, *Field Crops Res.*, 60, 143–163.

Müller, T., Feichtinger, H., Berger, H. and Müller, W. (1996). Endemic tytolean infantile cirrhosis: an exogenetic disorder, *Lancet*, 347, 877–880.

Müller, T., Müller, W. and Feichtinger, H. (1998). Idiopathic copper toxicosis, *Am. J. Clin. Nutr.*, Suppl. 67, 1082–1086.

National Academy of Sciences (1977). *Medical and Biological Effects of Environmental Pollutants: Arsenic.* Washington, D.C., 117–172.

Nriagu, J.O. and Azcue J.M. (1990). *Arsenic in the Environment. Part 1: Cycling and Characterization.* John Wiley and Sons, New York.

Philip, A. and Gearson, B. (1994a). Lead poisoning – part 1: incidence, etiology, and toxicokinetics, *Clin. Lab. Med.*, 14, 423–439.

Philip, A. and Gearson, B. (1994b). Lead poisoning – part 2: effects and assay, *Clin. Lab. Med.*, 14, 651–666.

Prasad, A.S. (1983). The role of zinc in gastrointestinal and liver disease, *Clin. Gastroenterol.*, 12, 713–741.

Sarkar, B. (1995). Copper, in Seiber, H.G. et al, eds., *Handbook of Metals in Clinical and Analytical Chemistry*, Marcel Dekker, New York, 339–347.

Saxena, A.K. (1987). Organotin compounds: toxicity and biomedicinal applications, *Appl. Organomet. Chem.*, 1, 39–56.

Schwartz, K., Milne, D.B. and Vinyard, E. (1970). Growth effects of tin compounds in rats maintained in a trace element-controlled environment, *Biochem. Biophys. Res. Comm.*, 40, 22–29.

Sedki, A., Lekouch, N., Gamon, S. and Pineau, A. (2003). Toxic and essential trace metals in muscle, liver and kidney of bovines from a polluted area of Morocco, *Sci. Total Environ.*, 317, 201–205.

Seiler, H.G., Sigel, A. and Sigel, H. *Handbook on Metals in Clinical and Analytical Chemistry.* Marcel Dekker, New York.

Shils, M.E., Olson, J.A. and Shike, M. (1994). *Modern Nutrition in Health and Disease.* Lea and Febiger, Malvern.

Silbergeld, E.K. (2003). Review. Facilitative mechanisms of lead as a carcinogen, *Mutation Res.*, 533, 121–133,

Sullivan, R.J. (1969). *Preliminary Air Pollution Survey of Arsenic and its Compounds.* National Air Pollution Control Administration Publication No. APTD 69-26, Raleigh.

Tanner, M., Kantarjian, A., Bhave, S. and Pandit, A. (1983). Early introduction of copper-contaminated animal feeds as a possible cause of Indian childhood cirrhosis, *Lancet*, 332, 992–995.

Valee, B.L. and Falchuk, K.H. (1993). The biochemical basic of zinc physiology, *Physiol. Rev.*, 73, 79–105.

Vreman, K., van der Veen, N.G., van der Molen, E.J. and Ruig, W.G. (1988). Transfer of cadmium, lead, mercury and arsenic from feed into tissues of fattening bulls: chemical and pathological data, *Neth. J. Agric. Sci.*, 36, 327–338.

WHO (1980). *Tin and Organotin Compounds.* Environmental Health Criteria, 15, World Health Organization, Geneva.

WHO (1989). *Evaluation of Certain Food Additives and Contaminants.* 33rd report of the Joint FAO/WHO Expert Committee on Food Additives, WHO Tech. Rep. Ser., 776. World Health Organization, Geneva.

WHO (1990). *Tributyltin compounds.* Environmental Health Criteria, 116, World Health Organization, Geneva.

WHO (1992a). *Cadmium.* Environmental Health Criteria, 134. World Health Organization, Geneva.

WHO (1992b). *Cadmium – Environmental Aspects.* Environmental Health Criteria, 135. World Health Organization, Geneva.

WHO (1993). *Evaluation of Certain Food Additives and Contaminants.* 41st report of the Joint FAO/WHO Expert Committee on Food Additives. WHO Tech. Rep. Ser., 837. World Health Organization, Geneva.

WHO (2001). *Arsenic Compounds.* Environmental Health Criteria, 224. World Health Organization, Geneva.

Ziemlański, S. (2001). *[Standards of human nutrition] Normy żywienia człowieka.* Wyd. Lek. PZWL, Warsaw, Poland.

11

Pesticides in Food

Carl K. Winter

CONTENTS

11.1 INTRODUCTION

Since the last part of the 20th Century, the issue of pesticides in foods has generated considerable public concern and debate. Pesticides are chemicals designed specifically for their toxicological effects on target pests, such as insects, weeds, and plant diseases. Public awareness that such chemicals are commonly detected in the food supply as residues contributes greatly to the debate.

Several widely-publicized events and reports have emerged in the past two decades to focus consumer, media, and regulatory attention upon pesticide residues in food. The illegal use of the insecticide aldicarb on watermelons in California in 1985 resulted in more than 1000 cases of probable or possible human pesticide poisoning (Goldman et al., 1990). This event was followed by the release of a landmark report by the U.S. National Research Council (NRC) that presented exaggerated estimates of potential human cancer risks from pesticides in the diet resulting from the use of worst-case human exposure assumptions (NRC, 1987). In 1989, an environmental advocacy group issued a report alleging "intolerable" risks to children from exposure to residues of neurotoxic and cancer-causing pesticides in food (Natural Resources Defense Council, 1989). A subsequent report by the U.S. NRC, published in 1993, concluded that the U.S. pesticide regulatory system did not adequately address the potential differences in exposure and susceptibility to pesticide residues of infants and children relative to adults, and recommended significant changes in pesticide risk assessment practices and pesticide regulation (NRC, 1993).

Such changes were widely adopted after the unanimous passage of the Food Quality Protection Act (FQPA) of 1996 by the U.S. Congress. The FQPA requires pesticide regulators to ensure that pesticides comply with a "reasonable certainty of no harm" statute before they can be allowed for use on food crops. In the determination of a "reasonable certainty of no harm," regulators are required to consider the potential increased susceptibility of infants and children, and the exposure to pesticides through food, water, and residential sources (aggregate exposure). In cases of families of pesticides that demonstrate a common mechanism of toxicological action, the EPA is required to ensure that exposure to the entire family of pesticides (cumulative exposure), rather than exposure to individual members of the family, constitute a "reasonable certainty of no harm."

The implementation of the FQPA dominated the pesticide landscape for several years as the scientific community struggled to develop the risk-assessment methodologies required by the U.S. Congress and the regulatory community faced the challenges of interpreting the new law. Several controversial pesticide regulatory decisions were made in the early years of FQPA implementation but most decisions were completed by 2002 when procedures for conducting aggregate and cumulative risk assessments were finalized.

Consumer demand for foods certified as "organic" rose greatly over the past two decades and much of the increased demand may be related to consumer concern over pesticide residues in foods. The organic foods industry benefited from the development of a U.S. national standard for organic foods, which was published in 2000. According to the U.S. organic standards, organic-food producers are typically not allowed to use synthetic chemicals, although they may use certain natural pesticides derived from mineral, botanical, and microbial sources. In a few cases, synthetic chemicals, such as sulfur, oil sprays, insecticidal soaps, and insect pheromones, are allowed.

11.2 PESTICIDES: TYPES, TOXICITY, AND USE

11.2.1 TYPES OF PESTICIDES

According to the U.S. Federal Insecticide, Fungicide, and Rodenticide Act (FIFRA), a pesticide is defined as "any substance or mixture of substances intended for preventing, destroying, repelling, or mitigating any pest, any substance or mixture of substances intended for use as a plant regulator, defoliant, or desiccant, and any nitrogen stabilizer..."

This comprehensive definition makes it clear that a wide number of substances may be considered to be pesticides, and that the commonality among all pesticides is their ability to provide control over pests. A variety of classifications for pesticides have been developed that are specific for the type of pest controlled. Insecticides, for example, are pesticides that control insects, while herbicides control weeds and fungicides control plant diseases (molds). In addition to these major classifications of pesticides, there are many other classifications. These include nematicides (for nematode control), acaracides (mite control), rodenticides (rodent control), molluscicide (snail and slug control), algacides (algal control), bacteriocides (bacterial control), and defoliants (leaf control).

11.2.2 PESTICIDE TOXICITY

11.2.2.1 Insecticides

The toxicity of insecticides to insects typically results from a variety of mechanisms, such as nerve damage, muscle poisoning, sterilization, and desiccation. The first major synthetic group of insecticides, developed in the 1930s and 1940s, is the chlorinated hydrocarbon family. This family includes DDT, aldrin, dieldrin, methoxychlor, and chlordane. Dramatic improvements in insect control were noted when the chlorinated hydrocarbons began to be used frequently due to their high insect toxicity. The chlorinated hydrocarbons are also noted for their high environmental persistence, which resulted in long-term insect control but also contributed to environmental buildup and biological magnification, leading to significant ecological and environmental impacts. Recent reports have indicated that some chlorinated hydrocarbon insecticides are associated with possible adverse effects on fertility and reproduction in non-target organisms, which may result from the enzyme-inducing or estrogenic properties of the chemicals. Because of the potential adverse impacts of chlorinated hydrocarbons on the environment and on non-target organisms, very few chlorinated hydrocarbon insecticides are currently allowed for use in the U.S.

In the 1960s and 1970s, the organophosphate and carbamate compounds replaced the chlorinated hydrocarbons as the most prominently used insecticides. These two families of insecticides share a common toxicological mechanism, the inhibition of cholinesterase enzymes in the nervous systems of both insects and mammals. They are typically far less persistent in the environment than are the chlorinated hydrocarbons but are much more acutely toxic.

A newer class of insecticides is the pyrethroids. These are synthetic derivatives of pyrethrins, which are natural extracts from chrysanthemums. Pyrethroids have been developed to be more stable (and thus more effective as insecticides) than the pyrethrins, which are particularly instable in light. Pyrethroids are frequently used as broad-spectrum insecticides. They have high insect toxicity, but lower mammalian toxicity than their organophosphate or carbamate counterparts. Pyrethroids are still limited in effectiveness due to their environmental lability, their high cost, and their potential for resistance development.

11.2.2.2 Herbicides

Herbicides are used widely throughout the world to control weeds and exist in a wide variety of different types. Examples of classes of herbicide include the triazine, sulfonylurea, phenoxy, and quaternary ammonium herbicides.

Herbicides exert their toxic action on weeds through a number of different mechanisms. Preplant herbicides are applied before a crop is planted, preemergent herbicides are applied after planting but prior to the development of weeds, and postemergent herbicides are used after weeds have appeared. Some herbicides, such as glyphosate, exert broad-spectrum weed killing effects making them toxic to virtually all forms of plant material, including the crop. Recently, many crops, such as soy, corn, and cotton, have been engineered through genetic modification to be resistant to damage by glyphosate or other herbicides.

In contrast to the broad-spectrum herbicides, others are more selective. The phenoxy herbicides, which include chemicals such as 2,4-D, 2,4,5-T, and MCPA, are toxic to broad-leaf plants but do not affect narrow-leaf plants such as grasses.

11.2.2.3 Fungicides

Molds and other plant diseases are controlled by fungicides, which act to affect the growth or metabolism of fungal pests. Many different fungicides exist, including sulfur, aryl- and alkyl-mercurial compounds, *bis*-dithiocarbamates, and chlorinated phenols.

11.2.2.4 Potentially Carcinogenic Pesticides

Public and regulatory concern over the potential cancer risks posed by pesticide residues in the diet has been significant over the past two decades. While the consumption of foods containing residues of pesticides has not been correlated with the development of human cancers, pesticide exposure has been linked to some cancers in agricultural workers. In most cases, however, pesticides that are listed as potential carcinogens are classified as such based upon the results of long-term cancer studies in rodents, such as mice and rats. Such studies are conducted using doses typically several orders of magnitude greater than humans would be expected to receive and are frequently performed in animal species that are predisposed to developing specific types of cancer.

A list of pesticides considered to be "probable" carcinogens by the U.S. Environmental Protection Agency (EPA) is provided in Table 11.1.

11.2.3 PESTICIDE USE

Pesticides are frequently applied in agriculture but are also extensively employed for industrial, commercial, and government uses, as well as in the home and garden sector. It has been estimated that in 1999 the agricultural use of pesticides represented an expenditure of \$7.6 billion dollars in the U.S. while industrial, commercial and government use represented \$1.5 billion and home and garden use, \$2.0 billion dollars (EPA, 2002). Of expenditure in 1999 on pesticides for agricultural uses, herbicides and plant growth regulators were responsible for \$5.0 billion, insecticides and miticides, \$1.4 billion, and fungicides, \$0.7 billion.

Estimates of the total world use of pesticides in 1999, in terms of kilograms of active ingredient applied, are provided in Figure 11.1. A total of approximately 5.7×10^9 kg of pesticides was estimated to have been used

Table 11.1
Some pesticides considered by the US Environmental Protection Agency to be 'probable' carcinogens.

Fungicides	Herbicides	Insecticides
Chlorothalonil	Acetochlor	Heptachlor
Cyproconazole	Aciflourfen sodium	Lindane
Folpet	Alachlor	Oxythioquinox
Iprodione	Amitrol	Propargite
Mancozeb	Cacodylic acid	Propoxur
Maneb	Lactofen	Thiodicarb
Metiram	Pronamide	
Pentachlorophenol		
Terrazole		
TPTH		
Vinclozolin		

Insect growth regulator	Wood preservative
Fenoxycarb	Creosote

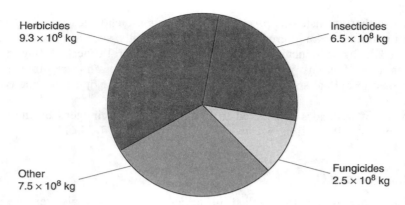

Figure 11.1 Worldwide pesticide use in1999 (kilograms of active ingredient applied). (Adapted from EPA (2002), *Pesticide Industry Sales and Usage. 1998 and 1999 Market Estimates*, U.S. Environmental Protection Agency, Washington, D.C.)

throughout the world in 1999. The most commonly used class of pesticides was herbicides (36%), followed by 'other pesticides' (which includes nematicides, fumigants, rodenticides, molluscicides, aquatic and fish or bird pesticides, other miscellaneous conventional pesticides, plus other chemicals used as pesticides, such as sulfur and petroleum)(29%), insecticides (25%), and fungicides (10%).

The estimated U.S. use of pesticides in 1999 is provided in Figure 11.2. It has been estimated that 5.7×10^8 kg of pesticides were used in the U.S. in 1999,

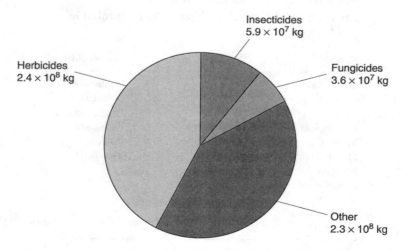

Figure 11.2 Pesticide use in the U.S. in 1999 (kilograms of active ingredient applied). (Adapted from EPA (2002), *Pesticide Industry Sales and Usage. 1998 and 1999 Market Estimates*, U.S. Environmental Protection Agency, Washington, D.C.)

led by herbicides (43%), 'other pesticides' (41%), insecticides (10%), and fungicides (6%).

Overall, the U.S. was responsible for 22% of worldwide pesticide use in 1999, including 30% of 'other pesticides,' 26% of herbicides, 14% of fungicides, and 9% of insecticides.

11.3 REGULATING PESTICIDES IN FOOD

11.3.1 INTRODUCTION

The use of pesticides in agriculture does not inevitably mean that food residues will result. In many cases, pesticides are applied to non-food agricultural crops, while in other instances pesticides may be applied around, but not directly on, food crops, such as the case in which a broad-spectrum herbicide is used. Even when pesticides are applied directly to food crops, food residues are often not detected. In some cases, pesticides may be applied prior to the development of edible portions of the crop, while in others the rapid environmental degradation of the pesticide between the time of application and the time of harvest may also avoid food residues.

11.3.2 U.S. REGULATION

When the normal use of a pesticide on a food crop may pose the potential to leave a food residue, the EPA establishes a tolerance. The tolerance represents the maximum level of a pesticide residue allowed on the food crop. Tolerances are pesticide and crop specific; different crops may have different tolerance levels for a particular pesticide, while a particular crop may have different tolerance levels for the different pesticides that may be used on it.

The processes that the EPA applies to establish pesticide tolerances are confusing and are frequently misunderstood. Readers interested in EPA's tolerance-setting practices should consider reading a comprehensive paper on the subject (Winter, 1992), however the following text gives a brief summary.

Pesticide tolerances are not based solely on safety, but rather are set to represent the maximum expected residue levels of a pesticide on a commodity as a result of the legal application of the pesticide. The maximum expected levels are derived from the results of controlled field studies conducted by the pesticide manufacturer, in which application conditions are chosen to provide the highest level of residue. Conditions include applying the pesticide at the maximum allowable rate, making the maximum number of applications per growing season, and harvesting the food after the minimum anticipated interval between application and harvest.

The manufacturer typically petitions the EPA to establish a tolerance at, or slightly higher than, the maximum residue encountered under the field studies. As such, one could consider the tolerance to represent a crude indicator of compliance with pesticide use conditions; it is possible that blatant misuse of a pesticide could result in residues being detected in excess of the established tolerance, while legal use of the pesticide should not result in residues over tolerance.

Pesticide residues will be considered illegal when pesticides are detected at levels that exceed the tolerance level, or when residues of a pesticide are detected, at any level, on a commodity for which a tolerance has not been established. Illegal residues should not be confused with 'unsafe' residues, however, since pesticide tolerances are most appropriately viewed as enforcement tools rather than as safety standards.

The EPA does consider health criteria when determining whether to approve or deny a manufacturer's petition to have a tolerance established. Human health risk assessment practices consider potential human exposure from all registered (and proposed) uses of the pesticide, and if the risk is deemed excessive, the EPA will deny the tolerance petition. In cases where the risks are deemed acceptable, the EPA will establish tolerances, as described in the previous paragraphs.

The practices used by EPA to assess the risks of pesticides to consumers became much more complicated following the passage of the FQPA in 1996. Prior to the passage of the FQPA, the EPA allowed tolerances to be established on a chemical-by-chemical basis and only considered exposure from food. Provisions of the FQPA require that the EPA now considers the aggregate exposure from pesticides in food, drinking water, and in residential settings. Additionally, the EPA must also consider the cumulative exposure from pesticide families possessing a common mechanism of toxicological action, such as the organophosphate and carbamate insecticides.

The FQPA also requires the EPA to consider the potential increased susceptibility of infants and children to pesticides. In the absence of any toxicological data suggesting that infants and children are no more susceptible to a specific pesticide than are adults, the EPA may set an acceptable level of exposure for infants and children. The EPA may consider the acceptable level (expressed on the basis of the amount of pesticide consumed relative to body weight per day) to be as much as ten times lower than a comparable acceptable exposure level for adults.

11.3.3 INTERNATIONAL REGULATION

While all nations of the world possess the sovereign right to establish their own acceptable levels for pesticide residues in foods, many lack the resources to develop their own regulatory programs and instead rely upon a set of international standards developed by the Codex Alimentarius Commission, frequently referred to as Codex. The Codex international standards are termed 'maximum residue limits' (MRLs) and, like U.S. tolerances, are established primarily as enforcement tools for determining whether pesticide applications are made according to established directions. While many countries have adopted Codex MRLs, others, such as the U.S. and several Asian countries, rely on their own standards. Thus, there is no uniformity among the world with respect to allowable levels of pesticides on foods. A pesticide–commodity combination may have different allowable levels in different countries, and the pesticide may be allowed for use on the commodity in some countries but not allowed on the same commodity in others.

In many cases, the U.S. tolerances and the Codex MRLs are similar, although there are other cases where they may be quite different. When U.S. tolerances and Codex MRLs can be compared directly, 47% have been shown to be equivalent, 34% of Codex MRLs were found to be lower (more restrictive), and 19% of U.S. tolerances were lower (General Accounting Office, 1991). There are a number of reasons that explain the differences; these include the use of different data sets, different methods to regulate pesticide metabolites, and different agricultural production and pest control practices.

11.4 PESTICIDE MONITORING

11.4.1 Introduction

Two regulatory agencies are responsible for the majority of pesticide residue monitoring in the U.S. The U.S. Food and Drug Administration (FDA) is the agency primarily responsible for enforcement of tolerances in domestic and imported foods shipped in interstate commerce. The U.S. Department of Agriculture (USDA) administers the Pesticide Data Program, which is designed to most-accurately capture actual resides of foods that reflect levels near the time of consumption of the food items. The USDA also administers the National Residue Program, which samples meat, poultry, and raw egg products for pesticide residues, animal drugs, and environmental contaminants.

11.4.2 FDA MONITORING

The FDA's monitoring activities rely on food sampling procedures in which the types of commodities to be sampled, and the origins of the samples, are chosen specifically to enhance the FDA's abilities to identify violative residues. FDA monitoring is therefore not a random process.

The majority of samples taken in the FDA monitoring program are from imported foods, which constitute approximately two thirds of all the samples taken. Imports are typically sampled at the point of entry into the U.S., while domestic samples are frequently collected close to the production source or at the wholesale level. Samples are usually analyzed using multiresidue techniques capable of the detection of approximately 200 pesticide active ingredients as well as several other pesticide metabolites, impurities, and alteration products.

Results from the FDA's 2001 pesticide regulatory monitoring program are shown in Table 11.2. Of the 2101 domestic samples analyzed for pesticide residues, 60.2% had no detectable residues, 38.7% had detectable residues within legal limits, and 1.1% had violative residues (FDA, 2003). The highest violation rate, 1.5%, was observed in vegetables, while fruits showed a violation rate of 1.1%, grains and grain products had a violation rate of 0.3%,

Table 11.2
US Food and Drug Administration regulatory
pesticide monitoring results, 2001.

	Domestic	Imported
Grains and grain products		
Number of samples	286	126
No residue found	58.4%	91.3%
Residue found, not violative	41.3%	8.7%
Residue found, violative	0.3%	0
Milk, dairy products, eggs		
Number of samples	33	15
No residue found	97.0%	100%
Residue found, not violative	3.0%	0
Residue found, violative	0	0
Fish, shellfish, other aquatic products		
Number of samples	114	326
No residue found	81.6%	94.2%
Residue found, not violative	18.4%	5.5%
Residue found, violative	0	0.3%
Fruits		
Number of samples	710	1203
No residue found	40.3%	67.8%
Residue found, not violative	58.6%	29.4%
Residue found, violative	1.1%	2.8%
Vegetables		
Number of samples	888	2506
No residue found	70.0%	69.1%
Residue found, not violative	28.5%	24.5%
Residue found, violative	1.5%	6.4%
Other		
Number of samples	70	198
No residue found	92.9%	82.3%
Residue found, not violative	7.1%	9.6%
Residue found, violative	0	8.1%
Totals		
Number of samples	2101	4374
No residue found	60.2%	72.0%
Residue found, not violative	38.7%	23.2%
Residue found, violative	1.1%	4.8%

Source: adapted from FDA (2003), *Food and Drug*
Administration Pesticide Program Residue Monitoring 2001.

and no violative samples were observed following the analysis of samples from the categories 'milk, dairy products, eggs', 'fish, shellfish, other aquatic products', and 'other.'

Results from imported foods were somewhat similar, although violation rates were higher and the rates of residue detection were lower. Of the 4374 imported samples analyzed for pesticide residues, 72.0% had no detectable residues, 23.2% had detectable residues within legal limits, and 4.8% had violative residues. Violations were observed in the 'other' category (8.1%), vegetables (6.4%), fruits (2.8%), and 'fish, shellfish, other aquatic products' (0.3%).

Pesticide residues are deemed violative if the residues encountered exceed the established tolerances or when residues for which no tolerance has been established are detected on the sampled commodity. In the case of imported food sample, the FDA noted that 92.9% of the violations occurred when pesticides were detected on commodities for which no tolerance was established, with the remaining 7.1% of violations occurring when residues exceeded tolerances. Violative residues from domestic food samples presented a different pattern, with 50% of the violations stemming from levels exceeding tolerance and the other 50% resulting from pesticides being detected on commodities for which no tolerance was established.

11.4.3 USDA Pesticide Data Program

The USDA's Pesticide Data Program (PDP) each year collects several thousand food samples, which are analyzed for pesticide residues. In contrast with the FDA's residue monitoring, the PDP is not an enforcement program. Instead, it has developed sampling procedures that are designed to use measurements of actual residue levels to determine residue levels near the time the food items are consumed. Pesticides and commodities sampled each year in the PDP are selected based upon the EPA's data needs. The EPA uses PDP data in its development of dietary pesticide risk assessments as required by the FQPA. PDP data are also employed to examine pesticide residue issues that may impact agricultural practices and U.S. trade, and may be used to identify crops where alternative pest management practices are needed and in promoting export of U.S. commodities in a competitive global market.

The PDP represents partnerships between the USDA and the states; in 2001, ten states (California, Colorado, Florida, Maryland, Michigan, New York, Ohio, Texas, Washington, and Wisconsin) participated in collecting and analyzing PDP samples.

In total, 12,264 samples were collected and analyzed for pesticide residues in the 2001 PDP (USDA, 2003). Specific fruits and vegetables analyzed in the 2001 PDP included apples, bananas, broccoli, carrots, celery, cherries, grapes, green beans, lettuce, mushrooms, nectarines, oranges, peaches, pineapples, potatoes, canned sweet corn, canned sweet peas, and canned tomato paste. Fruits and vegetable samples were taken most commonly (9903 samples), followed by beef (911 samples), enriched milled rice (689 samples), poultry (464 samples), and drinking water (297 samples). Domestic samples comprised 82% of the total and sampling was based on a statistical design to ensure that the data are reliable for use in exposure assessments.

In 2001, 44% of all samples contained no detectable residues, while 24% showed one residue and 32% showed more than one residue. In 0.1% of the samples, residues were detected that exceeded tolerances, while residues were found on commodities for which no tolerance was established on 1.8% of the samples.

11.4.4 RESIDUES IN ORGANIC FOODS

Much of the rapid growth in the consumption of foods labeled as 'organic' may result from the perception among consumers that organic foods may be healthier than conventional foods. While some pesticides are allowed for use on organic foods, it is logical to assume that the pesticide residue profiles for organic and conventional foods should differ, both qualitatively and quantitatively.

Analysis of PDP data from 1994 to 1999 showed that 73% of approximately 27,000 food samples that had no market claim (conventional or organic) showed detectable residues, while 23% of 127 fresh food samples designated as organic had detectable residue levels (Baker et al., 2002). Unavoidable contamination of some of the organic samples was due to the presence of persistent chlorinated hydrocarbon insecticides, which had been banned several years earlier, but 13% of the organic samples showed residues of pesticides other than the chlorinated hydrocarbon insecticides.

In addition to pesticide regulatory monitoring programs by the FDA and USDA, individual states have also developed monitoring programs. One such state is California, which analyzed more than 67,000 food samples for pesticide residues between 1989 and 1998. Pesticide residues were detected in 31% of approximately 66,000 samples for which no market claim was made, and in 7% of the 1097 samples claimed to be organic (Baker et al., 2002).

These results indicate that pesticide residues are less common in organic samples than in conventional samples, although residues are frequently detected in organic produce. Potential explanations for the greater-than-expected presence of pesticides in organic foods include mislabeling of products, misidentification of the samples during data entry, postharvest fungicide contamination, and inadvertent contamination from environmentally-persistent pesticides or from drift from pesticide applications made to adjacent crops.

11.5 DIETARY PESTICIDE RISK ASSESSMENT

11.5.1 BACKGROUND

The dietary risks from pesticides are frequently, although inappropriately, discussed in relation to the relative breakdown between legal and violative residues. It is commonly assumed that illegal residues represent 'unsafe' residues; data suggesting low violation rates is often used as evidence of the safety of the food supply with respect to pesticide residues, while data suggesting high violation rates frequently infers a lack of safety. Ironically, since the determination of what constitutes a high or a low violation rate is dependent upon the individual interpreting the data, the same data pools (such as FDA regulatory monitoring results) can be interpreted by some as a demonstration of safety but by others as an indication of unacceptable risk.

It is critical to realize that pesticide tolerances themselves are not safety standards but rather enforcement tools for indicating whether pesticides have been applied according to directions. Violative residues result when residue levels exceed the tolerance due to the misapplication of a pesticide, or when residues at any level are found on a commodity for which a tolerance was not established (which could result from product misuse). While a few isolated cases of violative residues have resulted in human harm, the vast majority of violative residues are of little or no toxicological consequence.

Contemporary risk assessment practices for pesticides in foods require far more data than simply the residue levels evaluated in government monitoring programs. Exposure to pesticides is determined by multiplying the residue levels on food by the amount of the food item consumed; once determined, exposure is compared with standard toxicological criteria derived from animal toxicology studies to determine the acceptability of the exposure.

11.5.2 TOXICOLOGICAL CRITERIA FOR SAFETY

The basic principle of toxicology, as first noted by the Swiss physician Paracelsus, is that "the dose makes the poison." While this principle is easy to understand, the processes used to understand the relationships between dose and biological response, and ultimately to determine what dose of a chemical poses 'a reasonable certainty of no harm', are much more complicated.

Models for determining the dose-response relationship vary based upon the type of toxicological hazard. In the dose-response for chemical carcinogens, it is frequently assumed that no threshold level of exposure (an exposure below which no effects would occur) exists, and, therefore, any level of exposure leads to some finite level of risk. As a practical matter, cancer risks of below one excess cancer per million members of the population exposed (1×10^6), when calculated using conservative (risk exaggerating) methods, are considered to represent a reasonable certainty of no harm (Winter and Francis, 1997).

For non-carcinogenic chemicals, it is usually assumed that a threshold dose does apply at low levels of exposure, implying that exposure below the threshold is not likely to be significant. The toxicity threshold dose for non-carcinogenic effects is largely theoretical, it is practical only in relation to the effects that occur at dose levels slightly above and slightly below the threshold. Toxicological studies are performed to identify the lowest dose level above which toxicological effects are observed, the 'lowest adverse effect level'

(LOAEL), and the highest dose at which no effects are observed, the 'no adverse effect level' (NOAEL). In the interest of prudence, the NOAEL is generally considered as a conservative estimate of the toxicity threshold.

NOAEL values derived from toxicology studies using small homogenous groups of laboratory animals may not adequately represent toxicity thresholds for large and non-homogenous human populations. As a result, uncertainty factors (frequently known as safety factors) are used to consider human variability and to guide the animal-to-human extrapolation. The most common uncertainty factor is 100; this is rationalized to consider that humans are ten times more sensitive to a chemical than are laboratory animals and that some humans are ten times more sensitive than the average population. The EPA may use an additional ten-fold uncertainty factor (resulting in a total uncertainty factor of 1000) if it finds that infants and children may be more sensitive to the toxic effects of a chemical than adults.

An estimate for the lowest level of toxicological concern for human exposure to a chemical is developed by dividing the appropriate NOAEL by the uncertainty factor. Historically, this estimate has been termed the 'acceptable daily intake' (or ADI) although it has been replaced by what EPA calls the 'reference dose' (or RfD). Both ADIs and RfDs are expressed in terms of the amount of chemical exposure per amount of body weight per day.

For carcinogen risk assessments, multiplying the proposed daily exposure by the unit cancer potency factor (derived from animal cancer studies) yields the cancer risk; cancer risks greater than 1×10^6 may trigger regulatory concern while those below 1×10^6 are frequently considered to be negligible. For non-carcinogenic risks, a comparison between the estimated exposure level and the RfD determines the significance of the risk.

11.5.3 EXPOSURE ASSESSMENT

11.5.3.1 Introduction

The determination of the estimated levels of exposure is obviously a critical component of the risk assessment process. Both pesticide residue levels and food consumption estimates must be considered. Methods for determining exposure are frequently classified as deterministic and probabilistic methods (Winter, 2003).

11.5.3.2 Deterministic Methods

Measurement of dietary exposure to pesticides has historically relied upon deterministic methods that assign finite values to both the pesticide residue level and the food consumption estimates to yield a 'point' estimate of exposure. The calculations are relatively simple, but consideration needs to be given to the accuracy of the assumptions concerning residue level and food consumption.

In the calculation of chronic risks from pesticides in foods, the EPA frequently uses a deterministic approach to yield the theoretical maximum residue contribution (TMRC) for a pesticide. This value represents the maximum legal exposure to a pesticide, and assumes that:

- the pesticide is always used on all commodities for which it is registered
- residues are always present at the tolerance level
- no reduction in residue levels occurs as a result of postharvest factors, such as transportation, washing, cooking, peeling, and processing
- the food is consumed at the average (50th percentile) daily rate

Such estimates yield an exaggerated level of exposure, but for many pesticides, exposure at the TMRC is far below the RfD and does not result in cancer risks greater than 1×10^6. In some cases, where the exaggerated levels of exposure for the TMRC exceed the RfD or cause the cancer risk to exceed 1×10^6, the exposure calculations may require refinements, such as using more realistic residue levels or adjusting pesticide use estimations. If these or other more comprehensive adjustments still do not result in acceptable levels of exposure, the EPA will not approve tolerances for the pesticide.

Because the use of deterministic approaches for estimating exposure frequently relies on worst-case or unrealistic levels, it is critical that the assumptions used in developing risk assessments are clearly specified and rationalized. Unfortunately, the communication of such risk assessments, particularly in the popular media, frequently occurs without reference to the potential degree of exaggeration and may therefore lead to an exaggerated perception of the degree of risk. As an example, the NRC, using the TMRC approach, estimated cancer risks from pesticides in the diet and considerable attention was focused upon the exaggerated levels of potential cancer risk (NRC, 1987). A comparative study using more refined estimates of pesticide exposure yielded risks 100 to 10,000 times lower than those reported in the NRC study (Archibald and Winter, 1990).

The FDA, in addition to conducting its pesticide regulatory monitoring program, also conducts its annual Total Diet Study to estimate dietary exposure to pesticides and other contaminants. In the Total Diet Study, FDA inspectors purchase market baskets of more than 200 food items and have the items prepared for consumption prior to analysis for pesticide residues. By making crude estimates of the consumption rates for the various foods, it is possible, using a deterministic approach, to use the results of the Total Diet Study to estimate the typical daily exposure to pesticides. In 1991 (the last year for which the FDA has used the Total Diet Study data to estimate human daily exposure to pesticides), exposure to most pesticides resulted in levels less than 1% of the RfD (FDA, 1992). To put such a finding in perspective, consider that the RfD is obtained by identifying the highest level of exposure that does not cause a noticeable adverse effect in the most sensitive animal species tested (NOAEL) and then dividing that by an uncertainty factor of 100 or more. As such, the RfD represents a level 100 times lower than a level that demonstrated no toxicological effect. Exposure at 1% of the RfD, therefore, results in an exposure 10,000 times lower than the level that does not produce noticeable effects in animals.

11.5.3.3 Probabilistic Methods

While deterministic methods are still quite useful in determining long-term, chronic exposures to pesticides, they are being replaced with probabilistic methods for the analysis of acute (short-term) exposures. These probabilistic methods take advantage of improvements in computational capabilities.

In reality, neither residue levels nor food consumption estimates exist as single values. They can better be depicted as distributions because residue patterns vary greatly, as do food consumption practices.

Probabilistic approaches take advantage of current computational capabilities to combine all of the data in a pesticide residue distribution (rather than a single 'expected' value) with food consumption data to develop a distribution of daily exposure. This approach is called a Monte Carlo simulation, although there are many ways to conduct this type of analysis.

In the case of a single pesticide found on a single commodity, a Monte Carlo analysis would randomly select a residue data point and a food consumption level value and multiply them together to yield an exposure level. By repeating this process, often thousands or tens of thousands of times, it is possible to develop a distribution of daily exposures that would allow a determination of which levels represent, for example, the 50th, 99th, and 99.9th percentiles of consumption.

Currently, the EPA considers acute pesticide exposures to represent a 'reasonable certainty of no harm' when exposure at the 99.9th percentile is below the RfD. When exposure at the 99.9th percentile exceeds the RfD, the EPA will generally conduct a sensitivity analysis to determine whether particular factors that drive the exposure, such as high residue or high consumption levels, are unusual and so may represent artifacts that artificially skew the exposure distribution curve.

More sophisticated probabilistic models are used by EPA to comply with the aggregate and cumulative risk provisions of the FQPA. These models consider 'rolling windows' of exposure, toxicological equivalence factors for pesticides that have common toxicological mechanisms, and include methods to incorporate exposure from drinking water and residential pesticide use into the pesticide exposure estimates.

11.6 SUMMARY AND CONCLUSIONS

It has been demonstrated that pesticides are frequently encountered in foods, although typically at levels not considered to cause concern from the regulatory community. When placed into perspective with other food safety risks, the dietary risks from exposure to pesticides are considered to be far lower than the risks from microbiological contamination, nutritional imbalance, environmental contaminants, and even naturally-occurring toxins.

The techniques used to establish the risks posed by pesticides are dynamic and evolving. The passage of the FQPA in 1996 paved the way for the development of sophisticated computational models for assessing pesticide exposure, and future refinement of such models is anticipated. Such advancements in pesticide risk assessment techniques should be applicable to the risk assessment of other chemicals in foods and in the environment.

11.7 REFERENCES

Archibald, S.O. and Winter, C.K. (1990). Pesticide residues and cancer risks, *California Agric.*, 43, 6, 6–9.

Baker, B.P., Benbrook, C.M., Groth, E. and Lutz Benbrook, K. (2002). Pesticide residues in conventional, integrated pest management (IPM)-grown and organic foods: insights from three US data sets, *Food Additives Contaminants*, 19, 5, 427–446.

EPA (2002). *Pesticide Industry Sales and Usage. 1998 and 1999 Market Estimates*, Biological and Economic Analysis Division, Office of Pesticide Programs, Office of Prevention, Pesticides, and Toxic Substances. U.S. Environmental Protection Agency, Washington, D.C.

FDA (1992). Pesticide program residue monitoring, 1991, *JAOAC* 75, 136A–158A.

FDA (2003). *Food and Drug Administration Pesticide Program Residue Monitoring 2001*, U.S. Food and Drug Administration, Washington, D.C.

General Accounting Office (1991). *International Food Safety: Comparison of U.S. and Codex Pesticide Standards*, GAO/PEMD-91-22, U.S. General Accounting Office, Washington, D.C.

Goldman, L.R., Beller, M., and Jackson, R.J. (1990). Aldicarb food poisonings in California, 1985-1988: toxicity estimates for humans, *Arch. Environ. Health*, 45, 141–147.

NRC (1987). *Regulating Pesticides in Food: The Delaney Paradox*, National Research Council, National Academy of Sciences, National Academy Press, Washington, D.C.

NRC (1993). *Pesticides in the Diets of Infants and Children*, National Research Council, National Academy of Sciences, National Academy Press, Washington, D.C.

Natural Resources Defense Council (1989). *Intolerable Risk: Pesticides in Our Children's Food*, National Resources Defense Council, Washington, D.C.

USDA (2003). *Pesticide Data Program Annual Summary Calendar Year 2001*, US Department of Agriculture, Agriculture and Marketing Service, Science and Technology, Washington, D.C.

Winter, C.K. (1992). Pesticide tolerances and their relevance as safety standards, *Reg. Toxicol. Pharmacol*, 15, 137–150.

Winter, C.K. and Francis, F.J. (1997). Assessing, managing, and communicating chemical food safety risks, *Food Technol.*, 51, 85–92.

Winter, C.K. (2003). Exposure and dose-response modeling for food chemical risk assessment, in Schmidt, R.H. and Rodrick, G.E., eds., *Food Safety Handbook*, Wiley-Interscience, Hoboken, pp. 73–88.

12

Antibiotic and Hormone Residues in Foods and their Significance

Stanley E. Katz and Paula-Marie L. Ward

CONTENTS

12.1   INTRODUCTION

Although it is hackneyed to quote the classical line of Paracelsus relating toxicity to dosage (Stillman, 1920), it is nevertheless appropriate. It can be strongly asserted that there is little to fear from antibiotic residues as a cause of acute poisonings. There are of course exceptions, such as the acute idiosyncratic reactions to chloramphenicol by a small segment of the population and allergic reactions to penicillin (which can be fatal, one case has been found in the literature of a death resulting from eating penicillin-containing meat [Tscheuschner,1972]), but these are extremely rare.

A great many antibiotics used in animal agriculture (for growth promotion and increased feed efficiency, subtherapeutic treatments, as well as for disease treatment) have also been used in human medicine, often at much higher levels then in agriculture. Many of those compounds that are not used in human medicine are either not absorbed from the intestinal tract or have analogs used in human medicine. Hormones exhibit different aspects of toxicity, but it is extremely difficult to document acute toxicity from overdoses. This chapter deals with the potential hazards from residues of antibiotics or antimicrobials and hormones (synthetic or natural) used in agricultural that are found in foods of animal origin.

12.2 ANTIBIOTIC USAGE IN ANIMALS

Considering the extensive use of antibiotics in animal agriculture, and the more modest usage in plants and aquaculture, it is axiomatic that residues will occur in foods. The use of any such potent and biologically active materials, in such vast quantities, will always result in some misusage, deliberate or accidental. Hence the occurrence of residues. It is the extent and the biological significance of these residues that is important.

Unfortunately, there is no truly accurate record of the quantities of antibiotics and antimicrobials used in animal agriculture. In the U.S., the Animal Health Institute estimated the amounts to be some 8.09 million kg per year, while the Union of Concerned Scientists estimated 11.2 million kg per year were fed to the three major livestock species (hogs, cattle, and poultry) for non-therapeutic purposes (Mellon et al., 2001). Worldwide usage is very difficult to estimate because in many parts of the world the feeding of antibiotics remains relatively unregulated and undocumented; therefore, figures on the amounts used for agricultural purposes are unavailable. These authors estimate that, at a minimum, total worldwide usage would be at least two times the estimates for the U.S., but it is likely that this low by a substantial amount.

The usual uses for antibiotics and antimicrobials in animal agriculture relate to subtherapeutic or growth promotional purposes, disease prevention, and disease treatment. The greatest amounts are used for subtherapeutic purposes, which are related to the economics of animal production. The proximate drug levels for these three usage patterns are, under 50 g per t (50 µg per g) for growth promotion, from 50 to 200 g per t (50 to 200 µg per g) for disease prevention, and greater than 200 g per ton (200 µg per g) for disease treatment. There is, of course, considerable variation and sometimes overlap to these proximate levels. Regardless of whatever the level is, residues would be minimized if there were strict attention to proper adherence to withdrawal times and use only at approved levels in designated species. Off-label use (as defined under the Code of Federal Regulations – 21 CFR 530.41) is always fraught with residue problems as withdrawal times are, at best, estimates.

The question as to whether residues can be avoided cannot be answered categorically, since there are no ways to control which antibiotics are used and how they are administered. There are no sampling or analytical systems that can definitively indicate that a product is residue-free; all analytical systems have finite limitations of sensitivity. All that can ever be said is that levels of specific drugs in a sample are below the levels of detection of the analytical method.

12.3 ANTIBIOTIC RESIDUES

What constitutes a residue is always open to discussion. Residues are defined in this chapter as any level of drug or its metabolites or degradation products that can be measured in a given product. This leads to a further subdivision related to whether the level found exceeds the maximum residue level (MRL) or tolerance level. Levels exceeding the MRL are defined as violative levels; levels below are legal residues (and in some quarters not defined as residues at all). The U.S. Food and Drug Administration (FDA) uses the designation 'safe level.' This level is defined more by the analytical methodologies than by toxicological parameters and is used primarily for residues in milk. More often than not, 'safe levels' are used when the legal tolerance is zero, levels below the analytical limit of detection.

12.4 ANIMAL RESIDUE DATA

Worldwide data are not readily available as many nations do not publish the results of their animal residue monitoring programs. The best available data are those published regularly by the Food Safety Inspection Service (FSIS) of the U.S. Department of Agriculture (USDA). It is possible to go back over data for many years and demonstrate improvements in the residue situation, however the records for the past few years are the important ones as they are representative of current or recent events. Since the publication of worldwide residue data is at best sparse and not consistent, this chapter has made use of the regularly published residue data from the FSIS/USDA surveys, which are available on the Internet. The assumption made in this chapter, and perhaps there is a certain naiveté to this assumption, is that international residue usage is similar to that found by the FSIS/USDA. This assumption is based upon the frequency of residues found in meat products imported into the U.S.

12.5 SAMPLING PROCEDURES

The number of animals sampled compared with the numbers produced will always astound the reader as relatively few animals are normally sampled and analyzed. It is impossible from both a logistical and cost point of view to sample huge numbers of animals. To accomplish a reasonable sampling program, an experience-based approach is both logical and realistic. This approach bases the sample size (number of animals analyzed) on what experience has shown the incidence of violative residues to be in that class of animal. Where a high incidence of violative residues is expected, a smaller number of samples is needed.

Based upon the FSIS/USDA experience, a statistically-based sampling plan determined that a minimum sample 299 animals should be sufficient to detect a violative incidence of 1%. By halving the incidence to 0.5%, the sample size for analysis would double. Similarly, an expected violative incidence of 0.1% would require a minimum sample size of 2990. If the probability of the presence of violative residues is greater than the 95th percentile confidence limit, the size of the sample must increase significantly (Table 12.1). It is obvious that the statistically-based sampling will only offer a snapshot, but there are no other practical approaches to the sampling and analyses.

The 1998 FSIS/USDA monitoring program analyzed approximately 7800 samples for antibiotics. Of that total, only 38 violative samples were detected in 37 animals, across all classes of animals (Table 12.2). Horses accounted for 21 of the 38 violative samples. This result shows that there was a very low frequency of violative samples, 0.21% for all classifications other than horses (USDA, 1998).

In addition to these monitoring studies, the FSIS performed on-site screening assays to measure the frequency of animals at slaughter having sulfonamide and antibiotic residues present in violative levels (1998 results are presented in Table 12.3). The results of both studies were consistent; both indicated a low frequency of violative antibiotic residues in a wide variety of animals used for food.

The question that must be asked is, given the total number of animals actually assayed was relatively small in comparison with the total number of animals produced, how significant are the results? Based on the statistical design and the observation that the range (95% confidence limits) will reflect closely the realities of the animal population sampled, the estimate of the frequency of residues in any given slaughter class is a good estimate.

Table 12.1
Sample sizes required to detect a residue problem within a sampled population.

Expected % violative	Confidence limits			
	90	95	99	99.9
1	230	299	459	658
0.5	460	598	919	1379
0.1	2303	2995	4603	6905
0.05	4605	5990	9209	13,813

Two years, 1998 and 2000 (the latest year available at this writing) will be used for this presentation (12.2).

Table 12.2

Incidence of residues of antibiotics and sulfonamides in the FSIS/USDA monitoring program, 1998.

Slaughter class	Number produced	Violations (%)	Range (95% confidence limits)	Non-violative (%) Antibiotic	Sulfa
Horses	68,783	4.5	2.8–6.9	0.00	0.00
Bulls	731,868	0.0	0.0	0.00	0.00
Beef/dairy cows	7,083,868	0.0/0.4	0.0–1.5	0.00	0.00
Heifers	12,871,623	0.3	0.0–1.8	0.00	0.00
Steers	19,818,380	0.2	0.0–1.2	0.00	0.00
Calves					
Bob	690,506	0.6	0.1–1.8	3.66	0.25
Formula-fed	727,677	0.8	0.2–2.0	6.86	0.54
Non-formula	24,592	1.2	0.2–3.4	1.56	0.00
Heavy	40,665	1.0	0.2–0.3	1.39	0.45
Sheep	214,892	0.0	0.0–1.2	0.00	0.00
Lambs	3,556,425	0.0	0.0–1.1	0.29	0.00
Goats	455,076	0.0	0.0–0.8	—	—
Market hogs	100,365,553	0.9	0.0–0.8	7.34	0.82
Boars/stags	736,616	0.5	0.0–2.5	0.00	0.92
Sows	3,578,225	0.0	0.0–0.7	(1)	(1)
Chickens					
Young	7,556,363,108	0.0	0.0–0.9	0.23	0.36
Mature	165,353,454	0.0	0.0–1.6	0.00	0.86
Turkeys					
Young	265,266,399	0.0	0.0–0.8	2.56	0.98
Mature	1,871,937	0.0	0.0–0.7	(2)	(2)
Ducks	23,050,277	0.0	0.0–0.7	0.76	0.00

Notes: (1) = combined with market hogs, (2) = combined all turkeys.

Source: USDA (1998). *1998 Domestic Residue Data Book*, FSIS, USDA, Washington, D.C.

The data from the 2000 FSIS/USDA monitoring program (Table 12.4) present very similar results to those found in the 1998 data (USDA, 2000). For the sake of simplicity, the data presented show the violations and the upper 95% confidence limits. These data confirm the consistently low incidence of antibiotic and sulfonamide residues in animals grown for food. Even in the worst-case situation, the upper range of the violative incidence remains relatively low, usually less than 2%. There are some 'hot spots,' namely in veal calves, hogs, and horses. Horses appear to be a special case because these animals are rarely used for food in the U.S. It may be that horses are treated with antibiotics or antimicrobials to ensure the animals or carcasses are in the best shape for marketing.

Undoubtedly, the actual level of violative residues is somewhere between the upper and lower levels of the statistical range, and is probably closer to the

Table 12.3
Incidence of violative samples found using on-site screening systems, 1998.

On-site assay system	Animal types	Total samples	Violative samples	%
STOP	Horses, cattle (undefined), sheep, lambs, goats, swine (undefined), ostriches	37,633	220	0.58
FAST	Cattle (undefined), sheep, goats, swine (undefined)	108,020	751	0.70
SOS	Swine (undefined), sheep, goats, cattle (undefined)	11,109	28	0.25

Notes: STOP = swab test on premises, measures antibiotic residues in the kidney; FAST = fast antimicrobial screen test, measures antibiotic and sulfonamide residue in kidney and liver; SOS = sulfa-on-site, measures for sulfonamide residues.
Source: USDA (1998). *1998 Domestic Residue Data Book*, FSIS, USDA, Washington, D.C.

measured incidence. The results reported for these two years (1998 and 2000) are very consistent with the results reported for 1996, 1997 and 1999.

12.6 ANTIBIOTIC RESIDUES IN IMPORTS

Earlier in this chapter, an assumption was made concerning the level of violative residues worldwide. It may be unwise to treat the residue levels in imports as an indicator of the worldwide picture, but there are few other sources of data available on which to base judgments. Fortunately, the data from the 2000 FSIS/USDA monitoring program (USDA, 2000) for imported meat products is available for easy comparison. Table 12.5 summarizes the results of residue screening for both antibiotic and sulfonamide residues in a wide spectrum of meat products from 28 countries.

The data in Table 12.5 are the result of a pooling of results from a number of different products that were spot-checked for a number of different residues (drugs, antibiotics, sulfonamides, pesticides, antimicrobials). As can be seen from these limited data, the number of samples is quite small in total but can be reflective of the residue status of various products. Overall, the data indicate a very low incidence of both antibiotic and sulfonamide residues in the imported products.

There is little available or published evidence to indicate that the antibiotic and sulfonamide residue profiles of similar products not used for export would be different. Until data can be found that indicate otherwise, the only assumption consistent with data is that residue levels and incidences are similar throughout the parts of the world where reasonable regulatory practices exist. However, for areas where regulatory monitoring is not considered important there is no system for estimating extent of residues. It may be prudent to make a worst-case situation assumption for these areas, namely that there would be a high frequency residues in products of animal origin.

Table 12.4

Incidence of residues of antibiotic and sulfonamides in the FSIS/ USDA monitoring program, 2000.

		Violations			
		Antibiotics		Sulfonamides	
Slaughter class	Numbers produced	%	Upper Limit	%	Upper Limit
Horses	50,449	15.2	18.0	0.4	2.0
Bulls	619,616	0.7	1.2	0.3	1.4
Beef/dairy cows	5,269,463	0.3/1.0	1.6/1.8	0.6/0.0	1.6/0.9
Heifers	11,789,720	0.0	0.6	0.0	0.9
Steers	17,457,463	0.0	0.6	0.4	1.3
Calves					
Bob	390,480	1.9	3.6	0.3	1.3
Formula-fed	655,056	0.6	1.3	0.0	1.2
Non-formula	16,321	2.2	1.4	0.0	4.4
Heavy	41,307	0.7	3.3	0.0	2.0
Sheep	163,756	0.0	1.9	0.0	7.0
Lambs	3,151,776	0.3	1.5	0.0	1.3
Goats	530,371	0.0	1.3	0.0	1.0
Hogs					
Market	90,082,453	0.8	1.6	1.2	2.4
Boars/stags	387,101	1.6	4.2	0.0	0.7
Sows	2,965,487	2.2	4.2	0.0	0.7
Chickens					
Young	8,082,061,151	0.4	1.1	0.0	0.7
Mature	169,679,149	0.2	1.9	0.0	5.8
Turkeys					
Young	259,906,886	0.0	0.7	0.0	0.7
Mature	1,871,937	0.0	2.1	0.0	1.7
Ducks	23,784,714	0.0	0.9	0.0	1.2
Rabbits	466,421	(a)	(a)	(a)	(a)
Geese	169,438	(a)	(a)	(a)	(a)
Other poultry	9,068,157	(a)	(a)	(a)	(a)

Source: USDA (2000). *2000 Domestic Residue Data Book*, FSIS, USDA, Washington, D.C.

12.7 ANTIBIOTIC RESIDUES IN MILK

Residues in milk occur primarily as the result of the treatment of lactating cows for mastitis and post partum prevention of infection. Antibiotic and antimicrobial residues in milk can pose significant problems in the making of milk products and cheeses. In the U.S., the primary drugs of concern are those of the β-lactam family, the sulfonamides and tetracyclines; the β-lactams because of their ability to inhibit the starter cultures used in cheese and cultured milk products; the tetracyclines and sulfonamides because of their

Table 12.5

Incidence of antibiotic and sulfonamide residues found in imported meat products in the FSIS/USDA monitoring program, 2000.

Country	Antibiotics		Sulfonamide	
	Samples	Non-detection	Samples	Non-detection
Argentina	11	11	52	52
Australia	254	254	3	260
Austria	–	–	3	2[a]
Belgium	–	–	9	9
Brazil	–	–	71	72
Canada	290	289[b]	422	422
Croatia	–	–	6	6
Costa Rica	12	12	15	15
Denmark	17	17	27	27
France	4	4	20	20
Germany	–	–	19	19
Honduras	6	6	5	5
Hong Kong	?	?	4	4
Hungary	–	–	126	126
Iceland	15	15	11	11
Ireland	3	3	3	3
Israel	–	–	28	27[a]
Italy	–	–	14	12[c]
Japan	3	3	1	1
Mexico	13	13	25	25
Netherlands	–	–	13	13
New Zealand	195	195	198	198
Nicaragua	18	18	13	13
Poland	15	15	?	?
Spain	?	–	16	16
Sweden	4	4	5	5
Switzerland	–	–	9	8[a]
United Kingdom	1	1	8	8

[a]One non-violative sample.
[b]Two violative samples.
[c]One violative sample.
Source: USDA (2000). *2000 Domestic Residue Data Book*, FSIS, USDA, Washington, D.C.

inappropriate wide-spread use and ability to select for resistance in bacteria (Table 12.6).

The data in Table 12.6 indicate the low incidence of antibiotic residues in market milk sampled and analyzed by both regulatory and industrial programs (FDA, 2001). An approximate 0.1% violation incidence is good considering

Table 12.6
Residue frequencies in milk from industrial and regulatory sampling and analysis, 1 October 1999 to 30 September 2000.

	Industrial samples			Regulatory samples			Total		
	Samples	Residue detected	%	Samples	Residue detected	%	Samples	Residue detected	%
Grade A	3,903,985	3565	0.09	223,352	274	0.12	4,1217,377	3839	0.09
Grade B	434,472	411	0.09	3519	0	0.00	437,991	411	0.09
Total	4,338,472	3976	0.09	226,871	274	0.12	4,565,328	4250	0.09

Note: Grade A and Grade B contain samples from bulk tanks, pasteurized milk, producer sources, and other sources.
Source: FDA (2001). *National Milk Drug Residue Data Base*, FDA, Washington D.C.

the volume of milk produced. Approximately 93.9% of the milk sampled was analyzed for the presence of the β-lactams. The percentage of residues found was for violative residues only, not for the total incidence of residues. In some circles, the only residues present are those that are violative. There are no data that indicate total incidence of violative and legal residues.

12.8 ANTIBIOTIC RESIDUES IN EGGS AND FISH

12.8.1 EGGS

Both in the U.S. and worldwide, there are no concerted or organized programs for determining the residue incidence in either eggs or fish. There is a report in the literature of the incidence of antibiotic residues in eggs in Canada. Quan (2000) sampled eggs produced in Canada and imported from the U.S. The survey assayed 3569 samples and found 33 positives, an incidence of 0.92%. However, if samples containing drugs other than antibiotics or sulfonamides are removed, the incidence dropped to 0.36%. Since the origin of all the samples was not defined exactly, the actual percentage of eggs produced in Canada that contain antibiotic or sulfonamide residues is somewhat unclear. However, the incidence does appear to be low, in the same general range as in meats or milk.

In the United Kingdom, the Veterinary Medicine Directorate (VMD) claimed that 97% of the eggs produced were free of detectable residues. Unfortunately, this still leaves 3% of eggs containing residues. The Soil Association believes the actual percentages were much higher, 2000% higher (Young and Craig, 2001). Without free access to all the data, it is difficult to make any unbiased assessment of the actual incidences of legal or violative residues. Regardless of the actual frequencies, it is obvious that concerted efforts by all governments should be made to monitor the residue levels of drugs and to publish these data on a yearly basis.

12.8.2 FISH

Fish, like eggs, is a protein food commodity. Fish and other seafood are produced under intensive rearing conditions and fed antibiotics and anti-microbials. These commodities may be monitored routinely for the corresponding residues but the results are not published routinely, if at all. There are many studies in the literature related to the feeding of antibiotics to fish and other seafood; unfortunately, there are no corresponding published monitoring data to indicate whether or not a residue problem exists for the consumer. It would require a large extrapolation of the residue patterns observed from controlled feeding studies to estimate what would be found in the product in the market place.

12.9 HORMONE RESIDUES IN FOODS OF ANIMAL ORIGIN

12.9.1 HORMONE USAGE

The issue of hormone residues in foods of animal origin is quite different to that of antibiotic residues in the same products. The great fear of growth abnormalities or sex-related changes is probably the reason for the emotional response. There is no doubt that hormones, in general, can have many untoward effects on humans, ranging from sexual changes in both male and females, precocious puberty in children, and effects on libido. At the same time, hormones have been employed as therapies to alleviate problems related to aging and sexuality. Hormones are used in various modalities as birth-control systems, worldwide. The dosages used for contraception are invariably much higher than the levels usually encountered in foods.

Although there are veterinary medical reasons for the treatment of animals with hormones, the majority of use in animal agriculture is for an economic reason, i.e., increased growth rate. The *Merck Veterinary Manual* (1991) presents a summary of some of the applications of hormones in various classes of cattle (Table 12.7).

As long as hormones are used as directed (as pellets or as prescribed ear implants) and proper treatment and withdrawal times are adhered to, the probability of unwanted residues is relatively low. If hormones are not correctly administered, there is little possibility of predicting either the presence or the concentration of residues in the food product.

Table 12.7
Summary of the use of growth regulating hormones in different classes of cattle.

Hormone	Application	Class of cattle	Response (%)	Effect days
Estradiol	Pellet	Steers	10–15	100–120
Progesterone	Pellet[a]	Heifers, cull cows	5–15	100–120
Testosterone	Pellet[a]	Veal calves	10–15	100–120
Trenbolone	Pellet	Heifer, steers, cull cows	5–10	60–90
Trenbolone	Pellet[a]	Steers, veal calves	10–20	60–100
Zeranol	Pellet	Cattle	10–15	–
Melengestrol	Pellet	Heifers, cull cows	5–10	As given

[a]In combination with estradiol.
Source: The Merck Veterinary Manual (reference 9)

12.9.2 HORMONE RESIDUES

The only effective manner by which the true incidence and possibly the significance of hormone residues in meats can be assessed is through the undertaking of formal surveys by regulatory agencies and the publication of the data. Unfortunately, there are all too few such readily available databases, although there are some such data in the literature that can give insights into the extent of the problem.

Neidert and Saschenbrecker (1996) of the Food Inspection Directorate Agriculture and Agri-Food Canada presented data as the part of a monitoring program "in support of setting Maximum Residue Limits (MRLs), to discern residue trends, to respond to international commitments, to identify potential problem areas for surveillance activities and to assess the effectiveness of control programs." The data, although modest in number overall, present a consistent profile (Table 12.8). All the samples met the residue standards for the compounds. Whether the number of samples seems sufficient, the same basis of sampling for hormone residues, as presented earlier, appears to be operative. Unfortunately, the actual residue levels (if any residue exceeded the limit of analytical detection) were not presented.

In a similar type of data collection, during 2000 to 2001 Woźniak (2002) examined the incidence of anabolic hormone residues in 5393 animals, consisting of cattle, pigs, horses, rabbits, chickens, geese, turkeys, ducks, and fish. Woźniak assayed for residues of diethylstibestrol, hexesterol, dienestrol, zeranol, trenbolone, and 19-noresterone. In addition, 632 cattle and swine were assayed for medroxyprogesterone and 1176 were assayed for natural 17-β-estradiol and testosterone. In only three heifers and two cows did serum testosterone exceed the MRL (EC: 0.5 μg per liter); two bulls and four cows had an increased content of 17-β-estradiol in their blood. A total of 11 animals of the 5393 examined (0.2%) had excessive quantities of hormone materials in their system. None of the other animals showed evidence of the presence of

Table 12.8
Number of compliant samples during monitoring for hormonal residues, 1990 to 1995.

Year	Zeranol	DES and stilbenes	Trenbolone	Melengestrol	Other anabolics
1990–1991	712	712	189	148	—
1991–1992	927	927	265	159	21
1992–1993	837	837	97	213	27
1993–1994	927	716	167	262	21
1994–1995	916	916	269	365	32

Notes: Animal samples included beef (beef and dairy cows), veal, pork (market hogs and sows), horse, and others. All samples were considered 'ok', indicating that the samples did not exceed MRLs and passed without need for further action.
Source: Neidert and Saschenbreker (1996). *EuroResidue III Residues of Veterinary Drugs in Foods. Overview of the Canadian Drug Residue Control Program,* 185–190.

hormone materials in their systems. Since 1989, the European Commission has prohibited the use of hormonal drugs for growth promotion in domestically-produced or imported meat. Theoretically, at least, no producer should use hormonal materials in the production of animals for human consumption. However, it is important to be aware that illegal and off-label uses of drugs are common. That is why studies such as that by Woźniak are of great importance. Regulatory or monitoring systems help to ensure that unwanted residues do not appear in foods of animal origin.

12.9.3 HORMONE LEVELS IN FOODS

Residue data from monitoring studies that is published in a form that can easily be retrieved and analyzed can help in the establishment of a scientific database that can be used for evaluation. Without such data, the scientific community and the public can be overwhelmed by opinion and overextrapolation of data. For example, there has been an extrapolation showing that since 1950, lifetime exposure to meat products from animals treated with hormone materials resulted in increases in breast cancers and other reproductive malignancies. The increases in those pathologies were related to hormone residues. Unfortunately, the advent of many other endocrine disrupters in the environment during the same time period was ignored. With the birth of the pesticide era, the explosion in the numbers and combinations of medicines being taken (especially by the more elderly portion of the population), increased exposure to chemicals, and the higher levels of both air and water pollution, it is too simplistic to focus on one factor as the cause of these human medical problems.

Advocates for the use of hormones in animal production claim that the levels of 'hormones' found in several common foods greatly exceed the levels at which hormones are found in beef from animals treated with hormone implants (Table 12.9, Ritchie, 1994).

Although on first inspection the data in Table 12.9 appear to be very impressive, showing no significance difference in hormonal residues in beef from ear-implanted steers versus non-implanted steers, they could be misleading. The assumption is that all steers are implanted in strict accordance with FDA clearance. Such an assumption must be considered invalid, since there are far too many reports (unfortunately not validated) that significant percentages of feedlot animals have hormone-containing pellets implanted in muscle tissue. Hence, the data from the few monitoring surveys that are available should be considered as presenting the best possible example. In the U.S., hormone pellets implanted in areas other than the ear can be a potentially serious hormonal residue problem. The extent of improper implantation of pellets is not definitively known because there is essentially no monitoring program for hormone residues and so no definition of the problem can be made because of lack of data. The report from Canada, where hormone use was legal (Neidert and Saschenbreker, 1996), and the report from Poland, where use was illegal (Woźniak, 2002), both indicated few, if any, violative samples; both reports showed minimal residue problems.

In 1988, the European Commission (EC) prohibited the use of hormones for growth promotion in animals to be used for food production. The ban also applied to imported of meat products. The result was a considerable amount of litigation, and trade disputes between North America and the European Union nations. The disputes led to tariff sanctions against the European Union nations. In 1998, the World Trade Organization (WTO) Appellate Body essentially condemned the EC for banning meat products from animals treated

Table 12.9
Estrogen content of various foods.

Food	Estrogen content (ng per 85g serving)
Soybean oil	170,000
Cabbage	2000
Wheat germ	1700
Eggs	1010
Ice cream	520
Peas	340
Potatoes	225
Milk	11
Beef implanted steers	1.9
Beef non-implanted steers	1.3

Source: Ritchie (1994). *How safe is our product – Beef? Do we have a story to tell?* www.msu.edu/~ritchieh/papers/ safebeefproduct.html

with hormonal growth promoters without undertaking a "state of the art scientific risk assessment of the risk associated with meat consumption." The WTO Appellate Body found the scientific assessment was too general and did not evaluate the risks from hormone residues in meat (European Commission, 2002). Following this decision, the EC reexamined the scientific information and agreed to remove the sanctions. It is expected that that the increased tariffs imposed by the U.S. and Canada will also be lifted (*Food Law News*, 2003).

This very unfortunate scenario reinforces the absolute need for continuous monitoring programs for residues of all types in animal products, and in particular for hormone materials used for growth promotion. There were no winners in this cautionary tale, the regulatory officials on both sides of the dispute did not monitor the situation and did not provide the proper scientific information for decision-making.

12.9.4 HORMONES IN MILK

No milk can be considered hormone free as natural hormones are always present. The question that has been under heated debate since approximately 1995 is whether the bovine somatotropin hormone (BST) injected into cows to increase milk production results in harmful levels of hormone in milk. The use of BST, which is based upon an economic return rather than any health benefit to the animal, raises two important questions; what are the health risks to the human consumer, primarily children? and what are the effects on the animals? It is fairly well accepted that the use of BST increases the incidence of mastitis and therefore the potential for increased residues of antibiotic and antimicro-bials in milk. Because of this Canada, Australia, Japan, the U.K., and other European Union countries decided that the health impact on animals was unacceptable and that BST was not to be used in their jurisdictions. Their decisions were not based upon any human health concerns, but strictly on concerns for animal health.

In the U.S., the debate is far more animated with concerns related to the possible health consequences of hormone levels in milk being higher than desirable, and to animal rights and animal health. There have been some reports, primarily by Epstein (1990a, 1990b, 1996), that state BST treatments have increased insulin growth factor-1 (IGF-1) content in milk. There have also been reports that indicate that IGF-1 is not completely broken down by digestive enzymes and that some may cross the intestinal wall into the bloodstream (e.g., Chan, 1998). Unfortunately, many of these reports extrapolate heavily from the effects of IGF-1 to the use of BST for increased milk production. Until there is substantive data on this argument, it will be necessary to accept the judgment of the FDA and the Food and Agriculture Organization/World Health Organization Joint Expert Committee on Food Additives, which find no evidence that the use of BST is a health risk.

The most recent arguments arise from the labeling of milk in the U.S. as 'hormone free.' This type of labeling has been declared as 'mislabeling' by the FDA on the ground that no milk is hormone free, which is true. Arguments on all sides of the issue will continue for the foreseeable future. However, with the excess of milk production in so many parts of the world, coupled with the increased mastitis and veterinary costs in the maintenance of treated animals and the possible increase in drug residues in the milk, use of BST seems somewhat illogical. The argument that the use of BST will make milk prices drop is incorrect, as prices have gone up, at least to consumers, in the U.S. Eventually the marketplace will dictate the success or failure of the use of BST.

12.10 REFERENCES

Chan, J.M. (1998). Plasma insulin-like growth factor 1 and prostate cancer risk: a prospective study, *Science*, 279, 563–566.

Epstein, S.S. (1990a). Questions and answers on synthetic bovine growth hormones, *Int. J. Heath Services*, 20, 573–582.

Epstein, S.S. (1990b). Potential public health hazards of biosynthetic milk hormones, *Int. J. Heath Services*, 20, 73–84.

Epstein, S.S. (1996). Unlabeled milk from cows treated with biosynthetic growth: a case regulatory abdication, *Int. J. Heath Services*, 26, 173–185.

European Commission (2002). *Opinion of the scientific committee on veterinary measures relating to public health on review of previous SCVPH opinions of 30 April 1999 and 3 May 2000 on the potential risks to human health from hormone residues in bovine meat and meat products* (adopted 10 April 2002).

FDA (2001). *National Milk Drug Residue Data Base*, Fiscal Year Annual Report October 1, 1999 to September 30, 2000. U.S. Food and Drug Administration, Washington D.C.

Food Law News – EU – 2003, European Commission press release IP/03/1393, 15 October 2003.

Mellon, M., Benbrook, C. and Benbrook, K.I. (2001). *Hogging It*, Union Concerned Scientist Publications, Cambridge, MA.

The Merck Veterinary Manual (1991). 7th ed., Merck and Co, Rahway.

Neidert, E. and Saschenbrecker, P.W. (1996). Overview of the Canadian Drug Residue Control Program, in *Haagsma, N. and Rviter, A., eds, Residues of Veterinary Drugs in Food. Proceedings of EuroResidue III Conference, Veldhoven, Netherlands, 6-8 May 1996, WPFC, Federation of European Chemical Societies*, pp. 185–190.

Quan, D.J. (2000). Monitoring of domestic and imported eggs for veterinary drug residues by the Canadian food inspection agency, *J. Agric. Food Chem.*, 48, 6421–6427.

Ritchie, H.D. (1994). *How safe is our product – Beef? Do we have a story to tell?* www.msu.edu/~ritchieh/papers/safebeefproduct.html

Stillman, J.M. (1920). *Paracelsus: His Personality and Influence as Physician, Chemist and Reformer*. The Open Court Publishing Company, Chicago.

Tscheuschner, I. (1972). Penicillin anaphylaxis following pork consumption. *Z. Haut. Geschlechtskr.*, 47, 591

USDA (1998). *1998 Domestic Residue Data Book*. Food Safety Inspection Service, U.S. Department of Agriculture, Washington, D.C.

USDA (2000). *2000 Domestic Residue Data Book*. Food Safety Inspection Service, U.S. Department of Agriculture, Washington, D.C.

Woźniak, B. (2002). Hormones residues control in slaughtered animals in Poland 2000–2001. *Bull. Vet. Inst. Puławy*, 46, 331–335.

Young, R. and Craig, A. (2001). *Too hard to swallow – the truth about drugs and poultry.* Soil Association, Bristol, U.K.

13

The Effect of Processing on the Nutritional Value and Toxicity of Foods

Zdzisław E. Sikorski

CONTENTS

13.1 INTRODUCTION

The preparation of food for consumption, as well as manufacturing of various products from different raw materials, usually involves the application of several discrete unit operations and processes. Many operations, such as washing, trimming, milling, leaching, disintegrating, mechanical separation, and use of membrane techniques, may decrease the natural toxicity of some raw materials by eliminating specific undesirable components. Examples include the removal of most of the fluorine compounds from Antarctic krill by peeling early after catch, or flushing pathogenic bacteria and viruses from live oysters by depuration in disinfected water. However, processing operations may also reduce the biological value of the products, by leaching or destroying essential ingredients, especially water-soluble vitamins.

Unit processes involving chemical changes may make some nutrients unavailable and decrease or increase toxicity. Different forms of wet or dry heating may reduce the concentration of pesticides and polychlorinated biphenyls (PCBs) in fatty fish by about 30 to 40% due to cooking losses. High temperature may also destroy some toxic compounds in food raw materials, such as paralytic shellfish poison in scallops, some heat labile microbial toxins, or the neurotoxic β-N-oxalyl-α,β-diaminopropionic acid found in the seeds of *Lathyrus sativus*. Thermal denaturation can also inactivate some allergens in salmon and tuna meat. Conversely, prolonged treatment at elevated temperature may lead to loss of sulfur containing amino acids and decrease the biological availability of essential nutrients by their reactions with other food components, e.g., lysine residues in proteins. It may also induce formation of harmful compounds, such as various mutagens, carcinogenic heterocyclic amines (HAs) or polycyclic aromatic hydrocarbons (PAHs). The effect depends on the temperature and time of heating, as well as on pH of the treated food material, presence of oxygen and other oxidizing agents, interactions with various food ingredients or additives, and application of chemical agents or ionizing radiation.

It is therefore apparent that when considering the different unit processes in food manufacturing and cookery, the risk and benefit concept must be observed (Miller Jones, 2002).

13.2 THE EFFECTS OF HEATING

13.2.1 Loss in Nutritive Value

Different forms of heating are applied in the food industry and in the kitchen, mainly in order to:

- remove fat, water, and volatile components
- extract sugar and lipids
- control enzyme reactions
- develop desirable sensory properties
- increase the digestibility of components
- inactivate toxins, parasites, and microorganisms

In most cases, the temperature of the inner parts of food during heating is well below 100°C (Table 13.1), even in a fish fillet that is fried in oil at 180°C. It may, however, reach about 130°C during several minutes of sterilization in canned products and be 160°C or higher in the dry surface layer of roasted or baked goods. Therefore, the extent of loss of nutritionally valuable food

Table 13.1
Temperature conditions during thermal processing of foods.

Treatment	Product	Temperature (°C) Core	Surface	Duration of treatment
Dewaxing	Vegetable oil	0–5	0–5	4–16 hours
Drying	Klipfish	20–25	20–25	6–8 days
Cold smoking	Salmon	20–30	20–30	4 hours
Hot smoking	Mild mackerel	up to 60	up to 60	3 hours
Hot smoking	Pork belly	30–80	30–80	22 hours
Pasteurization	Milk	62–65	62–65	30 minutes
	Milk	71–74	71–74	15–40 seconds
	Milk	85	85	2 seconds
Sterilization	Milk	110–120	110–120	10–20 minutes
Frying	Fish	65–80	up to 175	4–6 minutes
French fries		75–80	up to 170	2–3 minutes
Baking	Bread	93–97	up to 175	60 minutes
Deodorizing	Vegetable oil	245–260	245–260	15–45 minutes

components, such as vitamins and labile amino acids, and the formation of antinutritional compounds due to thermal changes and to chemical interactions is small in mildly heated products. It may, however, be extensive in the outer layers exposed to high temperatures. Nevertheless, in some cases, even small losses may decrease the nutritive value of foods substantially if they relate to components that are deficient in people's diets. Heat-induced changes in sterilized foods may decrease the availability of sensitive amino acids by a few percent, while severe heating, as performed in some laboratory experiments in exaggerated conditions, e.g., several hours at 130°C, by 30 to 70%.

The decrease in the biological value of proteins due to heating may, in part, be caused by the Maillard reaction, which involves a carbonyl compound and a non-ionized ε-NH_2 group of lysine residue or a terminal α-NH_2. The carbonyl group is usually that of a reducing saccharide, of a secondary product of lipid oxidation, or of a wood smoke aldehyde. As a result of a number of further reactions and rearrangements, different reactive products are created, including dicarbonyl and polycarbonyl unsaturated compounds, which also interact with amines and amino acids. Degradation of some reaction products yields various volatile compounds, which contribute to the flavor of the heated foods. Further changes and polymerization are responsible for the development of brown to black melanoidins.

A number of Maillard reaction products have been found to be mutagenic or carcinogenic (Lee and Shibamoto, 2002). Reactions of the lysine residue with other food components, including dehydroascorbic acid, result in crosslinking of the heated protein (Fayle et al., 2000).

The early products of the Maillard reaction involving the lysine residue can be nutritionally utilized in the human body. Later changes, however, make the lysine unavailable. During baking, lysine is mainly affected in the outer parts, e.g., crust of bread or rolls, exposed to high temperature, while in the body of the products the extents of the reactions are negligible. Such comparatively low loss of nutritional value can be regarded as compensated for by higher sensory quality of the product due to the desirable color and flavor. In roller-dried skimmed milk, however, the loss may reach 20 to 30%. The lysine availability of different liquid and powdered commercial enteral proteinaceous food formulations is about 75% of the total content of this essential amino acid (Castillo et al., 2002).

The extent of heat-induced changes in protein-rich foods can be measured by determining some early Maillard reaction products (O'Brien and Morrissey, 1989). Acid treatment of protein-bound or free N^ε-fructoselysine liberates lysine, with a yield of 50%, and two other amino acids, furosine (20%) and pyridosine (10%) (Figure 13.1). The three products that result from hydrolysis of N^ε-lactuloselysine are formed in the proportions of approximately 5:3 to 4:1 to 2, however the yield of different derivatives is variable. Therefore, in order to use these unique amino acids as indicators of changes in lysine content, the hydrolysis should be carried out in strictly-defined conditions. Furosine is present in various food products in a very wide range of concentrations (Table 13.2).

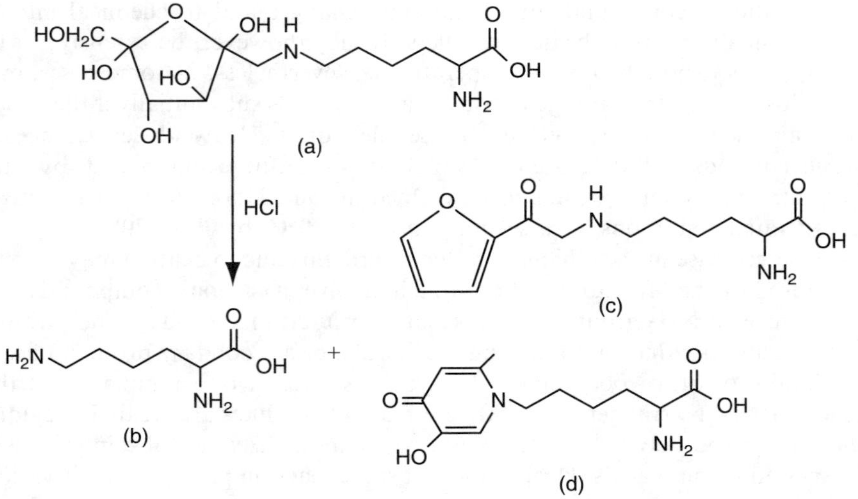

Figure 13.1 Acid treatment of N^ε-fructoselysine (a), liberates lysine (b) and two modified amino acids, furosine (c) and pyridosine (d).

In several foods, especially in dairy and meat products, N^ε-carboxymethyl-lysine (Figure 13.2) has also been found. Its content in meat homogenate (without additions) after heating for one hour at 100°C was about 17 μg per g

Table 13.2
Content of furosine in different food products.

Food	Furosine (µg/g protein)	Reference
Carrot		
raw	1	Kuncewicz et al., 2000
cooked	116	Kuncewicz et al., 2000
Potato, raw	7	Kuncewicz et al., 2000
Milk		
raw	35–55	Belitz et al., 2001
pasteurized	48–75	Belitz et al., 2001
	69–314	Villamiel et al., 1999
UHT	500–1800	Belitz et al., 2001
sterilized	5000–12000	Belitz et al., 2001
Egg		
raw	127	Kuncewicz et al., 2000
cooked	1400	Kuncewicz et al., 2000
Meat homogenate, raw	210	Hartkopf and Erbersdobler, 1995
Meat homogenate, 100°C, 1h		
without additives	600	Hartkopf and Erbersdobler, 1995
with glucose	1810	Hartkopf and Erbersdobler, 1995
with ascorbate	480	Hartkopf and Erbersdobler, 1995
Rice-corn-soy infant cereal		
raw	230	Guerra-Hernandez et al., 1999
roller-dried	8200	Guerra-Hernandez et al., 1999
Enteral formulae, sterilized	3840–4150	Rufian-Henares et al., 2002

protein, with added glucose or ascorbate it was 23 and 35 µg per g protein, respectively. N^ε-carboxymethyllysine can also be used as an indicator of lysine changes in formulated foods that have resulted from prolonged heating (Hartkopf and Erbersdobler, 1995). Pyrraline, another product of lysine modification (Figure 13.3), has been found in UHT milk, sterilized milk, and in the crust of white bread in concentrations of 2 to 5, 60 to 80, and 540 to 3680 µg per g protein, respectively (Belitz, Grosch and Schieberle, 2001).

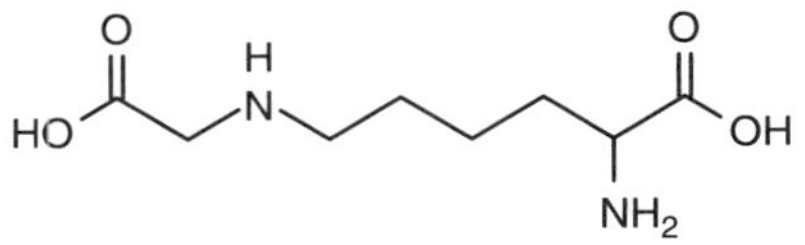

Figure 13.2 Structure of N^ε-carboxymethyllysine.

Maillard products are not only formed during cooking and other heat processing of foods, but also accumulate in some products that are rich in proteins and reducing sugars, e.g. condensed milk during months of storage at

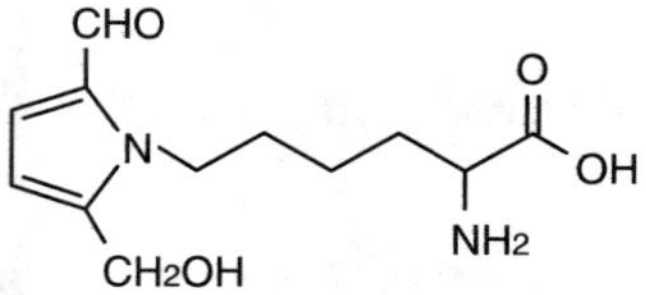

FIGURE 13.3 Structure of pyrraline.

ambient temperature. Although the rate of reaction is much slower, the content of available lysine may drop by several percent after prolonged storage.

Heating applied in pasteurization and sterilization may inactivate thermolabile milk immunoglobulins, which resist the treatment at 62.5°C for 60 minutes, but are inactivated above 75°C. It is therefore necessary to find protecting agents that will inhibit thermal inactivation of antibodies, which are added to infant formulae to act against specific enteropathogenic and enterotoxigenic *Escherichia coli* and other pathogenic microorganisms (Chen et al., 2000).

Denaturation of hemoproteins in cooked meats leads to liberation of the heme and oxidation of the porphyrin ring. Nonheme iron is less available nutritionally than heme iron and affects lipid oxidation more. In methemoglobin and metmyoglobin solutions heated for one hour at 78°C and 100°C the degradation of heme was about 22 to 26%, while after two hours at 120°C it increased to about 85 to 95% (Oellingrath, 1988). In meat cookery, however, such severe conditions do not apply.

Heating of foods rich in proteins may lead to formation of crosslinking isopeptide bonds between the ε-NH$_2$ group of lysine and the β- and γ-carboxyl groups of aspartic and glutamic acid residues or their amides.

13.2.2 UNNATURAL AMINO ACIDS AND PROTEIN CROSSLINKS

Hot NaOH solutions may be used for the extraction of proteins from different sources, e.g., oilseeds, grains, or bones from meat carcasses and poultry, the inactivation of mycotoxins and protein inhibitors, removal of nucleic acids from single-cell biomass, peeling of fruits and vegetables, and for other technological purposes. This treatment can, however, result in undesirable effects. Heating of protein-containing foods above 50°C at high pH causes the generation of unnatural amino-acid residues, racemization, and protein crosslinking.

The first reaction is β-elimination in cysteine, serine, phosphoserine, and threonine residues due to attack by hydroxide ion, leading to the formation of very reactive dehydroalanine (DHA). In a cystine residue, this results in rupturing of the disulfide bond and liberation of a sulfide ion and free sulfur (Figure 13.4). Nucleophilic additions of the ε-amino group of the protein-bound lysine to the double bond of DHA residue causes crosslinking of the polypeptide chain. After hydrolysis, a mixture of L-lysino-L-alanine and L-lysino-D-alanine, with probably a small proportion of DL and DD isomers,

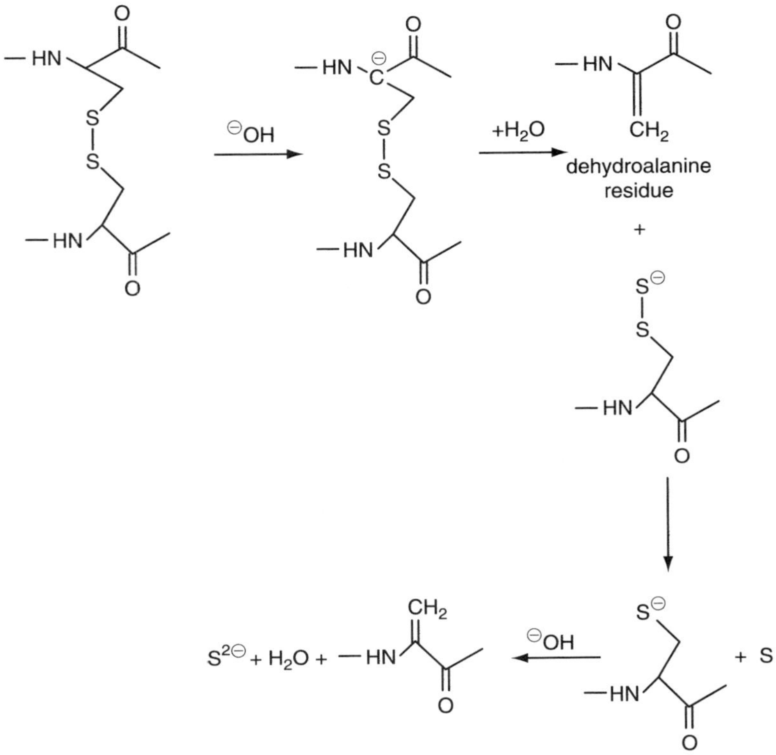

FIGURE **13.4** Formation of dehydroalanine.

appear (Figure 13.5). The concentration of lysinoalanine (LAL) in different food products depends on the pH as well as on the time and temperature of heating. Other reactions between amino-acid residues and DHA yield ornithinoalanine, lanthionine, and methyllanthionine. The products of reaction with ammonia and with phenylethylamine are diaminopropanoic acid and 3-(N-phenylethylamino)-alanine, respectively (Tucker et al., 1983). At a given temperature, the rate of formation of the modified amino-acid residues depends on the rate of β-elimination and on the accessibility of the DHA residue for the nucleophilic attack, which is related to the conformation of the protein. Therefore, various proteins differ in sensitivity to changes caused by heating at alkaline pH.

Due to recombination of the carboanion (see Figure 13.4) with a proton, both enantiomeres L and D of the amino acids can be formed. The rate of racemization depends on the properties of the amino-acid residues and of the proteins. It is generally about ten times higher in amino-acid residues in proteins than in free amino acids.

Prolonged heating of protein-rich foods in alkaline conditions may decrease the nutritional availability of proteins by loss of essential amino

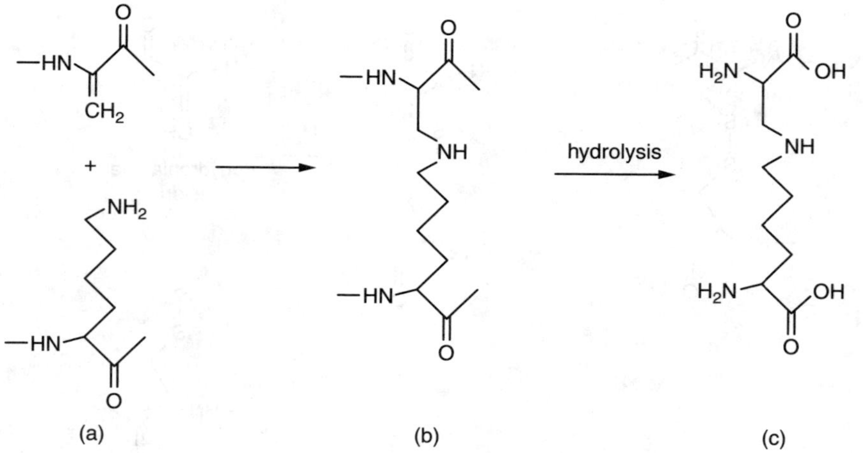

Figure 13.5 Formation of lysinoalanine: nucleophilic additions of the ε-amino group of the protein-bound lysine to the double bond of DHA residue (a) causes crosslinking of the polypeptide chain (b); lysinoalanine (c) is formed after hydrolysis.

acids, racemization, and impairing the digestibility due to crosslinking. The rate of absorption of the D-forms of essential amino acids is lower than that of the L-forms. LAL is known to chelate Cu^{2+}, Co^{2+}, and Zn^{2+}, inactivate metalloenzymes, and induce nephrocytomegaly in rats (Pearce and Friedman, 1988; Friedman and Pearce, 1989). Kidney damage may be caused also by other products generated due to the heating of proteins in alkaline conditions; diaminopropanoic acid and D-serine (Pearce and Friedman, 1988).

Cooking of food causes partial loss of thiamine, depending on the pH of the environment, as well as the temperature and duration of heating and on the presence of various reactive compounds. Thiamine is stable in acid foods, but decomposes readily at alkaline pH (Figure 13.6). The average loss of thiamine that occurs due to boiling of eggs is about 15%, baking of bread 15 to 20%, and cooking of vegetables 25 to 40%. In different cooked, canned, roasted, and fried meat and fish products, thiamine loss ranges from about 15 to 75%. Thiamine and its decomposition products may participate in the Maillard reaction.

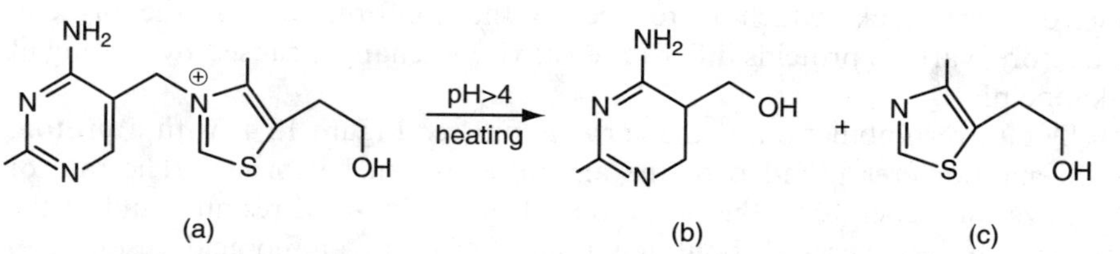

Figure 13.6 Degradation of thiamine (a) on heating in alkaline conditions, resulting in formation of (b) 2-methyl-4-amine-5-hydroxymethylpyrimidine and (c) 5-(2-hydroxy-ethyl)-4-methylthiazole.

13.2.3 MUTAGENIC AND CARCINOGENIC HETEROCYCLIC AMINES

Heating as applied in the canning industry and other commercial processes, as well as in culinary preparation of foods, may lead to formation of very small amounts of mutagens and, possibly, carcinogens. The mutagenicity of different canned meats and seafood may be several times higher than that of the raw material. There is, however, large variation in the mutagenicity, which may be due to differences in the natural composition of the foods, preliminary treatments that influence the concentration of different precursors of reactions involved in formation of mutagens, and temperature and duration of heating (Krone et al., 1986; Bartoszek, 2002; Jägerstad et al., 1998).

Presently about 20 different mutagenic and/or carcinogenic heterocyclic amines (HAs) have been isolated from various heat-processed foods. One class of these HAs is formed by pyrolysis of proteins or some amino acids. These HAs are amino-carbolines (Figure 13.7), and have been identified in grilled, broiled, baked, and fried meat and fish products, in meat sauces and bouillons, as well as in pyrolyzed proteins, glutamate, lysine, phenylalanine, tryptophan, ornithine, and creatine.

Carbolines are formed in model systems heated for several minutes to several hours in the temperature range 100 to about 225°C. Some of the carbolines are known to display mutagenic activity, however, they are usually weak carcinogens (Friedman and Cuq, 1988; Bartoszek, 2002).

The second group of mutagenic and carcinogenic HAs comprises compounds that are formed at lower temperature and have been found in cooked meat and fish dishes, gravies, pan residues, broiled and fried beef, and

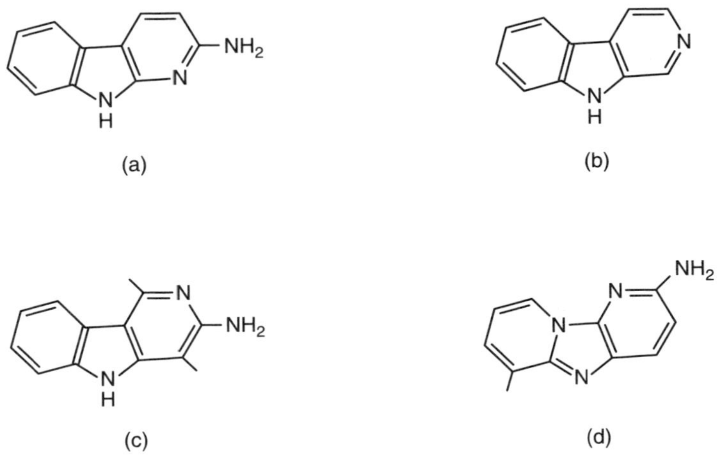

FIGURE 13.7 Mutagenic and carcinogenic heterocyclic amines of the carboline group; (a) AαC (2-amino-9H-pyrido[2,3,-b]indole), (b) norharman (9H-pyrido[4,3-b]indole), (c) Trp-P-1 (3-amino-1,4-dimethyl-5H-pyrido[4,3-b]indole), (d) Glu-P-1 (2-amino-6-methyl-dipyrido[1,2-a:3′,2′-d]imidazole).

in model systems in heated mixtures of amino acids, saccharides and creatine. They are derivatives of quinolines, quinoxalines, and pyridines (Figure 13.8). There is evidence that these compounds are formed from creatine and the products of the Maillard reaction. These HAs belong to the strongest mutagenic components of heated foods; some of them are carcinogenic in rodents. The published results of experiments seem to indicate that people who very frequently eat 'well-done' fried and roasted meats may be exposed to cancer risk from HAs.

The yield of HAs in food systems is affected by the concentration of substrates, enhancers and inhibitors, duration and temperature of heating, water activity, and pH. Some HAs are formed in mixtures of substrates heated for several weeks at relatively low temperature, about 37 to 60°C; at 150 to 200°C the rate of reaction is much higher. However, in model systems prolonged heating may also bring about a decrease of the concentration of some HAs. Low water activity in the surface layers of the heated products favors the formation of HAs. In presence of lipids, Fe^{2+}, and Fe^{3+}, the rate of reaction increases, probably due to oxidation and generation of radicals (Jägerstad et al., 2000).

The total contents of HAs in broiled, fried, and grilled protein-rich products is generally of the order of several ng per g wet weight (Bartoszek, 2002; Belitz et al., 2001; Gangolli, 1986). In fried fish fiber (a popular oriental commodity prepared by frying cooked, pressed, and shredded fish meat with

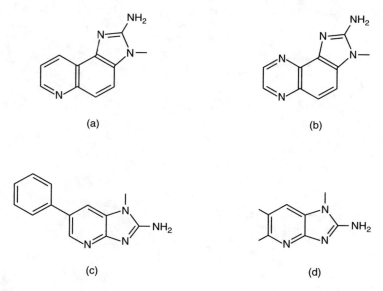

(a)   (b)

(c)   (d)

FIGURE 13.8 Mutagenic and carcinogenic heterocyclic amines; (a) IQ (2-amino-3-methylimidazo[4,5-*f*] quinoline), (b) IQx (2-amino-3-methylimidazo[4,5-*f*] quinoxaline), (c) PhIP, (2-amino-1-methyl-6-phenylimidazo[4,5-*b*] pyridine), (d) 1,5,6–TMIP (2-amino-1,5,6-trimethylimidazo[4,5-*b*] pyridine).

salt, sugar, soy sauce, monosodium glutamate, soybean flour, and antioxidants in oil at 120°C for 65 minutes), the total content of four different HAs ranged from about 1 to 85 ng per g, depending on the kind and quantity of added ingredients (Tai et al., 2001).

13.2.4 ACRYLAMIDE IN HEAT PROCESSED FOOD

Acrylamide (ACA) (Figure 13.9) is generated primarily in fried, grilled, and baked products at temperatures above 120°C. Its content can vary due to the composition of the food and the cooking conditions; the highest concentrations occur in potato chips, French fries, bread, and processed cereals. It has also been found in microwaved grated potato, fried beetroot, and fried spinach. In beef and chicken heated at high temperature, only low amounts of ACA have been detected. By using available analytical techniques, the detection limit of ACA in foods can be 10 ng per g (FAO/WHO 2002).

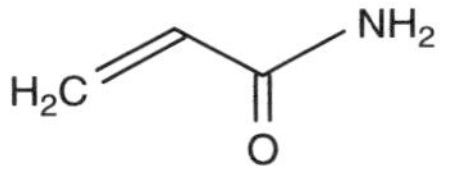

FIGURE 13.9 Structure of acrylamide.

The mechanisms of ACA formation in foods and its precursors are not known yet, although it is clear that the product yield increases with the duration and temperature of heating (Table 13.3). It has been suggested that ACA may be formed directly from amino acids, from lactic acid in dehydration and decarboxylation reactions, or from acrolein or acrylic acid, which might be derived from lipids, saccharides, or amino acids. Maillard-type reaction between glucose and asparagine may also be involved. ACA is a very reactive compound that interacts with the thiol group of cysteine, and, at a lower rate, with amino and hydroxyl groups of different food constituents. As a volatile and reactive substance, it can be partially lost after formation. The observed low concentrations of ACA in protein-rich foods may be due to volatilization, or to further interactions with other food components.

Since the mechanism of formation of ACA is not known, it is not yet possible to optimize conditions of formulation, processing, and cooking of food that would minimize the generation of this compound. However, it is known that the yield of ACA in fried and roasted potatoes increases with the content of fructose and glucose in the product. Therefore, it has been proposed that potatoes used for roasting and frying should contain less than 1 g per kg of reducing saccharides. By extracting the reducing sugars and asparagine from the surface of the cut potato in a water bath or spray, pre-frying at 140°C for 2.5 min, and frying at about 170°C, French fries with 40 to 70 ng per g ACA can be produced (Grob et al., 2003). German food processors have agreed to cook French fries at oil temperature not higher than 175°C.

Table 13.3
Acrylamide content in various foods.

Product	Acrylamide (ng/g)	Number of samples
Chips, potato	< 50–3500	39
Biscuits, crackers, toast, bread crisps	< 30–3200	58
Crisps, potato/sweet potato/corn	34–2287	45
Breakfast cereals	< 30–1346	29
Bakery products	< 50–450	19
Coffee powder	170–230	3
Chocolate powder	< 50–100	2
Instant malt drinks	< 50–70	3
Poultry, game, fish and seafood products, crumbed, battered	30–64	6

Source: data from FAO/WHO. *Health implications of acrylamide in food, Report of a joint FAO/WHO consultation*, Geneva, 25–27 June 2002.

ACA has been classified by the International Agency for Research on Cancer as "probably carcinogenic to humans." It has a carcinogenic potency in rats similar to that of other carcinogens in food. Furthermore, ACA has neurotoxic activity and may induce heritable damage.

13.3 HEALTH IMPAIRING OXIDATION PRODUCTS

13.3.1 Oxidized Lipids

Lipids are the food components that are most prone to oxidation. In food systems, oxidation of lipids starts as autoxidation, photooxidation, or lipoxygenase-catalyzed reactions, depending on the properties of the product and conditions of storage or processing (Kołakowska, 2002). The factors that affect the rate of oxidation of lipids in foods are high temperature, light, and the presence of oxygen and prooxidants. Polyenoic fatty acids oxidize at a very much higher rate than monoenoic fatty acids. Natural and added antioxidants, acting through various mechanisms, decrease the rate of reaction.

Cholesterol, present in animal fats, and phytosterols, the minor components of the unsaponifiable fraction of plant oils, turn into oxysterols in conditions known to promote the oxidation of fatty acids. A range of cholesterol oxidation products has been found in foods, mainly 7α- and 7-β-hydroxycholesterols, cholesterol-α- and -β-epoxides, cholestanetriol, 7-keto-cholesterol (Figure 13.10a), 20-α-hydroxycholesterol (Figure 13.10b), and 25-hydroxycholesterol. The total content of oxysterols ranges from trace amounts in fresh eggs, milk, and meat, through to several μg per g in fresh infant formulae, up to about 30 μg per g in sausages and powdered milk, and to

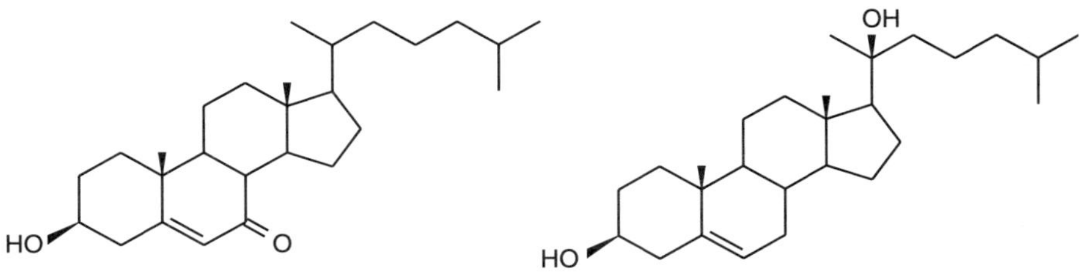

(a)   (b)

FIGURE 13.10 Examples of oxysterols; (a) 7-ketocholesterol, (b) 20-α-hydroxycholesterol.

as much as 200 µg per g in whole dried-egg powder. After storage in the dark at 4°C, the total content of oxysterols in liver pate type sausages increased from the initial value 12 µg per g of product to about 23 µg per g, while the concentration of cholesterol decreased by about 38 µg per g (Zaborowska et al., 2001).

The health impairing and toxic effects of oxidation of lipids are due to loss of vitamins, polyenoic fatty acids, and other nutritionally essential components; formation of radicals, hydroperoxides, aldehydes, epoxides, dimers, and polymers; and participation of the secondary products in initiation of oxidation of proteins and in the Maillard reaction. Different oxysterols have been shown *in vitro* and *in vivo* to have atherogenic, mutagenic, carcinogenic, angiotoxic, and cytotoxic properties, as well as the ability to inhibit cholesterol synthesis (Tai et al., 1999; Wąsowicz, 2002).

13.3.2 PROTEIN OXIDATION PRODUCTS

Oxidative changes also contribute to the loss of sensory and nutritional quality of protein-rich foods. During processing and prolonged frozen storage, the food proteins may be oxidized due to the activity of singlet oxygen ($^1O_2$), superoxide anion radical ($O_2^{-\cdot}$), and hydoxyl radical ($\cdot OH$). These reactive oxygen species are formed by enzymatic processes and catalytic action of cations, light, and ionizing radiation. Lipid radicals and lipid oxidation products also have an important impact. In some foods, the residues from H_2O_2 used in processing may oxidize the proteins. Polyphenols are readily oxidized to quinones by oxygen at neutral and alkaline pH. The quinones act as strong oxidizing agents in different products. The rate of change in proteins is controlled by the activity of the oxidizing agents and inhibitors, the presence of sensitizers, e.g., chlorophyll, methylene blue, erythrosine, and riboflavin, different prooxidants and antioxidants, temperature, and the sensitivity of various amino-acid residues. Abstraction of a hydrogen atom on the α-carbon, or in the amino acid side chain of a protein, generates radicals. These radicals may react with other protein or lipid radicals to yield polymers, or may undergo scission to various low-molecular products. The sulfur containing

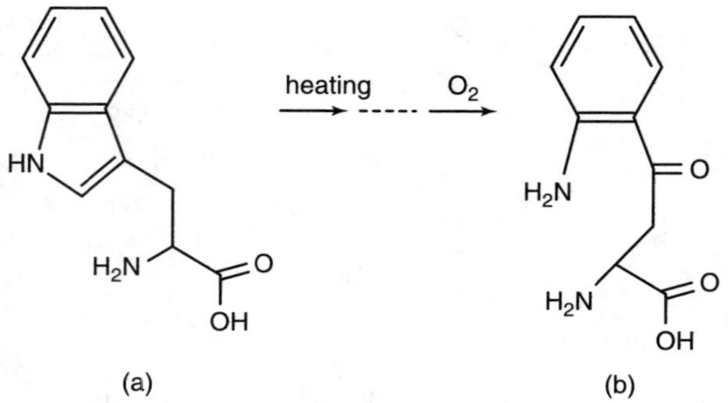

FIGURE 13.11 Oxidation of tryptophan (a) to kynurenine (b).

amino acids may be converted to cysteine sulfenic, sulfinic, and sulfonic acids, mono- and disulfoxides, and mono- and disulfones.

Other sensitive amino acids may also be oxidized, primarily histidine and tryptophan, yielding different products. Thermal degradation of tryptophan in the presence of oxygen leads in several steps to the formation of kynurenine (Figure 13.11). Moderate heating in the presence of air, as would occur during food processing, however, does not cause severe loss of tryptophan in protein-rich foods – from about 5 to 20%, depending on the product and the parameters of heat treatment (Friedman and Cuq, 1988). Oxidation may result in substantial loss in the nutritive value of proteins due to the unavailability of the oxidized amino acid, as well as decreased digestion of the protein hampered by stable crosslinking.

13.4   UNDESIRABLE EFFECTS OF CHEMICAL PROCESSING OF FATS

Chemical processes are used in industry to remove undesirable components of oils and modify their functional properties. Besides triacylglycerols (TAGs), unrefined vegetable oil also contains small quantities of other components that affect its sensory properties and stability. These constituents are removed during refining – the phosphatides by hydration and separation, free fatty acids by alkali refining or steam stripping, color bodies and decomposition products of peroxides by bleaching on mineral adsorbents, flavor and odor compounds by deodorizing in a high-temperature-steam distillation process, and waxy materials by chilling followed by filtration. Hydrogenation of double bonds in the fatty acid residues by using hydrogen gas in the presence of nickel catalysts, and chemical or enzymatic interesterification, are applied to modify the fatty acid composition of the TAGs (Chu and Hwang, 2002).

Refined, bleached, and deodorized oils may contain some nutritionally objectionable compounds – secondary oxidation products, di- and tri-enoic fatty acids containing conjugated double bonds, and fatty-acid polymers. Deodorization at 230°C in the presence of even minute amounts of oxygen leads to oxidation of the polyenoic fatty acids.

The aim of hydrogenation is selective saturation of a number of double bonds in the fatty-acid residues in order to increase the melting temperature of the TAGs, and thus turn the liquid oil into solid fat. However, hydrogenation destroys the essential polyenoic fatty acids (Figure 13.12). Furthermore, other undesirable side-effects may also appear – positional and geometric isomerization, as well as redistribution of the fatty-acid residues in TAGs. In natural rapeseed and soybean oil the TAGs contain about eight to twelve different fatty acids, while there are partially hydrogenated fats in over 100 saturated fatty acids and positional and geometric isomers of monoenoic fatty acids, including many *trans* fatty acids (Figure 13.13). In hydrogenated rapeseed oil, the positional isomerization applies to as much as 95% of all unsaturated fatty acids, and about 65% of the $C_{18:1}$ residues have the *trans* configuration.

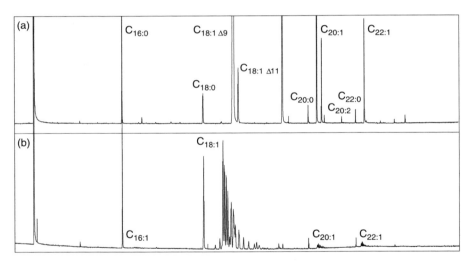

FIGURE 13.12 Fatty acid composition of rapeseed oil, (a) before and (b) after industrial partial hydrogenation. (Courtesy of A. Stołyhwo, Transfatty acids in the human diet and the human body. Paper presented at the First International Conference on Advanced Analysis – Exploring Biological Systems in Food. Olsztyn, September 6, 2003.)

Some of the unsaturated fats ingested by ruminants are partially hydrogenated by bacteria in the rumen. In consequence, milk fat, dairy products, as well as beef and mutton fat, also contain small amounts of *trans* isomers, about 2 to 9%. However, in fat from ruminants the main *trans* fatty acid is vaccenic (18:1 *t* 11), while in hydrogenated fats it is elaidic (18:1 *t* 9) (Figure 13.14).

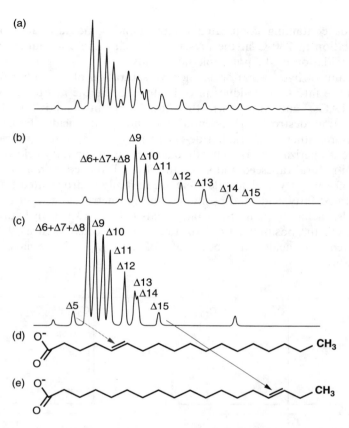

Figure 13.13 Fatty acid isomers in partially hydrogenated rapeseed oil; (a) all fatty acids, (b) C18:1 *cis* fatty acids, (c) C18:1 *trans* fatty acids, (d) structure of C18:1 Δ 5 *trans* fatty acid, and (e) structure of C18:1 Δ15 *trans* fatty acid. (Courtesy of A. Stołyhwo.)

The *trans* isomers are regarded as nutritionally undesirable. It is still not known precisely how the individual positional and geometric isomers of fatty acids are deposited or metabolized in the human body or what their health effects are (Figure 13.15). The results of metabolic investigations have shown that the *trans* fatty acids increase the concentration of low-density lipoprotein (LDL) cholesterol and decrease that of high-density lipoprotein (HDL) cholesterol in human blood, even twice as much as the saturated fatty acids. It has also been found that they increase the risk of coronary heart disease (Ascheiro et al.; Institute of Food Science and Technology, 1999). Results of model studies indicate that a diet low in Mg^{2+} and rich in *trans* fatty acids increases the risk of calcification of the endothelial cells. A further effect of partial hydrogenation is the appearance of a large number of unnatural TAGs,

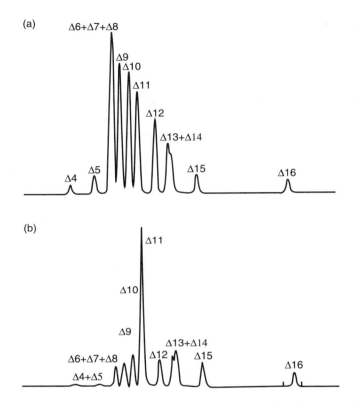

FIGURE 13.14 *Trans* isomers of C18:1 fatty acids of (a) partially hydrogenated rapeseed oil and (b) milk fat. (Courtesy of A. Stołyhwo.)

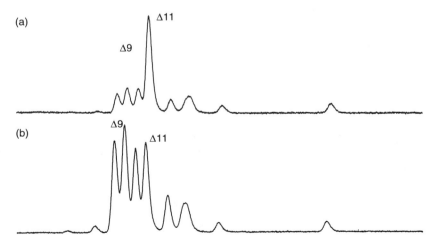

FIGURE 13.15 The effect of diet on the C18:1 *trans* fatty acids in the lipids of human milk; (a) diet rich in cows' milk fat, (b) diet rich in hydrogenated vegetable oil. (Courtesy of A. Stołyhwo.)

containing different saturated, *cis*-monoenoic, and *trans*-monoenoic fatty-acid residues. Some of these TAGs have melting temperatures as high as 55 to 58°C and are difficult to hydrolyze in the human alimentary tract.

13.5 TOXIC COMPOUNDS IN SMOKED FOODS

13.5.1 WOOD SMOKE AS A SOURCE OF CARCINOGENS

The possible health hazards associated with the smoking of food are caused by carcinogenic compounds from wood smoke that are found in smoked meats, fish, and cheese. These compounds include PAHs, *N*-nitroso-compounds (NNCs), and HAs.

Wood smoke contains PAHs with a wide range of molecular weights (mol wt), from indene (mol wt 116), to dibenzpyrenes (mol wt 302). Potthast (1979) isolated 61 different PAHs from wood smoke and presented positive identifications for 30 of them. According to Tilgner and Miler (1963), PAHs are not formed if the temperature of wood pyrolysis in a two-stage smoke generator does not exceed 425°C and the temperature of oxidation of the thermal decomposition products is below 375°C. Lowering the temperature of smoke formation to 300 or 400°C by using a smoldering-type generator, coupled with the use of filters, the PAH content of smoke can be decreased about ten-fold.

Several PAHs are mutagenic or carcinogenic. Among the PAHs found in smoke the following have the highest carcinogenic activity (Tóth and Potthast, 1984):

- 7,12-dimethylbenz[*a*]anthracene
- 3-methylcholanthrene
- benzo[*a*]pyrene
- dibenz[*ah*]anthracene
- dibenzo[*ai*]pyrene
- benzo[*c*]phenanthrene

The low-molecular weight hydrocarbons (mol wt < 216) are regarded as non-carcinogenic, unlike many heavy PAHs. Furthermore, the degree of carcinogenic activity depends on the structure of the compound. The maximum limits for PAH concentration in air and water samples, therefore, have been established for individual PAHs. Benzo[*a*]pyrene (BaP, Figure 13.16) is

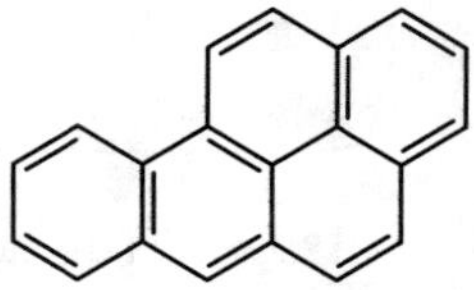

FIGURE 13.16 Benzo[*a*]pyrene.

regarded as an indicator of carcinogenic PAHs in wood smoke and smoked products. In many investigations on PAHs in smoked foods the following compounds are also determined:

- fluoranthene
- pyrene
- benzo[*b*]fluorene
- 3,6-dimethylphenanthrene
- benz[*a*]anthracene
- perylene
- dibenz[*ac*]anthracene
- dibenz[*ah*]anthracene
- picene
- indeno[1,2,3-*c*,*d*]pyrene
- anthanthrene
- 9,10-diphenylanthracene
- dibenzo[*ae*]pyrene
- dibenzo[*ai*]pyrene
- dibenzo[*ah*]pyrene
- dibenzo[*al*]pyrene
- chrysene
- benzo[*a*]fluoranthene
- benzo[*k*]fluoranthene

13.5.2 POLYCYCLIC AROMATIC HYDROCARBONS IN SMOKED MEATS

The PAHs isolated from smoked products are mainly compounds with mol wt less than 216. In smoked meat products, their total mass may be about 30 to 250 times larger than that of BaP, while that of the heavy PAHs about 10 times larger. According to German regulations, which have been in force since 1973, and the Slovakian directive from 1996, the content of BaP in smoked meat products should not exceed 1 ng per g. However, for meat products treated with smoke preparations, the European Union has set an upper limit of 0.03 ng per g (Hartmann, 2000; Simko, 2002). In Germany in the years 1962 to 1991, about 71% of samples of meat products sent by consumers (who suspected the BaP content being too high) for analysis, values did not exceed the limit set for smoked meats. However, in about 1.5% of the investigated samples, high levels of BaP, even as much as 40 ng per g, were found (Potthast, 1992).

The range of concentration of BaP in different smoked meat products, including ham, bacon, frankfurters, salami, and mutton, has been reviewed recently by Simko (2002) and found to be 0.4 to 56.5 ng per g. The lowest content of BaP, in smoked ham has been given by Potthast (1978) as 0.01 ng per g. According to various published data, the contents of BaP in hot-smoked sausages is usually below 1 ng per g and in different sausages smoked according to traditional methods 1.3 to 1.5 ng per g (Obiedziński and Olkiewicz, 1982). However, in some black smoked products it may reach

55 ng per g in the surface layer (Tóth, 1982). In flame-grilled sausages, BaP was found in concentrations of 18 to 42 ng per g. The contents of BaP in barbecued pork and beef may be in the range 1.5 to 10.5 ng per g, and in charcoal-broiled steaks, 5 to 8 ng per g. Samples of Icelandic smoke-cured mutton contained BaP levels from 0.1 to 5.6 ng per g (Dennis et al., 1984).

13.5.3 Polycyclic Aromatic Hydrocarbons in Fishery Products

13.5.3.1 Fresh Fish and Marine Invertebrates

Seafood may naturally contain small amounts of various PAHs, absorbed from the sea water. The aquatic environment is contaminated with PAHs due to oil spills, incomplete combustion of fossil fuels, industrial and urban effluents, extraction from creosoted wharfs and pilings, as well as from biosynthesis by plants and marine microorganisms.

The natural background level of PAHs is generally lower in the muscles of fish than in fish livers or in mollusks. This is because fish, unlike bivalve mollusks, have been reported to excrete PAHs rapidly, in the form of water-soluble metabolites. The content of BaP in mollusks is generally less than 10 ng per g wet weight; however, in samples taken from creosote polluted areas, as much as 215 ng per g was found. Seventeen PAHs were isolated from oysters taken from a gulf contaminated with petroleum hydrocarbons. The total average PAH content in 57 samples was about 90 ng per g wet weight, while the contents of carcinogenic PAHs were 19 ng per g, and BaP, 0.8 ng per g (Iosifidou et al., 1982).

In the edible parts of crabs, lobsters, prawns, and shrimps, the content of BaP is either not detectable or does not exceed a few ng per g. However, lobsters taken from a commercial storage facility made of creosoted timber have been found to contain levels of BaP up to 280 and 2300 ng per g in the tail meat and in the digestive gland, respectively (Dunn and Fee, 1979). In the meat of fish from unpolluted seas, BaP is generally below the detectable level (Rainio et al., 1986).

Zabik et al. (1996) determined 26 different PAHs in the flesh of raw trout from Lakes Michigan and Superior. The total concentration of 15 PAHs found in the samples ranged from 1.2 to 2.2 ng per g in lean fish to 5.2 to 7.6 ng per g in fat trout.

13.5.3.2 Smoked Fish

Smoked fish contains much more BaP than fresh – about 0.05 to 60 ng per g of product. The BaP levels in smoked fish depend on the contamination and composition of the raw material, parameters of smoking, quality of smoke, and protection of the edible parts by the skin (Petrun and Rubenchik, 1966; Tilgner and Daun, 1969; Wierzchowski and Gajewska, 1972; Steinig and Meyer, 1976; Steinig, 1976; Lawrence and Weber, 1984; Nistor, 1985).

The surface layers of fish, which are exposed to the smoke – especially the skin of eel, may contain up to five times more BaP than the main body of the product (Steinig, 1976). Smoke-dried bonito, a typical Japanese food (katsuobushi), is produced by repeated cycles (up to nine) of smoking for several hours at 80 to 120°C followed by overnight drying. The layer of tar that forms on such products makes up about 3% of the total fish weight. The meat under the surface contains about 10 ng BaP per g, while the tar fraction 20 to 40 times more (Kikugawa et al., 1986).

In the edible parts of fish smoked in a modern, automatic kiln with external smoke generation, the content of BaP is about 0.1 ng per g, while in products from traditional smoking ovens it is up to several ng per g (Table 13.4). The critical factors are the temperature of smoke generation, the density of smoke, and the duration of smoking. Suggestions that electrostatic smoking "may become a method which significantly reduces or completely controls the development of BaP in fish products" (Petrun and Rubenchik, 1966) are not substantiated, since in the experiments of the cited authors the very low levels of BaP in electrostatically smoked kilka (*Cluponella delicatula*), 0.1 to 1.7 ng per g, was not caused by electrostatic smoke deposition, but rather by using smoke generated at 275 to 300°C.

Table 13.4
The content of benzo[a]pyrene in fish, hot-smoked in traditional kiln or smokehouse with external smoke generator.

Smoked fish	Benzo[a]pyrene (ng/g wet weight of product)	
	Traditional kiln	**Smokehouse**
Eel		
Muscle	2.6–3.3[a]	0.3–0.5[a]
Muscle	0.3–3.9[b]	n.d.–0.1[b]
Skin	49–74[a]	1.8–4.0[a]
Mackerel		
Muscle	0.5–2.4[a]	0.5–0.9[a]
Muscle	0.5–2.4[b]	0.2–2.0[b]
Skin	19–30[a]	1.3–2.4[a]
Dogfish, skinned	2.6–3.7[a]	1.1[a]
Halibut, muscle	1.5–3.7[a]	0.6–0.8[a]
Bückling		
Muscle	0.5–1.4[a]	0.3[b]
Skin	22–43[a]	
Sprat		
Muscle	1.1–2.4[a]	1.6–6.8[b]
Skin	9–28[a]	

Note: n.d. = not detectable.
Sources: [a]Steinig (1976), *Lebensm.-Wiss. U. Technol.*, 9, 215–217; [b]Karl and Leinemann (1996), *Z. Lebensm. Unters. Forsch.*, 202, 458–464.

Oil sardines, smoked at 45 to 70°C for a total of six hours in a traditional kiln, in smoke generated at 400 to 600°C, contained BaP levels of about 12 ng per g wet weight. In comparison, the BaP content of product smoked for three and a half hours at 45°C in filtered smoke generated at 300 to 400°C, and subsequently dried in the sun four to five hours was only about 1.6 ng per g (Chandrasekhar and Kaveriappa, 1985). Hot smoked trout from Lakes Michigan and Superior contained 132 to 320 ng per g of total PAH and 6.2 to 10.3 ng per g of BaP (Zabik et al., 1996).

The concentration and distribution of BaP in smoked products may change during storage due to degradation, depending on the environmental factors, and as a result of diffusion. In experiments by Simko (1991), the BaP content of smoked fish that was hung freely at 18°C with unlimited air access and daylight decreased after four days from 0.6 to 0.1 ng per g. Immediately after smoking, the BaP contents of the surface and internal layers of the fish were 10.6 and 0.0 ng per g, respectively, while after seven day's storage the levels were 1.3 and 0.1 ng per g.

13.5.4 OTHER CARCINOGENS IN SMOKED PRODUCTS

Nitropolycyclic aromatic hydrocarbons have recently been identified in various foods. In smoked sausages, 1-nitropyrene, 2-nitronaphthalene, and 2-nitro-fluorene have been found in concentrations of about 4.2, 8.4, and 19.6 ng per g, respectively; this is comparable with the levels found in roasted coffee beans (2.4, 4.0, and 30.1 ng per g).

In very heavily smoked products there may also be small amounts of HAs, usually less than 1 ng per g. The smoke-dried bonito (baikan) contains 2 to 3 ng HAs per g (Kikugawa et al., 1986). Smoke-dried mackerel, produced by smoke-drying at 80 to 140°C for two hours, repeated several times, has been found to contain 2-amino-3,8-dimethylimidazo[4,5-*f*]quinoxaline (0.8 ng per g), and a smaller quantity of 2-amino-3,4,8-trimethylimidazo[4,5-*f*]quinoxaline (Kato, Kikugawa and Hayatsu, 1986).

13.6 THE EFFECT OF OTHER CHEMICAL REACTIONS

In meat curing, nitrite is traditionally used for developing the pink, heat-stable pigment. Its other important role is the inhibition of the outgrowth of *Clostridium botulinum* spores in pasteurized products and, in some countries, in several types of smoked fish. Nitrite also serves as an antioxidant and contributes positively to the development of the flavor of cured-meat. The undesirable side-effect, however, is the reaction of nitrite with amino groups of food constituents, leading to the formation of NNCs.

Nitrites added to meat or fish products decompose easily in an acid environment, forming very reactive nitrosating agents:

$$O=N^+, \ O=N-O-N=O,$$

and

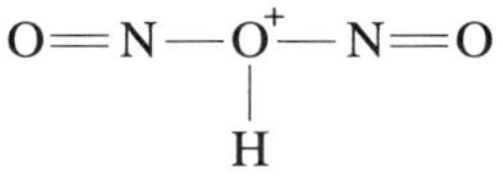

$$O{=}N{-}\overset{+}{\underset{H}{O}}{-}N{=}O$$

These compounds react with amines and amides present in foods, forming different NNCs. The rate of nitrosation of the secondary amines is about 20 times higher than that of tertiary amines and generally increases with the temperature of processing. However, NNCs are also formed, albeit at a low rate, in frozen stored products. Conversely, some decompose or volatilize during cooking or other thermal treatment. These reactions can be inhibited by additives capable of binding the nitrosating agents, e.g., ascorbate. The main NNCs present in foods are *N*-nitroso-dimethylamine, *N*-nitroso-diethylamine, *N*-nitrosopyrrolidine, and *N*-nitroso-piperidine. In smoked meat products, NNCs may be generated by reactions of the aldehydes from smoke with the constituents of meat in the presence of nitrite. Glycolaldehyde from smoke may participate in reactions leading to the formation of 2-(hydroxymethyl)-*N*-nitrosothiazolidine (Figure 13.17) and 2-(hydroxymethyl)-*N*-nitrosothiazolidine-4-carboxylic acid. Foods low in nitrates and amines usually contain NNCs at levels up to 10 ng per g, while cured and heavily smoked meat and fish products may contain up to several hundred ng per g.

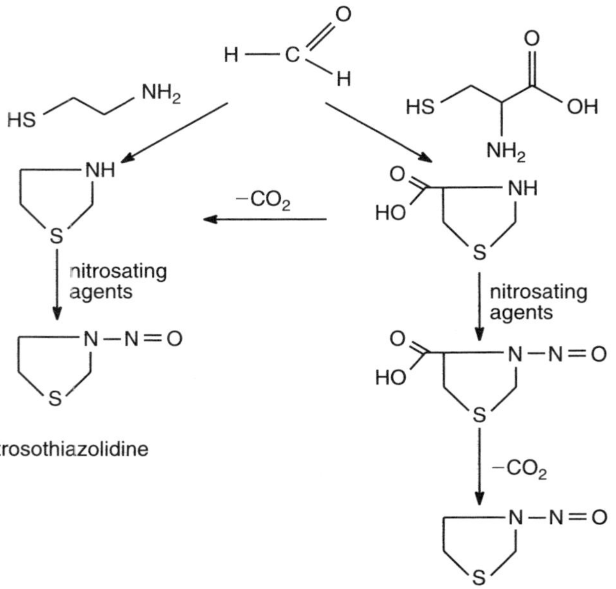

FIGURE **13.17** Formation of *N*-nitrosothiazolidine.

Of about 300 NNCs tested, some 90% have been found in animal experiments to be carcinogenic. N-nitroso-dimethylamine is among the most carcinogenic NNCs, while the activity of N-nitroso-pyrrolidine is about 100 times lower.

Chemical or enzymatic modification may be used to improve the functional properties of food proteins. This can be achieved by increasing the net negative or positive charge or by changing the hydrophobicity or the steric parameters of protein molecules and complexes. Among the modifications, predominantly made in laboratory experiments, are acylation and alkylation of amino-acid residues. Acylation generally results in decreased rate of enzymatic release of the modified amino acids. The effect increases with the size of the acylating moiety and the degree of change. The nutritional value of alkylated proteins depends on the properties of the alkylating compound and decreases with the increase of the degree of alkylation. The initial rate of enzymatic hydrolysis of the alkylated molecules is generally significantly lower than that of the unmodified proteins. However, after prolonged incubation the difference in the degree of hydrolysis is lower (Sikorski, 2002).

13.7 TOXIC RESIDUES AFTER TREATMENT WITH FUMIGANTS

Many food raw materials and products have to be treated with chemical insecticides to prevent losses due to damage caused by fly larvae, beetles, and other insects. This applies to, for example, dried fish, dried fruits, raisins, almonds, nuts, cocoa beans, and grain.

One of the fumigants used for this purpose is methyl bromide. Its residual content in the treated food material should not exceed 50 ng per g. Most of the methyl bromide escapes during subsequent aeration and storage, while part of it reacts with the food components, predominantly proteins. Roasting of fumigated almonds and cocoa beans brings about almost total elimination of free methyl bromide, partially due to increased rate of reaction with the components of the beans (Franz et al., 1992).

13.8 CONCLUDING REMARKS

Operations and processes applied in industrial processing and culinary preparation of foods may have beneficial or detrimental effects on the safety and biological value of the products. When setting the parameters for processing, the risk and benefit concept should be observed.

Generally, short-term storage and mild heating, not more severe than adequate to eliminate or destroy toxic components and develop desirable sensory properties, do not cause substantial loss of the nutritional value of foods. Prolonged treatment at high temperature, however, may bring about significant degradation of essential food components and generation of toxic compounds. The detrimental effects occur primarily in the surface layers exposed to direct flame or in contact with hot oil or metal surfaces.

It is recommended that the exposure of humans to genotoxic and carcinogenic substances should be as low as reasonably achievable. In order to reduce the concentration of various undesirable compounds in foods by rational changes in formulation, processing, and other practices, it is necessary to have a deep understanding of the mechanisms of formation of various toxygenic compounds in food systems, of their interactions with other components, and of their stability during storage.

Thanks to the great developments in analytical techniques, it is possible to detect different toxic compounds at very low concentrations, of the order of 1.0 or even 0.1 ng per g wet weight of the product. However, there is a need for interlaboratory validation of various methods applied to different products to make the results comparable, as well as for the development of simple, low-cost procedures for routine monitoring of many toxic compounds in foods.

13.9 REFERENCES

Ascheiro, A., Stampfer, M.J. and Willett W.C., Trans *fatty acids and coronary heart disease. Background and scientific review,* www.hsph.harvard.edu/reviews/transfats.pdf

Bartoszek, A. (2002). Mutagenic, carcinogenic and chemopreventive compounds in foods, in Sikorski, Z.E., ed., *Chemical and Functional Properties of Food Components,* 2nd ed., CRC Press, Boca Raton, 307–336.

Belitz, H.-D., Grosch, W. and Schieberle, P. (2001). *Lehrbuch der Lebensmittelchemie.* Fünfte, vollständig überarbeitete Auflage, Springer-Verlag, Berlin.

Biedermann-Brem, S., Noti, A., Grob, K., Imhof, D., Bazzocco, D. and Pfefferle, A. (2003). How much reducing sugar may potatoes contain to avoid excessive acrylamide formation during roasting and baking? *Eur. Food Res. Technol.,* 271, 3, 185–194.

Changrasekhar, T.C. and Kaveriappa, K.M. (1985). A process for reduction of benzo(a)pyrene content in smoked oil sardine, in Reilley, A., ed., *Spoilage of Tropical Fish and Product Development,* FAO Fisheries Rep. No. 317, FAO, Rome, 262–266.

Castillo, G., Ángeles Sanz, M., Ángeles Serrano, M. and Hernández, A. (2002). Influence of protein source, type and concentration and product form on the protein quality of commercial enteral formulas, *J. Food Sci.,* 67, 1, 328–334.

Chen, C.-C., Tu, Y.-Y. and Chang, H.-M. (2000). Thermal stability of bovine milk immunoglobulin G (IgG) and the effect of added thermal protectants on the stability, *J. Food Sci.,* 65, 188–193.

Chu, Y.H. and Hwang, L.S. (2002). Food lipids, in Sikorski, Z.E., ed., *Chemical and Functional Properties of Food Components,* 2nd ed., CRC Press, Boca Raton, 115–132.

Dennis, M.J., Cripps, G.S., Tricker, A.R., Massey, R.C. and McWeeny, D.J. (1984). *N*-nitroso compounds and polycyclic aromatic hydrocarbons in Icelandic smoked cured mutton, *Food Chem. Toxic.,* 22(4), 305–306.

Dunn, B.P. and Fee, J. (1979). Polycyclic aromatic hydrocarbon carcinogens in commercial seafood, *J. Fish. Res. Board Can.,* 36, 1469–1476.

FAO/WHO (2002). Health implications of acrylamide in food, *Report of a joint FAO/WHO consultation*, Geneva, 25–27 June, 2002.

Fayle, S.E., Gerrard, J.A., Simmons, L., Meade, S.J., Reid, E.A. and Johnston, A.C. (2000). Crosslinking of proteins by dehydroascorbic acid and its degradation products, *Food Chem.*, 70, 193–198.

Franz, A., Reichmuth, Ch. and Wohlgemuth, R. (1992). Brommethan- und Bromidgehalte in Samenkernen nach Vorratsschutz-Begasung und verschiedenen Verarbeitungsverfahren, *Z. Lebensm. Unters. Forsch.*, 194, 148–151.

Friedman, M. and Cuq, J. L. (1988). Chemistry, analysis, nutritional value and toxicology of tryptophan in food, A review, *J. Agric. Food Chem.*, 36, 1079–1093.

Friedman, M. and Pearce, K.N. (1989). Copper(II) and cobalt(II) affinities of LL- and LD-lysinoalanine diastereomers: Implications for food safety and nutrition, *J. Agric. Food Chem.*, 37, 123–127.

Gangolli, S.D. (1986). The toxicology of smoked foods. *IFST Proceedings*, 19, 2, 69–78.

Guerra-Hernandez, E., Corzo, N. and Garcia-Villanova, B. (1999). Maillard reaction evaluation by furosine determination during infant cereal processing, *J. Cereal Sci.*, 29, 171–176.

Hartkopf, J. and Erbersdobler, H.F. (1995). Model experiments with sausage meat on the formation of N^{ε}-carboxymethyllysine, *Z. Lebensm. Unters. Forsch.*, 201, 27–29.

Hartmann, K. (2000). Benzo[*a*]pyren–Bestimmung bei mit Raucharoma geräucherten Fleischerzeugnissen. *Deutsche Lebensmittel-Rundschau*, 96, 163–166.

Institute of Food Science and Technology (1999). *Trans* fatty acids, *Position Statement*, 23 June 1999, Public Affairs and Technical and Legislative Committees.

Iosifidou, H., Kilikidis, S. and Kamarianos, A. (1982). Concentration of PAH in mussels (*Mytilus galloprovincialis*), *Food Technol. Hygiene Rev.*, 4, 1, 20–23.

Jägerstad, M., Skog, K., Arvidsson, P. and Solyakov, A. (1998). Chemistry, formation and occurrence of genotoxic heterocyclic amines identified in model systems and cooked foods, *Z. Lebensm. Unters. Forsch A*, 207, 419–427.

Karl, H. and Leinemann M. (1996). Determination of polycyclic aromatic hydrocarbons in smoked fishery products from different smoking kilns, *Z. Lebensm. Unters. Forsch.*, 202, 458–464.

Kato, T., Kikugawa, K. and Hayatsu, H. (1986). Occurrence of the mutagens 2-amino-3,8-dimethylimidazo[4,5-*f*]quinoxaline (MeIQx) and 2-amino-3,4,8-trimethylimidazo[4,5-*f*]quinoxaline (4,8-Me₂Iqx) in some Japanese smoked, dried fish products, *J. Agric. Food Chem.*, 34, 810–814.

Kikugawa, K., Kato, T. and Hayatsu, H. (1986). Formation of mutagenic substances during smoking-and-drying (baikan) of bonito meat, *Eisei Kakagu*, 32, 5, 379–383.

Kołakowska, A. (2002). Lipid oxidation in food systems, in Sikorski, Z.E. and Kołakowska, A., eds., *Chemical and Functional Properties of Food Lipids*, CRC Press, Boca Raton, 133–166.

Krone, C.A., Yeh, S.M.J. and Iwaoka, W.T. (1986). Mutagen formation during commercial processing of foods, *Environ. Health Perspect.*, 67, 75–88.

Kuncewicz. A., Panfil-Kuncewicz, H. and Michalak, J. (2000). Lactulose and furosine as indices of the degree of heating of milk and other food products, *Przemysł Spożywczy*, 5, 20–22.

Lawrence, J.F. and Weber, D.F. (1984). Determination of polycyclic aromatic hydrocarbons in some Canadian commercial fish, shellfish and meat products by liquid chromatography with confirmation by capillary gas chromatography-mass spectrometry, *J. Agric. Food Chem.*, 32, 789–794.

Lee, K.-G. and Shibamoto, T. (2002). Toxicology and antioxidant activities of non-enzymatic browning reaction products: review, *Food Rev. Int.*, 18, 2&3, 151–175.

Miller Jones, J. (2002). Food safety, in Sikorski, Z.E., ed., *Chemical and Functional Properties of Food Components*, 2nd ed., CRC Press, Boca Raton, 291–305.

Nistor, C. (1985). Prezenta unor hidrocarburi policiclice aromatice in peştele afumat, *Igiena*, 34, 3, 227–230.

Obiedziński, M. and Olkiewicz, M. (1982). Investigations on the amount of benzo(a)pyrene in selected food products, *Roczniki Instytutu Przemysłu Mięsnego i Tłuszczowego*, 19, 65–75.

O'Brien, J. and Morrissey, P.A. (1989). Nutritional and toxicological aspects of the Maillard reaction in foods, *Crit. Rev. Food Sci. Nutrition*, 28, 3, 211.

Oellingrath, J.M. (1988). Heat degradation of heme in methemoglobin and metmyoglobin model systems measured by reversed-phase ion-pair high performance liquid chromatography, *J. Food Sci.*, 53, 40–42.

Pearce, K.N. and Friedman, M. (1988). Binding of copper(II) and other metal ions by lysinoalanine and related compounds and its significance for food safety, *J. Agric. Food Chem.*, 36, 707–717.

Petrun, A.S. and Rubenchik, B.L. (1966). On the possibility of appearance of the carcinogenous agent 3,4-benzpyren in electrostatically smoked fish, *Vrachebnoe Delo*, 2, 93–95.

Potthast, K. (1978). Einfluss der Räuchertechnologie auf die vollständige Zusammensetzung der polycyklischen Kohlenwasserstoffe in geräucherten Fleischwaren, in Rauchkondensaten und in den Abgasen von Räucheranlagen, *Die Fleischwirtschaft*, 58, 10, 1515–1523,

Potthast, K. (1992). Räucherarten von Fleischerzeugnisse, *Fleisch Lebensmittel Markt*, 5, 9–11.

Rainio, K., Linko, R.R. and Routsila, L. (1986). Polycyclic aromatic hydrocarbons in mussel and fish from the Finnish archipelago sea, *Bull. Environ. Contam. Toxicol.*, 37, 337–343.

Rufian-Henares, J. A., Guerra-Hernández, E. and Garcia-Villanova, B. (2002). Maillard reaction in enteral formula processing: furosine, loss of *o*-phthaldialdehyde reactivity and fluorescence, *Food Res. Intl.*, 35, 527–533.

Sikorski, Z.E. (2002). Chemical reactions of proteins in food systems, in Sikorski, Z.E., ed., *Chemical and Functional Properties of Food Proteins*, CRC Press, Boca Raton, 191–216.

Simko, P. (1991). Changes of benzo(a)pyrene contents in smoked fish during storage, *Food Chem.*, 40, 293–300.

Simko, P. (2002). Determination of polycyclic aromatic hydrocarbons in smoked meat products and smoke flavouring food additives, *J. Chromatogr. B*, 770, 3–18.

Steinig, J. (1976). 3,4-Benzpyren-Gehalte in geräucherten Fischen in Abhängigkeit von der Räuchermethode, *Z. Lebensm. Unters-Forsch.*, 162, 235–242.

Steinig, J. and Meyer, V. (1976). 3,4-Benzpyren-Gehalte in geräucherten Fischen, *Lebensm.-Wiss. U. Technol.*, 9, 215–217.

Tai, C.-Y, Chen, Y.C. and Chen, B. H. (1999). Analysis, formation and inhibition of cholesterol oxidation products in foods: An overview (Part I): *J. Food Drug Anal.*, 7, 4, 243–257.

Tai, C.-Y., Lee, K. H. and Chen, B. H. (2001). Effects of various additives on the formation of heterocyclic amines in fried fish fibre, *Food Chem.*, 75, 309–316.

Tilgner, D.J. and Daun, H. (1969). Polycyclic aromatic hydrocarbons (polynuclears) in smoked foods, *Residue Rev.*, 27, 19–41.

Tilgner, D.J. and Miler, K. (1963). The possibilities of eliminating carcinogens from curing smoke, *Przemysł Spożywczy*, 17, 2, 85–90.

Tóth, L. (1962). Geräucherte Lebensmittel – ernstzunehmende gesundheitliche Gefahren? *Deutsche Apotheker-Zeitung*, 122, 46, 2366–2368.

Tóth, L. and Potthast, K. (1984). Chemical aspects of the smoking of meat and meat products, in Chichester, C.O., Mrak, E.M. and Schweigert, B.S., eds., *Advances in Food Research*, Academic Press, New York, 87–158.

Tucker, D.J., Jones, G.P. and Rivett, D. E. (1983). Formation of β-phenylethylaminoalanine in protein foods in the presence of added amine, *J. Sci. Food Agric.*, 34, 1427–1433.

Villamiel, M., Arias, M., Corzo, N. and Olano, A. (1999). Use of different thermal indices to assess the quality of pasteurized milks, *Z. Lebensm. Unters. Forsch. A.*, 208, 169–171.

Wąsowicz, E. (2002). Cholesterol and phytosterols, in Sikorski, Z.E. and Kołakowska, A., eds., *Chemical and Functional Properties of Food Lipids*, CRC Press, Boca Raton, 93–107.

Wierzchowski, J. and Gajewska, R. (1972). Determination of 3,4-benzpyrene in smoked fish, *Bromat. Chem. Toksykol.*, 5, 4, 481–486.

Zabik, M.E., Booren,A., Zabik, J., Welch, R. and Humphrey, H. (1996). Pesticide residues, PSBs and PAHs in baked, charbroiled, salt boiled and smoked Great Lakes lake trout, *Food Chem.*, 55, 3, 231–239.

Zaborowska, Z., Uchman, W., Bilska, A., Jeleń, H., Rudzińska, M., Wąsowicz, E. and Kummerow, F.A. (2001). Effect of storage on oxidation of cholesterol and lipids in liver pate type sausage, *Electron. J. Polish Agricu. Universities, Series Food Sci. Technol.*, 4, 2.

14

Toxic Components of Food Packaging Materials

Barbara Piotrowska

14.1 INTRODUCTION

Packaging is an indispensable element in the food manufacturing process. Nowadays, plastics are used preferentially for packaging foodstuffs. They are capable of retarding and sometimes preventing the detrimental changes that may occur in packed products due to external influences, e.g., oxygen, light, and microorganisms. Plastics are also able to reduce greatly the loss of components, such as water or flavor, from packed material. Therefore, plastic packages extend the shelf-life of many products. Various materials and additives can be used in packaging, as long as they have the desirable functional properties and do not pose health hazards after being in contact with food. Such concerns may occur when some substances migrate from the packaging into the food.

Plastics contain low-molecular components, such as monomers and oligomers, as well as additives, e.g., plasticizers, stabilizers, antioxidants, lubricants, or slip additives, which are necessary for the processing and stability of the final materials. Plastic additives and residual monomers or oligomers are not chemically bound to the polymer molecules and therefore can move freely within the polymer matrix. Recently, migration of low-molecular weight compounds has become one of the most important problems for plastic packaging intended to come into contact with foodstuffs. Migration is the only factor that originates from the packaging itself, and may inadvertently affect the food or pose health concerns to the consumer. The safety of food packaging materials is therefore generally dictated by the lack of potential toxic substances and the absence of migration of such substances.

The assurance of safety of packaging material encompasses all components, both those added to foods intentionally and those ending up in the food from the food-contact material or processing equipment.

14.2 REGULATORY CONTROL

Plastic materials represent a source for contamination through mass transfer, i.e., the migration of substances from the packaging into the food. Identification of the potential migrants or contaminants and assessing their toxicological potency is currently one of the crucial steps in the public safety monitoring processes. It is also very important to determine the levels of residual monomers or additives in food-contact materials and in foods, and to identify the factors affecting the migration of contaminants. Based on this knowledge, it is possible to estimate the maximum likely intake of the contaminants resulting from the contact of food with plastic packaging materials.

In order to protect consumers from harmful substances migrating from packaging into foodstuffs, special directives have been implemented within the European Union. The European Directives harmonize legislation, propose analytical test methods to enable limits to be observed, introduce overall migration limits (OML) for migration from food-contact materials into food and food simulants, and set specific migration limits (SML) or composition limits for free monomers in the final articles. An SML is the maximum allowed concentration of a migrating compound in a food, and is determined according to a compound's individual toxicity. An OML determines the inertness of a material and prevents an unacceptable change in the composition of a food. It reduces the need for a large number of SMLs or other restrictions, thus giving effective control.

European Directives can be divided into three categories: Framework Directive, Specific Directives, and Individual Directives. The Framework Directive 89/109/EEC applies to all materials and articles in contact with foodstuffs, such as packaging materials, forks, cups, processing machines (in factories or at home), transportation pipes, and containers. The Directive states that food-contact materials must be manufactured in compliance with good manufacturing practice, so that, under their normal or foreseeable conditions of use, they do not transfer their constituents to foodstuffs in quantities which could endanger human health or induce unacceptable changes in the sensory properties of foods. It implies not only that any danger for human health shall be avoided, but also that a substantial contamination of foods due to massive migration of substances is forbidden, even if the substances released were demonstrated to be harmless. The Directive establishes also that if an article is intended for food use it shall be labeled "for food use" or bear the symbol of a glass and fork as established by Directive 80/590/EEC.

Specific directives exist for three groups of materials and articles: ceramics, regenerated cellulose film, and plastics. Ceramics are regulated by Council Directive 84/500/EEC. The Directive sets migration limits for cadmium and lead which might be released from the decoration or glazing. Regenerated cellulose film is regulated by Commission Directive 93/10/EEC as amended by Directive 93/111/EC. Plastics are regulated by Commission Directive 2002/72/EC.

Directive 2002/72/EC establishes an OML of 60 mg (of constituents) per kg (of foodstuff or food simulant) for all substances migrating from a material into foodstuffs. It also establishes a positive list of authorized monomers and other starting substances and a list of authorized additives, with restrictions on their use (such as SML), where applicable. The Directive also lays down the procedures for adapting, revising, and completing the lists of authorized substances. For the purposes of the Directive, 'plastics' are the organic macromolecular compounds obtained by polymerization, polycondensation, polyaddition, or any other similar process from molecules with a lower molecular weight or by chemical alteration of natural macromolecules. This term does not include varnished or unvarnished regenerated cellulose films, elastomers, natural and synthetic rubber, and paper and paperboard, whether or not modified by the addition of plastics, surface coatings obtained from paraffin waxes, mixtures of the waxes, ion-exchange resins, and silicones.

Three groups of substances are regulated individually, i.e. vinyl chloride monomer in plastics (78/142/EEC), nitrosamines in rubber teats and soothers (93/11/EEC), and bisphenol A diglycidyl ether, bisphenol F diglycidyl ether, and novolac glycidyl ethers in plastics and coatings (2002/16/EC).

Packaging materials have not received much attention within the Codex Alimentarius Commission supported by the Food and Agriculture Organization and World Health Organization. The Codex specifies that packaging materials should provide adequate protection for products to minimize contamination, prevent damage, and accommodate proper labeling. Packaging materials must be nontoxic and not pose any threat to the safety and suitability of food under the specified conditions of storage and use (Codex Alimentarius, 1997). The Codex Alimentarius contains only guideline levels for vinyl chloride monomers and acrylonitryl in food and packaging material (Codex Alimentarius Commission, 1991, 2003).

14.3 TOXIC MATERIALS EMPLOYED IN PROCESSING AND PACKAGING

14.3.1 POLYMERS AND THEIR CONSTITUENTS

14.3.1.1 Introduction

Plastic materials are the main components of food packages used for dairy products, baked goods, breads, beverages, breakfast cereals, confectionery, pasta, and other miscellaneous food products (Table 14.1).

Plastics can be classified as thermoplastic or thermosetting. Thermoplastics are materials that can be repeatedly softened by heat and hardened by cooling. Typical of the thermoplastic family are the styrene polymers and copolymers, acrylics, cellulosics, polyethylenes, polypropylenes, vinyls, and nylons. Thermoset polymers are those that undergo chemical reactions induced by heat, pressure, catalysts, and ultraviolet (UV) light, leading to an infusible state. Typical plastics in the thermosetting family are amines (melamine,

Table 14.1
Polymers commonly used in food packaging applications.

Material	Packaging
Laminated polyethylene-fibreboard-printed polyethylene	Milk carton
Laminated aluminum polyethylene	Chip bag, soup pack
Polystyrene	Yogurt tub, cheese tray, biscuit inner tray
Printed polyethylene	Biscuit, ice cream, bread and chocolate bar wrappers, chip bag, milk shake cup, milk thick shake straw, soy milk tetra pack, pasta, noodles, shredded cheese, outer cheese, carrot slice, coffee, lecithin, green beans, and brown rice packs
Printed fibreboard	Ice cream, biscuit outer, rolled oats, cereal outer, cocoa outer, tea, apricot pie, and jelly outer packs
Polyethylene	Cheese wrapper, cereal contents pack
Polyethylene terephthalate	Ice cream lid, juice container, soft drink bottle
High-density polyethylene	Ice cream tub, milk jug
Low-density polyethylene	Food-freeze and ice bags
Cellophane	Biscuit contents pack, cocoa, and jelly inner packs
Polyvinyl chloride	Lemon squeeze container
Polypropylene	Ketchup bottle

Source: data from Balafas et al. (1999), *Food Chem.*, 65, 279–287.

benzoguanamine, and urea), most polyesters, alkyds, epoxides, polyurethanes, and phenolics. Thermoset polymers, after crosslinking, drying, curing, and hardening solidify to a three dimensional crosslinked matrix, cannot be melted without destroying their original characteristics. The most common thermoset plastics are epoxy resins, derived from reaction of bisphenol A and epichlorhydrin.

To achieve the desirable functional properties of the finished products, additives have to be incorporated with the polymers. Emulsifiers, surfactants and buffering agents are also used to provide a suitable medium for polymerization.

The largest controversy relating to safety of plastic packaging arises not from the actual use of polymers, but rather from the presence and possible migration of monomers (e.g., vinyl chloride) and other starting substances. This group consists of substrates undergoing polymerization, natural or synthetic macromolecular compounds used in the manufacture of modified macromolecules, and chemicals used to modify natural or synthetic macro-molecular components. Monomers or oligomers are not chemically bound to the polymer molecules and can therefore move within the polymer matrix. Consequently, at the interface between packaging material and food they can dissolve in the food product. Monomers are reactive substances with respect to living organisms, and are therefore toxic to some degree.

A lot of concern also focuses on additives from packaging materials ending up in food (e.g., phthalate plasticizers, which are accused of many serious, chronic health effects).

14.3.1.2 Polyethylene Terephthalate

Polyethylene terephthalate (PET) is a copolymer of ethylene glycol with either terephthalic acid or dimethyl terephthalate. PET is used in packaging applications for soft drinks and mineral water, and for the bottles that are collected by curbside or deposit systems. As it does not thermally deform below about 220°C, PET is also used for trays and dishes for microwave and conventional cooking.

PET itself is biologically inert if ingested and is dermally safe during handling. No adverse effects have been observed at exposures anticipated to occur from the use of PET packages (International Life Sciences Institute, 2000). It poses no hazard if inhaled and no evidence of toxicity has been detected in feeding studies using animals.

SMLs have been established for the monomers commonly used in making PET (Table 14.2). Studies conducted using monomers and PET intermediates indicated that these materials are essentially non-toxic and pose no threats to human health. The chemistry of compounds that are used to manufacture PET shows no evidence of estrogenic activity (International Life Sciences Institute, 2000).

Cause for concern arose from the presence of antimony trioxide (SML = 0.02 mg per kg), a catalyst widely used in the manufacture of PET. Studies

Table 14.2

Monomers commonly used in the manufacture of polyethylene terephthalate (PET) and copolyesters for food packaging.

Monomer	SML[a] (mg/kg)
1,4-Bis(hydroxymethyl) cyclohexane	No SML
Diethyleneglycol	30 (alone or with ethyleneglycol or stearic acid esters of ethylene glycol)
Ethyleneglycol	30 (alone or with diethyleneglycol or stearic acid esters of ethylene glycol)
Isophthalic acid	5
Isophthalic acid dimethyl ester	0.05
Terephthalic acid	7.5
Terephthalic acid dimethyl ester	No SML

[a]Specific migration limit, Directive 2002/72/EC.

designed to detect migration of metal additives showed trace levels of antimony, less than 5 mg per g. The results of a detailed animal feeding study have led to the conclusion that a diet containing up to 20 g per kg of antimony trioxide had no detectable toxic effects (International Life Sciences Institute, 2000).

The migration of di(2-ethylhexyl) phthalate and carbonyl compounds, such as formaldehyde, acetaldehyde, and acetone, from PET mineral-water bottles was reported (Nawrocki et al., 2002; Biscardi et al., 2003). Recently, new chemical and biological studies have also indicated that genotoxic and carcinogenic compounds are present in PET bottles used for storing mineral water (Evandri et al., 2000; Biscardi et al., 2003). Water samples stored in PET bottles induced cytogenetic aberrations. The finding that chromosomal aberrations were particularly apparent after exposure of the water bottles to direct sunlight suggest that storage conditions are very important (Evandri et al., 2000). Studies on the influence of stored water on macroscopic (root length, color, and form) and microscopic (root tip, mitotic index, chromosome aberrations) parameters were conducted using the *Allium cepa* test. However, plant systems are not considered as primary screening tools by current international guidelines for mammalian systems. Therefore, any extrapolation of the results from this test system to other systems, and to humans, should be based on results from a battery of assays covering various metabolic pathways.

Food-grade PET essentially contains only very high molecular weight molecules. However, PET is known to contain cyclic oligomers, predominantly cyclic trimers, which can diffuse to the surface of the packaging, e.g., in metallized PET (Gollier and Bertrand, 2002). Migration of cyclic oligomers from an aluminized PET film to microwaveable French fries, popcorn, fish sticks, waffles, and pizza was reported by Begley et al. (1990).

14.3.1.3 Nylon Resins

Polyamides, commonly known as 'nylons,' may safely be used to produce articles intended for application in processing, handling, and packaging of food, including for products intended to be cooked directly in their packages. Nylon resins are manufactured by condensation of hexyamethylenediamine and adipic acid (nylon 66) or sebacic acid (nylon 610), by the polymerization process, e.g., of ω-laurolactam (nylon 12), or by condensation and polymerization, e.g., nylon 66 salts and ε-caprolactam.

Nylon microwave and roasting bags were reported to release, at cooking temperatures, volatile compounds, such as Nylon 6,6 cyclic monomer and cyclic oligomers up to the tetramer, and Nylon 6 monomer and cyclic oligomers up to the octamer. The same non-volatile compounds (except Nylon 6 heptamer and octamer) were extracted from the same packages (Soto-Valdez et al., 1997).

Loss of up to 1.5% of the original weight of nylon films used for boil-in-the-bag food packaging, and migration of caprolactam and cyclic oligomers up to the nonamer into the cooking water take place during boiling (Barkby and Lawson, 1993). Caprolactam is an important intermediate used in the production of nylon 6, but it is not especially toxic (National Institutes of Health, 1982a).

14.3.2 MONOMERS, OLIGOMERS AND OTHER STARTING SUBSTANCES

14.3.2.1 Bisphenol-Type Contaminants

Food and beverage cans often have an internal polymeric coating, used to protect the product and prevent undesirable interactions between the metal from the can and the content. Such polymeric coatings are usually highly crosslinked thermoset resins, which can withstand typical processing conditions. Among the coating varnishes or lacquers used in food cans, epoxyphenolic, vinyl organosols (novolacs), and polyester phenolic are the most widely used. Of these, the epoxyphenolic and vinylic organosols find most frequent application.

Bisphenol A (BPA) (Figure 14.1a) is a starting substance utilized in the manufacture of most types of epoxy resins, which are then crosslinked and used to coat food cans. Another application of BPA is in the manufacture of plastic materials, in particular polycarbonates. BPA serves also as an antioxidant or stabilizing material for many types of plastics, e.g., polyvinyl chloride (PVC).

Bisphenol F (BPF) is a mixture of three isomers: 2,2'-, 2,4'-, and 4,4'-dihydroxydiphenylmethane, in the ratio 15%, 50% and 35%, respectively. It has also found application in the manufacture of epoxy resins, but as a fully crosslinked polymer it is rarely used in food-contact materials. Residues of

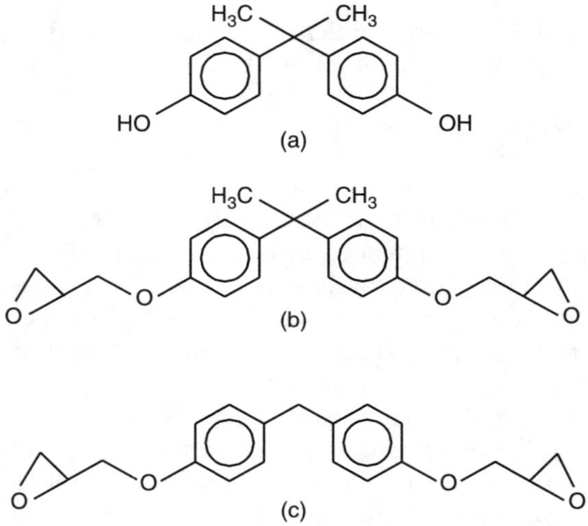

FIGURE 14.1 Structures of (a) bisphenol A, (b) bisphenol A diglycidyl ether, and (c) bisphenol F diglycidyl ether.

BPF isomers (Novolac) may arise from their application in the manufacture of Novolac glycidyl ethers (NOGE), which serve as scavengers for hydrogen chloride in PVC organosol coatings.

Vinylic organosols include in their composition epoxy resins such as bisphenol A diglycidyl ether (BADGE) (Figure 14.1b) and bisphenol F diglycidyl ether (BFDGE) (Figure 14.1c). These resins are obtained from the monomers: BPA and BPF, respectively. BPA is not normally present in PVC organosol coatings, but if BADGE is applied as an additive to scavenge hydrogen chloride in these coatings, residues of BPA may occur.

All the bisphenol-type compounds mentioned have the potential to migrate into the packaged food. Migration of BPA can occur from can coatings into food (Goodson et al., 2002) or food simulants (Nerín et al., 2002). BPA migration has been identified in canned commodities, including vegetables, fish in aqueus media, and meat products (Goodson et al., 2002), and from cans containing coffee and caffeine (Kang and Kondo, 2002). PVC stretch films used for food packaging may also be a source of BPA (Lopez-Cervantes and Paseiro-Losada, 2003). The monomer can be leached when canned food is heated at typical can processing temperatures. Kawamura et al. (2001) reported that BPA migration from the can coating required heating to more than 105°C. Migration of BADGE and BFDGE has been reported, e.g., in canned fish (Hammarling et al., 2000; Theobald et al., 2000).

Directive 2002/72/EEC lists BPA in the positive list, with an SML of 3 mg per kg. The amount of BADGE, BFDGE, and NOGE in plastics, coatings, and adhesives are regulated by Commission Directive 2002/16/EC. For BADGE and BFDGE, as well as their derivatives, SMLs have been set at 1 mg per kg. The Directive also sets a very strict limit for NOGE and its derivatives as there are no sufficient data available on the toxicity of this group of substances. This limit in practice rules out their use as additives in coatings.

Recent research has identified environmental chemicals that disrupt reproductive processes by altering the actions of endogenous steroid hormones. BPA is mentioned among them (Hoyer, 2001). BPA stimulates, with a relatively low potency, cell proliferation and induces expression of estrogen-responsive genes *in vitro*. *In vivo*, BPA increases prolactin release and stimulates uterine, vaginal, and mammary growth and differentiation. BPA shares similarities in structure, metabolism, and action with diethylstilbestrol, a known human teratogen and carcinogen (Ben-Jonathan and Steinmetz, 1998). Hence, human exposure to BPA may be significant, given that BPA-based products are common in food utensils.

14.3.2.2 Isocyanates

Fourteen isocyanates are currently permitted for use in food-contact materials:

- cyclohexyl isocyanate
- dicyclohexylmethane-4,4'-diisocyanate
- 3,3'-dimethyl-4,4'-diisocyanatobiphenyl
- diphenylether-4,4'-diisocyanate
- diphenylmethane-2,4'-diisocyanate
- diphenylmethane-4,4'-diisocyanate
- hexamethylene diisocyanate
- 1-isocyanato-3-isocyanatomethyl-3,5,5-trimethylcyclohexane
- 1,5-naphthalene diisocyanate
- octadecyl isocyanate
- 2,4-toluene diisocyanate
- 2,6-toluene diisocyanate
- 2,4 toluene diisocyanate dimer
- 1,6-diamino-2,2,4-trimethylhexane (mixture of 40% w/w) (2,4,4-trimethylhexane-1,6-diisocyanate (mixture of 60% w/w)

As they are considered to be toxic compounds, their use in the manufacture of plastic materials and articles that are intended to come into contact with foods is regulated by Directive 2002/72/EC. Their residual levels in the finished plastics must not exceed 1.0 mg per kg, expressed as isocyanate moiety (NCO).

Isocyanates are used in polyurethane polymers and adhesives. In production of multilayer plastic materials, it is common to apply reactive adhesive mixtures containing aromatic isocyanate monomers. However, in cases of incomplete curing, primary aromatic amines (PAAs) may be produced from residues of the aromatic isocyanates and water. PAAs can be transferred from packaging into food. Some PPAs, including 2,4-diaminotoluene and 4,4'-methylenedianiline, are classified as "possibly carcinogenic to humans" by the International Agency for Research on Cancer (IARC). According to European legislation, the total concentration of PAAs migrated into food should not be detectable using an analytical method with detection limit of 20 µg per kg. Detectable levels of 2,4-diaminotoluene, 2,6-diaminotoluene and 4,4'-methylenedianiline were found in water simulant, that migrated from multilayer packages, e.g., materials that were intended for high-temperature use. None of these packages produced PAA levels above the EU limit (Brede et al., 2003).

14.3.2.3 Styrene

Styrene is a commercially important monomer that is used extensively in the manufacture of polystyrene resins and in co-polymers with acrylonitrile and 1,3-butadiene (reinforced plastics). Exposure to styrene occurs due to intake of food that has been in contact with styrene-containing polymers. IARC has determined that styrene is possibly carcinogenic to humans. There is no restriction on using styrene within the European Union (i.e., there is no SML).

Styrene migration depends strongly on the fat content of the food and storage temperature. The level of styrene migration from polystyrene cups to water is significantly lower then to fatty foods. In 15% ethanol, the migration level is equivalent to that in milk or soup containing 3.6% fat. Maximum observed migration was 0.025% of the total styrene in the cup for cold or hot beverages and take-away foods (Tawfik and Huyghebaert, 1998). Migration of styrene monomers and styrene dimers was detected in some styrene polymers used in food packaging. The 'global migration,' however, turned out to be lower than the overall migration limit fixed by current legislation (Brunelli et al., 2002). There was also no detectable migration of styrene into margarine (Varner et al., 1983).

Results of studies on animals have indicated that styrene treatment (0.5 g per kg body weight) alters dopaminergic function in some brain regions that are important in the initiation and control of movement. However, the deficits in motor function resulting from styrene exposure were not permanent and the functions returned to control levels after cessation of such treatment (Chakrabarti, 2000).

14.3.2.4 Vinyl Chloride

Vinyl chloride monomer (VCM) is the main substrate for the manufacture of polymers used as packaging materials for food. Since VCM is considered by IARC to be a human carcinogen, monomer levels in PVC food packaging materials are strictly controlled. To ensure a safe product, the residual content of VCM in the finished material or article is limited to one mg per kg in the final product (Council Directive 78/142/EEC). Furthermore, VCM should not be detectable in foodstuffs. Commission Directives 80/766/EEC and 81/432/EEC give the method of analysis for official control of the VCM level in food packaging materials and in foods – gas-phase chromatography using the 'headspace' method, after dissolution or suspension of samples in N,N-dimethylacetamide. Both residual monomer content of the polymer and migration levels to foods or food simulant are regulated (Directive 80/766/EEC, Directive 81/432/EEC).

14.3.3 ADDITIVES IN POLYMERIC PACKAGING

14.3.3.1 Antioxidants, Light Stabilizers and Thermal Stabilizers

Plastics generally age rapidly and undergo polymer degradation when exposed to UV light and in the presence of oxygen. The rate of oxidation is decreased by adding stabilizing additives, such as antioxidants or light stabilizers. These compounds stabilize the polymers by being preferentially degraded. Antioxidants can be divided into two major classes, based on their mechanisms of action: primary and secondary antioxidants. The primary antioxidants are radical scavengers, hydrogen donors, or chain reaction breakers, and include hindered phenols and secondary aryl amines. The secondary antioxidants are peroxide decomposers, mainly composed of organophosphites and thioesters. To take advantage of synergistic effects, various combinations of primary and secondary antioxidants are often used.

Commonly used antioxidants include:

- mixtures of the isomers 3-*tert*-butyl-4-hydroxyanisole and 2-*tert*-butyl-4-hydroxyanisole (BHA)
- 2,6-di-*tert*-butyl-4-methyl-phenol (BHT)
- 2-(2'-hydroxy-5'methylphenyl)benzotriazole (Tinuvin P)
- 2-(5-chloro-2*H*-benzotriazole-2-yl)-6-(1,1-dimethylethyl)-4-methylphenol (Tinuvin 326)
- bis(2,2,6,6-tetramethyl-4-piperydyl)sebacate (Tinuvin 770 DF)
- 2-[2-hydroxy-3,5-bis(1-methyl-1-phenyl)phenyl]benzotriazole (Tinuvin 234)
- 2-hydroxy-4-*n*-octyloxybenzophenone (Chimasorb 81)
- octadecyl-3-(3,5-di-*tert*-butyl-4-hydroxyphenyl)propionate (Irganox 1076)
- 1,3,5-trimethyl-2,4,6-tris(3,5-di-*tert*-butyl-4-hydroxyphenyl)propionate (Irganox 1330)
- pentaerythrityl-tetrakis-3-(3,5-di-*tert*-butyl-4-hydroxyphenyl)propionate (Irganox 1010)
- tris-(2,4-di-*tert*-butylphenyl)phosphite (Irgafos 168)
- tetrakis(2,4-di-*tert*-butylphenyl)-4,4'-biphenylene diphosphonite (Irgafos P-EPQ)

Some of these antioxidants appear in the list of additives that may be used in the manufacture of plastic materials intended to come into contact with food. For example, Irganox 1010 and Irgafos 168 are allowed without SML, Tinuvin P and Tinuvin 234 with SML of 30 mg per kg, and Irganox 1076 with SML of 6 mg per kg.

Determination of the migration levels of antioxidants from low-density polyethylene (LDPE) commercial samples showed that there is no significant antioxidant migration into food simulants, i.e., migration does not exceed SML (Dopico-Garcia et al., 2003). However, application of arylsubstitued phosphites in packaging materials is only allowed if the respective packaging material is not in contact with fat-containing foods. Hydrophobic antioxidants, such as Irganox 1010 or Irgafos 168, migrate into the oils. The rate of their migration is greater from polyolefins with high content of amorphous fraction. The loss of these antioxidants is reduced when polypropylene or high-density polyethylene are selected for the oil containers (Marcato et al., 2003).

The migration/sorption behavior test for BHT and α-tocopherol in LDPE packaging materials in contact with fatty food simulants has indicated that the rate of migration of α-tocopherol into food simulants is lower than that for BHT. Since α-tocopherol was transferred from the film to the simulant to a lesser extent, it is considered a more stable antioxidant than BHT (Wessling et al., 1998). BHT has also been found to migrate more rapidly than Irganox 1010 into dry food stored in LDPE wraps (Schwope et al., 1987a).

The differences in the migration rates of antioxidants depend on the food simulants used in tests and on the properties of the polymer-containing packaging. The rate of migration of Irganox 1010 to fatty food simulants was greater from ethylene-vinyl acetate (EVA) films than from LDPE. In contrast, a low migration rate of this antioxidant was recorded on exposure of the EVA film to aqueous media, whereas migration from LDPE into such media was relatively high (Schwope et al., 1987b).

Light stabilizers improve the long-term durability of plastics, especially polyolefins. Polymeric hindered amines, such as Tinuvin 622, and Chimasorb 944, are commonly used in polyolefins as light stabilisers.

The poor thermal stability of some polymers, e.g., PVC, requires the use of thermal stabilizers in the processing of the polymer. The stabilizers protect PVC during the compounding and processing stages, prevent dehydrochlorination and discoloration, and maintain stability during use. The highly effective lead-based and cadmium-based additives were applied for many years as thermal stabilizers, but they have now been replaced by less-toxic equivalents. Epoxidized seed and vegetable oils, such as epoxidized soybean oil (ESBO), find application as heat stabilizers in a range of food-contact plastics.

14.3.3.2 Plasticizers

Plasticizers are used in the polymer industry to improve flexibility, workability, and general handling properties. Dibutyl sebacate and phthalates, such as dibutyl phthalate, diethyl phthalate, dicyclohexyl phthalate, butylbenzyl phthalate, and diphenyl-2-ethylhexyl phosphate, serve widely as plasticizers in vinylidene chloride copolymers, nitrocellulose-coated regenerated cellulose film, and cellulose acetate (Castle et al., 1988a). In PVC, di(2-ethylhexyl) phthalate (DEHP) and di(2-ethylhexyl) adipate (DEHA) are used in the largest quantities.

Butyl stearate, acetyltributyl citrate, alkyl sebacates, and adipates are typical low-toxicity plasticizers and are commonly used. Results of studies conducted by the U.S. National Toxicology Program indicated that DEHP and DEHA cause carcinogenic effects at high doses in mice and rats of both sexes (National Institutes of Health, 1980, 1982b). Although these phthalates are animal carcinogens, there are suggestions that their mechanisms of carcinogenessis may not be relevant to human systems (Shea, 2003). It was also reported that phthalates might interrupt the natural hormonal process of the body and therefore might impair human fertility, e.g., by reducing sperm counts (Rozati et al., 2002).

As the plasticizers are not bound to the base polymer by covalent linkages, they may be leached from packaging materials into foods and beverages. Migration of DEHA from plasticized PVC films into cheese, cooked meats, cakes, and microwave-cooked foods has been reported (Startin et al., 1987). The following levels of DEHA were found in retail foods wrapped in plasticized PVC films: from 1.0 to about 75 mg per kg in uncooked meat and poultry, from about 9.5 to about 50 mg per kg in cooked chicken portions, from about 30 to 135 mg per kg in cheese, less than 2.0 mg per kg in fruit and vegetables, and 11 to about 215 mg per kg in baked goods and sandwiches (Castle *et al.*, 1987). The presence of phthalates in packaging materials made from printed polyethylene, polystyrene, polyethylene terephthalate, or polyethylene has been confirmed by Balafas et al. (1999). Surveys conducted on baby-food containers indicated the presence of dibutyl phthalate and DEHP in the products (Ozaki et al., 2002).

The correct labeling of plasticized PVC is important for avoiding risk of significant consumer intakes of DEHA through use of film directly in contact with fatty foodstuffs (Petersen et al., 1997). PVC should not be used in direct contact with food in microwave ovens (Badeka and Kontominas, 1996).

ESBO is also widely applied as plasticizer. ESBO is a mixture of triacylglycerols, with linoleic, oleic and linoleic acids being the major unsaturated fatty acid components. ESBO also serves as a secondary heat stabilizer, especially in PVC products. Studies on embryotoxicity of ESBO using an *in vitro* battery system indicate that it is not embriotoxic (Rhee et al., 2002). However, contamination with ESBO by migration from PVC film to cheeses, sandwiches, cakes, and microwave-cooked meals has been reported (Castle et al., 1988b). The presence of ESBO in baby food, due to migration from PVC gasket lids of glass jars containing ready-cooked food, has also been reported (Hammarling et al., 1998).

14.3.3.3 Lubricants and Slip Additives

While plasticizers change the physical properties of a polymer, lubricants are added to change the processing properties of the material. Lubricants are widely used in thermoplastic polymers to increase the overall rate of processing or to improve surface release properties during extrusion, injection, molding or compression molding.

Lubricants may be categorized by their chemical nature (Table 14.3), or may be classified according to their action into two basic groups: external lubricants and internal lubricants.

Slip additives act at the surface of a polymer film or article to reduce the friction between it and another surface. In a variety of plastics, such as polyolefins, polystyrene, and polyvinyl chloride, fatty-acid amides are applied as slip additives. Fatty-acid amides, such as oleamide, stearamide, erucamide, and oleyl palmitamide, are added to plastic formulations where they gradually tend to bloom to the surface, imparting useful properties including lubrication, prevention of films sticking together, and reduction of static charge.

Within the European Union there are no restrictions regarding these additives. However, primary fatty-acid amides have been shown to have hormone-like activity, e.g., oleamide (*cis*-9,10-octadecenoamide) is an endogenous bioregulator that acts like a sleep-inducing factor (Cravatt et al., 1995; Bezuglov et al., 1998).

14.3.3.4 Nonylphenol

Alkylphenols, e.g., *p*-nonyl-phenol (NP), serve widely as antioxidants and surfactants for plastics such as PVC and polystyrene. NP, like BPA and some phthalic acid esters, belongs to the group of anthropogenic endocrine disruptors. It has estrogen-like properties when tested in the human breast tumor MCF_7 cell line and in the castrated rat models (Soto et al., 1991). NP may be leached from PVC food packaging films in domestic applications, such as wrapping of food and reheating in a microwave oven. Its migration to samples heated in a microwave oven for one minute ranged from not detectable (< 1 µg per kg) to 410 µg per kg (Inoue et al., 2001).

Table 14.3
Commonly used lubricants.

Lubricant	Examples of use
Saturated hydrocarbons	Paraffin waxes, microcrystalline wax, earth wax, polyethylene waxes, oxidized polyethylene waxes
Fatty acids	Stearic acid
Metallic soaps	Zinc and calcium stearate
Fatty acid esters	The butyl stearate, octyl stearate, fatty acid glyceryl esters
Fatty acid amides	Stearamide, erucamide, ethylene bisstearamide (EBS), ethylene bisoleamide (EBO)

Source: data from Wang and Buzanowski (2000), *J. Chrom. A.*, 891, 313–324.

14.4 MIGRATION OF TOXIC COMPONENTS

A large amount of research has been conducted into the migration of contaminants and toxic additives from plastic packaging materials into food and food simulants (Brede et al., 2002). Estimates of the exposure to contaminants in the diet are determined by combining migration data with information on the uses of food packaging that may contain additives or contaminants (Simoneau et al., 1999). Traditionally, migration data are obtained from tests in which plastics are brought into contact with a food simulant (e.g., vegetable oil, alcoholic or acidic solution) under established time and temperature limits (Commission Directive 97/48/EC, Council Directive 85/572/EEC).

The European Commission has mandated the European Committee for Standardization to establish a validated method of analysis for the determination of OMLs and SMLs. If a product complies with the compositional requirements of the directives, i.e., it is produced from authorized monomers and additives, then it may be tested for any desired application. If it meets the migration requirements, it is acceptable for use in cases covered by that test method. Typical food simulants used in the tests are hot water, acetic acid, ethyl alcohol and olive oil. The choice of an appropriate simulant depends on the type of food expected to come into contact with the packaging.

Analysis of migrants in a foodstuff or simulant may be very expensive, time-consuming and complicated because of the low concentrations of migrating substances in the foods and the complexity of the matrix. To overcome these difficulties, migration evaluation procedures based on theoretical prediction of migration from plastic food-contact material were recently introduced. Using data from migration studies under controlled conditions it is possible to establish mathematical models of the migration process specific to different food-contact materials and foods. Such models are indispensable in the prediction of the extent of migration, and could be crucial for helping regulatory authority to set up guidelines regarding the use of food-contact materials (Baner et al., 1996; Begley 1997; Lau and Wong 1997; Helmroth at al., 2002). The rate and extent of migration are mainly affected by the properties listed in Table 14.4.

The process of migration of additives or contaminants from polymeric food packaging to food may be separated into three stages: diffusion within the polymer, solvation at the polymer–food interface, and dispersion into bulk food.

The rate of migration of additives or contaminants is controlled primarily by diffusion within the polymer lattice. Because the migrants pass through voids and other gaps between the polymer molecules, the migration rate depends on the size and shape of the migrants and on the size and number of the gaps. It also depends on polymer's properties, such as density, crystalinity, and degree of crosslinking and branching. The glass transition temperature (T_g) of the polymer, which determines the flexibility of the polymer molecules, is also important. Below T_g, the polymer molecules are stiff (glassy state) and

Table 14.4
Factors affecting rate and extent of migration in packaged foods.

- Concentration and properties of the migrant in the packaging materials
- Concentration and properties of the migrant in the printing ink
- Properties of polymer used to produce the food packaging materials
- Maximum solvent absorption in the polymer
- Storage period
- Storage temperature
- Fat content in the food
- Contact area

the chance of a migrant finding a sufficiently large gap is limited. Above T_g, the polymer molecules are highly flexible (rubbery state), which makes the migration rate higher. In general, the lower the T_g of a polymer, the higher the migration rate from that polymer. Irrespective of the T_g, the higher the flexibility of the polymer molecules, the higher is the migration rate.

In the second stage, the migrant moves by way of solvation into the food. In the third stage, the solvated migrant diffuses away from the interface and moves into the bulk of the food. Thermodynamic properties, such as polarity and solubility, influence the migration rate due to interactions between polymer, migrant, and food simulant. If a migrant has a poor solubility in the food simulant, it will remain in the polymer rather than migrate into the food simulant.

The possibility of basing approval of packaging materials on predictions rather than on experiments is being discussed at European level. In the Commission Directive 2001/62/EC the use of "generally recognized diffusion models" as an alternative test method has been approved. The key point of predicting migration is how to obtain values for the model parameters that are specific for each combination of migrant, polymer, and food simulant. However, reliable use of such a method requires a certain insight in the scientific background and application area of these models.

14.5 CONCLUDING REMARKS

Packaging materials made of plastics are necessary for the food industry, and it would be a major problem if they were suddenly abandoned. Most of the plastics used are almost inert towards food constituents, however a small amount of toxic additives or unbound monomers and oligomers may migrate into food. Migration may occur during storage of food in plastic packages, and may be particularly extensive when fatty food surfaces are in direct contact with plastic packaging. Heating food in plastic containers, e.g., in microwave ovens, increase the rate and extent of migration.

Human exposure to migrating substances (e.g., di(2-ethylhexyl)phthalate) may result in reproductive disorders. There is a hazard that vinyl chloride monomers or bisphenol A migrating into food may induce carcinogenic, mutagenic, and teratogenic episodes.

Good knowledge and understanding of the mechanisms involved in the interaction between food packaging materials and food is an indispensable element. These are parts of the driving process towards innovation of plastic packages and are the means of ensuring that regulatory control is based on reliable science. Safety of food packaging materials is controlled around the world. Legislative agencies in many countries assess migration levels of plastic constituents. Such levels are well within the margin of safety, and thus levels of the migrants that might be consumed, e.g., as a result of plastic film use, are below the threshold showing no toxic effect in animal studies.

Risks associated with plastic packages may be increased by human behavior and lifestyle. It is common to get into the habit of eating only some kind of foods, but this may increase the risk of continuous exposure to a specific migrant from the packaging used for these favored foodstuffs. Frequent consumption of 'fast foods' or 'microwave meals' packaged in plastic films may also exert negative effects in the long term.

14.6 REFERENCES

Badeka, A.B. and Kontominas, M.G. (1996). Effect of microwave heating on the migration of dioctyladipate and acetyltributylcitrate plasticizers from food grade PVC and PVDC/PVC films into olive oil and water, *Z. Lebensm. Unters. Forsch.*, 202, 4, 313–317.

Balafas, D., Shaw, K.J. and Whitfield, F.B. (1999). Phthalate and adipate esters in Australian packaging materials, *Food Chem.*, 65, 279–287.

Baner, A., Brandsch J. Franz, R. and Pringer, O. (1996). The application of a predictive migration model for evaluating the compliance of plastic materials with European food regulations, *Food Addit. Contam.*, 13, 5, 587–601.

Barkby, C.T. and Lawson, G. (1993). Analysis of migrants from nylon 6 packaging films into boiling water, *Food Addit. Contam.*, 10, 5, 541–553.

Begley, T.H. (1997). Methods and approaches used by FDA to evaluate the safety of food packaging materials, *Food Addit. Contam.*, 14, 6-7, 543-553.

Begley, T.H., Dennison, J.L. and Hollifield, H.C. (1990). Migration into food of polyethylene terephthalate (PET) cyclic oligomers from PET microwave susceptor packaging, *Food Addit. Contam.*, 7, 6, 797–803.

Ben-Jonathan, N. and Steinmetz, R. (1998). Xenoestrogens: the emerging story of bisphenol A, *Trends Endocrinol. Metab.*, 9, 124–128.

Bezuglov, V.V., Bobrov, M.Yu. and Archakov, A.V. (1998). Bioactive amides of fatty acids, *Biochem.*, 63, 1, 22–30.

Biscardi, D., Monarca, S., De Fusco, R., Senatore, F., Poli, P., Buschini, A., Rossi, C. and Zani, C. (2003). Evaluation of the migration of mutagens/carcinogens from PET bottles into mineral water by *Tradescantia*/micronuclei test, Comet assay on leukocytes and GC/MS, *Sci. Total Environ.*, 302, 101–108.

Brede, C., Skjevrak, I. and Herikstad, H. (2003). Determination of primary aromatic amines in water food simulant using solid-phase analytical derivatization followed by gas chromatography coupled with mass spectrometry, *J. Chrom. A*, 983, 35–42.

Brede, C., Skjevrak, I., Herikstad, H., Ånensen, E., Austvoll, R. and Hemmingsen, T. (2002). Improved sample extraction and clean-up for the GC-MS determination of BADGE and BFDGE in vegetable oil, *Food Addit. Contam.*, 19, 5, 483–491.

Brunelli, N., Nocci, R. and Magno, F. (2002). Global migration from styrenics to liquid food simulants, *Ann. Chim.*, 92, 7–8, 637–648.

Castle, L., Mercer, A.J., Startin, J.R. and Gilbert, J. (1987). Migration from plasticized films into foods. 2. Migration of di(2-etylhexyl) adipate from PVC films used for retail food packaging, *Food Addit. Contam.*, 4, 4, 399–406.

Castle, L., Mercer, A.J., Startin, J.R. and Gilbert, J. (1988a). Migration from plasticized films into foods. 3. Migration of phthalate, sebacate, citrate and phosphate esters from films used for retail food packaging, *Food Addit. Contam.*, 5, 1, 9–20.

Castle, L., Sharman, M. and Gilbert, J. (1988b). Gas chromatographic-mass spectrometric determination of epoxidized soybean oil contamination of foods by migration from plastic packaging, *J. Assoc. Off. Anal. Chem.*, 71, 6, 1183–1186.

Chakrabarti, S.K. (2000). Altered regulation of dopaminergic activity and impairment in motor function in rats after subchronic exposure to styrene, *Pharm. Biochem. Behavior.*, 66, 3, 523–532.

Codex Alimentarius (1997). Joint FAO/WHO Food Standards Programme. International code of practice – general principles of food hygiene, in *General Requirements (Food Hygiene)*, Codex Alimentarius (supplement to volume 1B), FAO/WHO, Rome.

Codex Alimentarius Commission (1991). *Report of the 19th Session of the Joint FAO/ WHO Codex Alimentarius Commission*, FAO, Rome.

Codex Alimentarius Commission (2003). *Schedule 1 of the Proposed Draft Codex General Standard for Contaminants and Toxins in Food.* Joint FAO/WHO Food Standards Programme. Codex Committee on Food Additives and Contaminants, Thirty-fifth Session, Arusha, Tanzania.

Commission Directive 2002/72/EC, *O.J.E.C.*, L220, 15.08.20002.

Commission Directive 2002/16/EC, *O.J.E.C.*, L51, 22.02.2002.

Commission Directive 2001/62/EC, *O.J.E.C.*, L221, 17.08.2001.

Commission Directive 93/10/EEC, *O.J.E.C.*, L93, 17.04.1993.

Commission Directive 81/432/EEC, *O.J.E.C.*, L167, 24.06.1981.

Commission Directive 80/766/EEC, *O.J.E.C.*, L213, 16.08.1980.

Commission Directive 80/590/EEC, *O.J.E.C.*, L151, 19.06.1980.

Commission Directive 97/48/EC, *O.J.E.C.*, L222, 12.08.97.

Commission Directive 93/111/EC, *O.J.E.C.*, L310, 14.12.1993.

Commission Directive 93/11/EEC, *O.J.E.C.*, L93, 17.04.1993.

Council Directive 89/109/EEC, *O.J.E.C.*, L40, 11.02.1989.

Council Directive 85/572/EEC, *O.J.E.C.*, L372, 31.12.1985.

Council Directive 84/500/EEC, *O.J.E.C.*, L277, 20.10.1984.

Council Directive 78/142/EEC, *O.J.E.C.*, L44, 15.02.1978.

Cravatt, B.F., Prospero-Garcia, O., Siuzdak, G., Gilula, N.B., Henriksen, S.J., Boger, D.L. and Lerner, R.A. (1995). Chemical characterization of a family of brain lipids that induce sleep, *Science*, 268, 1506–1509.

Dopico-García, M.S., López-Vilariño, J.M. and Gonzáles-Rodríguez, M.V. (2003). Determination of antioxidant migration levels from low-density polyethylene films into food simulants, *J. Chromatogr. A*, 1018, 53–62.

Evandri, M.G., Tucci, P. and Bolle, P. (2000). Toxicological evaluation of commercial mineral water bottled in polyethylene terephthalate: a cytogenetic approach with *Allium cepa*, *Food Addit. Contam.*, 17, 12, 1037–1045.

Gollier, P.-A. and Bertrand, P. (2002). Cyclic oligomer segregation at the metallized poly(ethylene terephthalate) surface, *J. Adhesion Sci. Technol.*, 16, 1, 1–13.

Goodson, A., Summerfield W. and Cooper I. (2002). Survey of bisphenol A and bisphenol F in canned foods, *Food Addit. Contam.*, 19, 8, 796–802.

Hammarling, L., Gustavsson, H., Svensson, K., Karlsson, S. and Oskarsson, A. (1998). Migration of epoxidized soya bean from plasticized PVC gaskets into baby food, *Food Addit. Contam.*, 15, 2, 203–208.

Hammarling, L., Gustavsson, H., Svensson, K. and Oskarsson, A. (2000). Migration of bisphenol-A diglycidyl ether (BADGE) and its reaction products in canned foods, *Food Addit. Contam.*, 17, 11, 937–43.

Helmroth, E., Rijk, R., Dekker, M. and Jongen, W. (2002). Predictive modelling of migration from packaging materials into food products for regulatory purposes, *Trends Food Sci. Tech.*, 13, 102–109.

Hoyer, P.B. (2001). Reproductive toxicology: current and future directions, *Biochem. Pharmacol.*, 62, 1557–1564.

Inoue, K., Kondo, S., Yoshie, Y., Kato, K., Yoshimura, Y., Horie, M. and Nakazawa, H. (2001). Migration of 4-nonylphenol from polyvinyl chloride food packaging films into food simulants and foods, *Food Addit. Contam.*, 18, 2, 157–164.

International Life Sciences Institute (2000). *Report on Packaging Materials: 1. Polyethylene terephthalate (PET) for food packaging applications.* ILSI Europe Packaging Material Task Force, Brussels.

Kang, J.-H. and Kondo, F. (2002). Bisphenol A migration from cans containing coffee and caffeine, *Food Addit. Contam.*, 19, 9, 886–890.

Kawamura, Y., Inoue, K., Nakazawa, H., Yamada, T. and Maitani, T. (2001). Cause of bisphenol A migration from cans for drinks and assessment of improved cans, *Shokuhin Eiseigaku Zasshi (J. Food Hyg. Soc. Japan)*, 42, 1, 13–17.

Lau, O.-W. and Wong, S.-K. (1997). Mathematical model for the migration of plasticisers from food contact materials into solid food, *Anal. Chim. Acta*, 347, 249–256.

Lau, O.-W. and Wong, S.-K. (2000). Contamination in food from packaging material, *J. Chrom. A*, 882, 255–270.

Lopez-Cervantes, J. and Paseiro-Losada, P. (2003). Determination of bisphenol A in, and its migration from, PVC stretch film used for food packaging, *Food Addit. Contam.*, 20, 6, 596–606.

Marcato, B., Guerra, S., Vianello, M. and Scalia, S. (2003). Migration of antioxidant additives from various polyolefinic plastics into oleaginous vehicles, *Int. J. Pharm.*, 257, 217–225.

National Institutes of Health (1980). *Carcinogenesis bioassay of DEHA (CAS No. 103-23-1) in F334/N rats and B6C3F₁ mice (feed study).* NTP Technical Report Series No. 212, NIH Publ. No. 81–1768, Research Triangle Park, NC.

National Institutes of Health (1982a). *Carcinogenesis bioassay of caprolactam (CAS No. 105-60-2) in F334/N rats and B6C3F₁ mice (feed study).* NTP Technical Report Series No. 212, NIH Publ. No. 81–1770, Research Triangle Park, NC and Bethesda, MD.

National Institutes of Health (1982b). *Carcinogenesis bioassay of DEHP (CAS No. 171-81-7) in F334/N rats and B6C3F₁ mice (feed study)*. NTP Technical Report Series No. 217; NIH Publ. No. 82–1773, Research Triangle Park, NC, and Bethesda, MD.

Nawrocki, J., Dąbrowska, A. and Borcz, A. (2002). Investigation of carbonyl compounds in bottled waters from Poland, *Water Res.*, 36, 4893–4901.

Nerín, C., Philo, M.R. Salafranca, J. and Castle, L. (2002). Determination of bisphenol-type contaminants from packaging materials in aqueous foods by solid-phase miceoextraction-high-performance liquid chromatography, *J. Chrom. A*, 963, 375–380.

Ozaki, A., Yamaguchi, Y., Okamoto, A. and Kawai, N. (2002). Determination of alkylphenols, bisphenol A, benzophenone and phthalates in containers of baby food, and migration into food simulants, *Shokuhin Eiseigaku Zasshi (J. Food Hyg. Soc. Japan)*, 43, 4, 260–266.

Petersen, J.H., Lillemark, L. and Lund, L. (1997). Migration from PVC cling films compared with their field of application, *Food Addit. Contam.*, 14, 4, 345–353.

Rhee, G.S., Kim, S.H., Kim, S.S., Sohn, K.H., Kwack, S.J., Kim, B.H. and Park, K.L. (2002). Comparison of embriotoxicity of ESBO and phthalate esters using an *in vitro* battery system, *Toxicol. in Vitro*, 16, 443–448.

Rozati, R., Reddy, P.P., Reddanna, P. and Majtuba, R. (2002). Role of environmental estrogens in the deterioration of male factor fertility, *Ferti. Steril.*, 78, 6, 1187–1194.

Schwope, A.D., Till, D.E., Ehntholt, D.J., Sidman, K. R., Whelan R.H., Schwartz P.S. and Reid R.C. (1987a). Migration of BHT and Irganox 1010 from low-density polyethylene (LDPE) to foods and food simulating liquids, *Food Chem. Toxicol.*, 25, 4, 317–326.

Schwope, A.D., Till, D.E., Ehntholt, D.J., Sidman, K. R., Whelan, R.H., Schwartz, P.S. and Reid, R.C. (1987b). Migration of Irganox 1010 from ethylene-vinyl acetate films to foods and food-simulating liquids, *Food Chem. Toxicol.*, 25, 4, 327–330.

Shea, K.M. (2003). Pediatric exposure and potential toxicity of phthalate plasticizers, American Academy of Pediatrics, Technical Report, *Pediatrics*, 111, 6, 1467–1474.

Simoneau, C., Theobald, A., Wiltschko, D. and Anklam, E. (1999). Estimation of intake of bisphenol-A-diglicidyl-ether (BADGE) from canned fish consumption in Europe and migration survey, *Food Addit. Contam.*, 16, 11, 457–463.

Soto, A.M., Justicia, H., Wray, J.W. and Sonnenschein, C. (1991). *p*-Nonyl-phenol: an estrogenic xenobiotic released from "modified" polystyrene, *Environ. Health Perspect.*, 92, 167–173.

Soto-Valdez, H., Gramshaw, J.W. and Vandenburg, H.J. (1997). Determination of potential migrants present in Nylon 'microwave and roasting bags' and migration into olive oil, *Food Addit. Contam.*, 14, 3, 309–318.

Startin, J.R., Sharman, M., Rose, M.D., Parker, I., Mercer, A.J., Castle, L. and Gilbert, J. (1987). Migration from plasticized films into foods. 1. Migration of di(2-etylhexyl) adipate from PVC films during home-use and microwave cooking, *Food Addit. Contam.*, 4, 4, 385–398.

Tawfik, M.S. and Huyghebaert, A. (1998). Polystyrene cups and containers: styrene migration, *Food Addit Contam.*, 15, 5, 592–599.

Theobald, A., Simoneau, C., Hannaert, P., Roncari, P., Roncari, A., Rudolph, T. and Anklam, E. (2000). Occurrence of bisphenol-F-diglycidyl ether (BFDGE) in fish canned in oil, *Food Addit. Contam.*, 17, 10, 881–887.

Varner, S.L., Breder, C.V. and Fazio, T. (1983). Determination of styrene migration from food-contact polymers into margarine, using azeotropic distillation and headspace gas chromatography, *J. Assoc. Off. Anal. Chem.*, 66, 5, 1067–1073.

Wang, F.C.-Y. and Buzanowski, W.C. (2000). Polymer additive analysis by pyrolysis – gas chromatography. III. Lubricants, *J. Chromatogr. A*, 891, 313–324.

Wessling, C., Nielsen, T., Leufven, A. and Jagerstad, M. (1998). Mobility of α-tocopherol and BHT in LDPE in contact with fatty food simulants, *Food Addit. Contam.*, 15, 6, 709–715.

15

Epidemiological and Medical Impact of Toxins in Foods

Elżbieta Kucharska

CONTENTS

15.1 INTRODUCTION

Disease syndromes caused by ingestion of endotoxin or exotoxin from food, by bacteria that produce poisonous substances in a patient's gastrointestinal system, and by xenobiotics present in food products, are a major challenge for medical personnel.

The most frequent causes of diseases are toxins produced by bacteria. It is estimated that between three and five billion people suffer from poisonings or toxicoinfections annually and about three million die. Bacteria mainly affect children and in most cases water is the source of infection (bacterial waterborne diseases). Children mostly die due to dehydration and electrolyte imbalance. The majority of children's diarrheas affect infants fed infant formula and so who are not protected by elements of specific immunity transmitted from their mothers.

Symptoms of food poisoning may be difficult to distinguish from protozoan or worm infestation and viral infections, and so the relative proportions of gastrointestinal poisonings and infections remain unknown. In practice, a short-duration gastrointestinal infection, which does not require medical treatment, may also be diagnosed as poisoning. Every disease that starts with sudden vomiting, diarrhea, stomachache, and increased body temperature should be identified as a possible poisoning. A common set of symptoms may affect a group of people after consumption of the same meal.

In Poland, 24,393 cases of bacterial food poisonings were recorded in 2001. In the same year, 19,822 cases of foodborne and waterborne infections were diagnosed, a number close to that for bacterial food poisonings. In total there were 44,546 cases of foodborne poisonings (including chemical and drug poisonings) and infectious and contagious diseases, which led to a morbidity rate of up to about 63 cases per 100,000 people (Przybylska, 2003).

According to the U.S. Centers for Disease Control and Prevention (CDC, a), the total number of laboratory-confirmed cases of foodborne infections in the U.S. in 2002 was 16,580, including (rates per 100,000 people): salmonellosis (16.1), campylobacteriosis (13.3), and shigellosis (10.3). *Escherichia coli* O157, *Listeria*, *Vibrio*, *Yersinia*, *Cryptosporidium*, *Cyclospora*, and hemolytic-uremic *E. coli* were also found to be the causes of infections. The morbidity rate reached about 46 cases per 100,000 people.

15.2 FOODBORNE POISONINGS AND INFECTIONS

15.2.1 TRAVELERS' DIARRHEA

The most frequent cause of gastrointestinal disorders among adults is travelers' diarrhea (TD), affecting on average from 12 to 20 million people traveling from industrialized countries to developing tropical and subtropical areas. TD episodes occur during the first three to five days, and usually do not require medical treatment. There are many causes of travelers' diarrhea. Symptoms occur within six to sixteen hours from ingestion of food containing toxins produced by enterotoxigenic and enteropathogenic *E. coli*, some *Salmonella*, *Shigella*, or *Vibrio*. Toxins produced by *Staphylococcus aureus* and *Bacillus cereus* may also be responsible for TD (Butterton and Claderwood, 2001). *Salmonella*, *Shigella*, or *Campylobacter* are isolated in about 15% of poisoning or gastroenteritis cases, occurring with varying frequencies in different regions.

Especially risky foods include lettuce, vegetable, or egg salads prepared from improperly handled ingredients (Butterton and Claderwood, 2001). Tap water and ice made from tap water are also associated with an increased risk of acquiring TD.

15.2.1.1 Enterotoxigenic *E. coli*

Enterotoxigenic *E. coli* (ETEC) is the main cause of TD in Latin America, whereas in Asia it is reported in only 15% of cases. Enteroinvasive *E. coli* (EIEC) strains are recorded with even less frequency. ETEC is isolated in 0 to 5% of cases. Symptoms of poisoning develop after 16 hours from consumption of contaminated water, salads, cheeses, or meats. The outgrowth of ETEC rods takes place in a patient's gastrointestinal tract, where they produce thermo-stable and thermolabile toxins that imitate *Vibrio cholerae* infections. Stimulation of intestinal guanylcyclase and interruption of ion transport leads to watery stools, which do not require medical treatment or only need simple replacement of fluids and salts by means of multielectrolyte solutions. If a co-infection with EIEC strains occurs, the symptoms of enteritis will develop, with the presence of leukocytes, erythrocytes, and mucous in stools due to a cytotoxic influence of bacteria (Butterton and Claderwood, 2001).

15.2.1.2 Dysentery

In the U.S. and in Europe, the majority of dysentery cases are caused by *Shigella sonnei*, while in developing countries infections caused by *Sh. dysenteriae* and *Sh. boydii* are dominant. In 2001 in Poland, 128 cases of dysentery (0.3 cases per 100,000 people) were reported, of which 116 cases were caused by *Sh. sonnei* (Stypułkowska-Misiurewicz and Gonera, 2003).

Toxins produced by dysentery rods injure the colon's epithelium and bacteria may penetrate the submucous layer. Non-intestine syndrome affects patients with deeply impaired immune systems. Mucous and bloody stools, which lead to a dehydration in a short time, are a predominant symptom. Infections most frequently occur during the summer among groups of children, such as in nursery schools, kindergardens, or summer camps (Keusch, 2001). According to Centers for Disease Control and Prevention (CDC, b), the frequency of dysentery among U.S. children aged one to four years is 27 cases per 100,000 children and dysentery primarily affects children from low-income families. Among adults, the morbidity rate is six incidents per 100,000 people, with seasonal increase in epidemic periods.

15.2.1.3 Salmonellosis

Salmonella rods are present on the surfaces of eggs and may penetrate into eggs via shell pores. They are also found in poultry and milk, and may contaminate meat during jointing. Foodborne toxicoinfections caused by *Salmonella* rods, but not involved in typhus or paratyphus, are named salmonellosis. In 2001 in Poland, the morbidity rate reached 51.2 per 100,000 (19,788 cases) (Gonera,

2003). Toxins produced by rods in patient's intestines are responsible for emerging symptoms. Risky food products include, poultry salads, mayonnaise, meat salads, unpasteurized milk and milk products, salami, sausages, ready-to-eat meat products, smoked or marinated fish, and cakes and pastries with creams Bacteria may survive in dried or frozen products. The disease most frequently affects long-distance travelers between 20 and 39 years of age. The onset of salmonellosis starts within 6 to 72 hours, and commonly associated symptoms include nausea, vomiting, frequent stools (sometimes a bit bloody if the large intestine is attacked), abdominal cramps, and fever. It is very difficult to distinguish salmonellosis from dysentery based on such symptoms. Diagnosis may be facilitated by the fact that salmonellosis usually affects children under twelve months of age whereas dysentery attacks children between six months and four years of age (CDC, b).

15.2.1.4 *Vibrio parahaemolyticus* Infections

Vibrio spp. contaminate water (especially salt water due to the halophilic properties of bacteria), seafood, mollusks, crustaceans, and undercooked vegetables. In Asia, infections frequently accompany floods and other natural disasters. In the Far East and in Japan, *V. parahaemolyticus* infections are endemic. The causative factor is achlorhydria (often iatrogenic). The onset of *Vibrio* infection acquired via the orofecal pathway resembles dysentery due to frequent bloody stools (Butterton and Claderwood, 2001).

15.2.2 STAPHYLOCOCCAL INTOXICATION

Ingestion of semi-liquid, spoiled milk products, such as cream, yogurts, refrozen ice-creams, improperly stored ready-to-eat products, confections with cream, as well as salads, may be a cause of intoxication with staphylococcal enterotoxin. The morbidity rate observed in Poland in 2001 reached 1.6 per 100,000 (647 cases)(Przybylska, 2003a). Predominant symptoms include nausea, frequent vomiting (sometimes bloody), and abdominal cramps, and an accompanying symptom is a non-fever diarrhea. Dehydration may lead to a hypovolemic shock. The presence of enterotoxin in patients' blood and vomits may be diagnosed by means of antibodies using a precipitation method in agarose gels.

15.2.3 BACILLUS CEREUS TOXIN POISONING

Bacillus cereus exotoxin is produced in the gastrointestinal tract after ingestion of improperly stored boiled or fried rice. *B. cereus* toxin is thermoresistant, as is staphylococcal enterotoxin. Symptoms of food poisoning occur up to six hours after food ingestion and are not characteristic (Butterton and Claderwood, 2001).

15.2.4 BOTULISM

Botulism, also known as sausage poisoning, results from the ingestion of food containing *Clostridium botulinum* spores that have germinated and produced botulin. In Poland in 2001, the morbidity rate was 0.1 per 100,000 and two deaths were reported (Przybylska, 2003b). Each year in the U.S., 110 cases are recorded, and it has been found that 25% of botulism is of food origin, 72% affects infants, and the rest is caused by wound infections among drug addicts. The onset of botulism starts up to 18 hours after ingestion of contaminated food. Symptoms do not include vomiting or diarrhea, whereas paresis or oculogyric, facial or other nerve paralysis will occur. Anisocoria and double or blurred vision, dropping eyelids, salivation, slurred speech, difficulty in swallowing, bloating, abdominal pains, and increasing symptoms of paralytic occlusion are typical for botulism. Headaches and trouble with urination are also observed. Symptoms are usually not accompanied by fever.

15.3 SELECTED NON-BACTERIAL POISONINGS

15.3.1 MARINE TOXINS POISONING

Foodborne poisoning may result from the ingestion of food contaminated with marine toxins (Butterton and Calderwood, 2001; CDC, c).

Consumption of improperly stored scombroid fish may cause symptoms of histamine poisoning due to the outgrowth on their surfaces of microflora excreting histidine. The main symptoms include skin redness, headache, vomiting, diarrhea, lip and throat burning, and tachycardia. Scombrotoxic poisoning begins from two minutes to two hours after ingestion of marine toxins. (Phycotoxins of marine food are exhaustively treated in Chapter 7 of this volume.)

15.4 XENOBIOTIC POISONINGS

15.4.1 INTRODUCTION

In addition to bacterial endotoxins and exotoxins, food additives and contaminants are also significant agents of acute and chronic poisonings. Their maximum permissible concentrations are evaluated based on toxicological studies. In 2001 in Poland, only three cases of poisonings caused by fruit contaminated by pesticides were reported, suggesting an incidental occurrence of such poisonings (Przybylska, 2003c).

15.4.2 NITRATES AND NITRITES

Nitrates and nitrites used for curing meat or accumulated in vegetable roots demonstrate the potential to cause poisoning. Poisoning may develop after ingestion of vegetables grown in overfertilized and overnitrated soil. Another source is water from wells improperly protected against dropped leaves. An excess of nitrogen dioxide in the human body results in formation of methaemoglobin, especially fetal (HbF), and nitrosamines (known for their carcinogenic effects). Methaemoglobin does not act as an oxygen carrier and hinders oxygen release in tissues. Symptoms resemble that of increasing anemia: fatigue, headaches and dizziness, tachycardia, weakness, progressing dyspnoea, cyanosis (a gray-brownish skin discoloration), coma, and death. Besides nitrites and nitrates in food, aniline preparations, analgesic drugs, malaricidals, and nitrobenzene may promote methaemoglobinaemia.

15.4.3 ANTIOXIDANTS

Antioxidants applied to fats to protect against rancidity do not cause immediate acute poisonings. However, such substances may accumulate in the human body due to their ability to dissolve in fats. Butylated hydroxyanisole may undesirably influence their production process and cause cirrhosis of liver in experimental animals. Esters of gallate are known to inhibit enzymes, such as alcaline phosphatase, lipase, tetrapeptidase, cause degenerative changes in testicles, and in animal experiments, inhibit the growth of young animals.

15.4.4 MYCOTOXINS

Mycotoxins are a widely distributed group of substances present in moldy food. They are thermoresistant, carcinogenic, and cause dysfunction of parenchymatous organs, inflammatory and thrombotic changes in the central nervous system, leading to embolism and hemorrhage. They were proven to cause increased morbidity of primary liver cancer diagnosed endemically in the Far East, Philippines, Thailand, and Mozambique.

15.4.5 HEAVY METAL POISONINGS

15.4.5.1 Introduction

Contamination of food with heavy metals is constantly reduced due to the intensification of technical controls in industry, which is the primary producer of contaminants found in soil and aquatic environments.

15.4.5.2 Lead

Lead contamination of soil is a result of introduction of trilead tetroxide, present in petrol and combustion gas. Lead may also be released from incorrectly enameled plates and old plumbing (Galal-Gorchev, 1993). Lead may accumulate in vegetables, fruit, and herbs. About 50% of the lead intake of children and 20% of intake by adults is absorbed from the gastrointestinal tract. It is distributed through the human body via the bloodstream and is deposited in soft and hard tissues. About 90% of lead is deposited in the skeleton, where it may remain for up to 25 years. In soft tissues, the half-life is 40 days. Lead accumulates in hair, nails and body fluids, and is excreted with urine. Early symptoms of lead poisoning in adults include abdominal and joint pains, headaches, motorial neuropathy, short-term memory loss, concentration disorders, and hyperactivity. A gray 'lead line' may appear on the border between teeth and gums. Lead accumulated in the skeleton may be released during periods of increased resorption, such as pregnancy, lactation, and menopause, causing anemia, hypertension, and hyperthyroidism. In acute cases of lead poisoning, a renal insufficiency may occur (Hu 1991, 2001; Hu et al., 1996).

15.4.5.3 Mercury

Mercury is a chemical element present in organic and inorganic compounds. Methylmercury, which contaminates seafood, is the most frequent cause of mercury poisoning. Seafood contamination may be a result of industrial sewage being dumped into seas and leading to accumulation of mercury compounds in tuna and swordfish, as happened in Minamata Bay, Japan, in 1955 (Harada, 1995). The other main source of food contamination is seed that has been preserved using phenyl-mercuric ethanoate. Flour can be also contaminated with N-(ethylmercuric)-p-phenylsulphaniline.

Methylmercury is a compound that can be absorbed from the gastro-intestinal tract, is soluble in fats, and easily penetrates natural body barriers, such as the blood–brain, placenta, and female milk. The central nervous system and kidneys accumulate any methylmercury that has not been bound to cysteine and glutathione in the liver. The onset of foodborne poisoning includes bloody vomits, diarrheas, rectal tenesmus, painful swallowing (caused by burning of the upper part of gastrointestinal tract), and abdominal pains. Such symptoms are followed by bleeding gums and tooth loss, as well as bradycardia, conduction disorders (observed in electrocardiogram), and neurological disorders. These neurological disorders include paraesthesia, vision and speech abnormalities, motorial instability, hyperactivity, depressions, and memory disorders. In case of acute poisonings, symptoms of increased renal insufficiency, circulation disorders, and, frequently, non-reversal shock may also appear.

If a pregnant woman is affected by mercury poisoning, the consequences may affect the child. As a result, the child may suffer from profound mental deficiency, atrophy of cerebral cortex, commisure and cerebellum neuron destruction. Acrodynia is a syndrome that affects children exposed to organic and inorganic mercury compounds. Symptoms include itchy, measles-like rash followed by desquamation of palm and foot skin, essential tachycardia, generalized swellings, hypertension and salivation (Harada, 1995).

15.4.5.4 Arsenic

This ion is a chemical component released during volcanic eruptions. However, most contamination is of industrial origin, resulting mainly from the processing of the colored metal ores.

Inorganic arsenic salts are also present in pesticides, herbicides, fungicides, paints, and tobacco plants. If transmitted to water, they accumulate in fish, mollusks, crustaceans, and algae (Johansen et al., 2000). Transformed into organic salts, they reach the gastrointestinal tract via food and are delivered to liver, spleen, kidneys, and lungs. Arsenic is deposited in skin, nails, and hair.

Acute arsenic poisonings lead to enteritis and intestine necrosis and may cause bleeding in the gastrointestinal tract. The onset of arsenic poisoning includes vomiting, diarrhea, and abdominal pains. A smell of garlic from a patient's mouth is the most characteristic symptom. Other symptoms such as increasing cardiomyopathy, renal insufficiency, hemolysis, and central nervous system damage, appear during a disease course. In milder cases, hyperpigmentation and skin hyperkeratosis, multinervous inflammations, paraesthesia, and inflammations of the upper and lower respiratory tracts occur. Quadriplegia and 'black-foot disease,' caused by increasing inefficiency of peripheral blood vessels, may also appear. Disorders in peripheral circulation are connected with drinking mineral waters containing arsenic at concentration from 10 to 1820 ppm. Chronic exposition to arsenic salts increases morbidity from gastrointestinal, liver, and skin cancers (Bates et al., 1992; Guo et al., 1997; Hopenhayn-Rich et al., 1998).

15.4.5.5 Cadmium

Cadmium is released into the atmosphere during the production of plastics, combustion of wastes (especially cadmium-nickel batteries), and as a result of tinctorial and galvanic processes. It is accumulated by plants and so is found in leafed plants and cereals (Galal-Gorchev, 1993). Symptoms of poisoning include gastrointestinal disorders, anosmia, yellow discoloration of teeth, liver injury, microcytic anemia resistant to treatment with iron, dysfunction of renal tubules, and decalcification leading to bone damage. In Japan, in the basin of the Jintzu river, mine waters contaminated drinking water and led to 'itai-itai' disease (known also as 'ouch-ouch' disease due to painful fractures caused by osteomalacia) (Johansen et al., 2000; Hu 1991, 2001; Hu et al.,1996).

15.5 REFERENCES

Bates, M.N., Smith, A.H. and Cantor, K.P. (1995). Case-control study of bladder cancer and arsenic in drinking water, *Am. J. Epidemiol.*, 141, 523–30.

Butterton, J. and Calderwood, S. (2001). Acute infectious diarrheas and bacterial intoxications, in *Harrison's Principles of Internal Medicine*, 14th ed., Lublin, Czelej, 1181–1188.

CDC (a). *www.cdc.gov/mmwr/preview/mm5215a4.htm*, Centers for Disease Control and Prevention website.

CDC (b). *www.cdc.gov/travel/food-drink-risks.htm*, Centers for Disease Control and Prevention website.

CDC (c). *www.cdc.gov/ncidod/dbmb/diseaseinfo/marinetoxins_g.htm*, Centers for Disease Control and Prevention website.

Galal-Gorchev, H. (1993). Dietary intake, levels in food and estimated intake of lead, cadmium, and mercury, *Food Addit. Contam.*, 10, 1, 115–128.

Gonera, E. (2003). Salmonellosis in 2001, *Przegląd Epidemiologiczny*, 57, 1, 67–80.

Guo, H.R., Chiang, H.S., Hu, H., Lipsitz, S.R. and Monson, R.R. (1997). Arsenic in drinking water and incidence of urinary cancers, *Epidemiol.*, 8, 545–550.

Harada, M. and (1995). Minamata disease: Methylmercury poisoning in Japan caused by environmental pollution, *Crit. Rev. Toxicol.*, 25, 1–25.

Hopenhayn-Rich, C., Biggs, M.L. and Smith, A.H. (1998), Lung and kidney cancer mortality associated with arsenic in drinking water in Cordoba, Argentina, *Int. J. Epidemiol.*, 27, 561–569.

Hu, H. (1991). Knowledge of diagnosis and reproductive history among survivors of childhood plumbism, *Am. J. Public Health*, 81, 1070–1072.

Hu, H. et al. (1996). The relationship of bone and blood lead to hypertension. The normative aging study, *JAMA*, 275, 1171–1176.

Hu, H. (2001). Heavy metals poisoning, in, *Harrison's Principles of Internal Medicine*, 14th ed., Lublin, Czelej, 3861–3868.

Johansen, P., Pars, T. and Bjerregaard, P. (2000). Lead, cadmium, mercury and selenium intake by Greenlanders from local marine food, *Sci. Total Environ.*, 245, 1–3, 187–194.

Keusch, G. (2001). Shigellosis-dysentery, in, *Harrison's Principles of Internal Medicine*, 14th ed., Lublin, Czelej, 1441–1446.

Przybylska, A. (2003a). Foodborne poisonings and infections in 2001, *Przegląd Epidemiologiczny*, 57, 1, 85–99.

Przybylska, A. (2003b). Botulism in 2001, *Przegląd Epidemiologiczny*, 57, 1, 99–107.

Przybylska, A. (2003c). Herbicides poisonings in 2001, *Przegląd Epidemiologiczny*, 57, 1, 107–115.

Stypułkowska-Misiurewicz, H. and Gonera, E. (2003). Dysentery in 2001, *Przegląd Epidemiologiczny*, 57, 1, 77–85.

Index